Postgraduate Medical Education
at
The University of the West Indies

STEMMING THE BRAIN DRAIN FROM THE CARIBBEAN

Reform and Expansion of the Faculty of Medicine, UWI
in the restless decade 1965-75

Professor Mohan M. S. Ragbeer,

MD, DCP (Lond.), LMCC, FRCPC, FRCPath, FSMT,WI (Hons.)
First full-time Dean, Medical Faculty, UWI, 1971-5

A synopsis of this account was presented at Mona, UWI, Jamaica. on Dec 5, 2004, with the aid of PowerPoint, as the Dr Jeffrey Wilson Memorial Lecture, sponsored by the Association of Consultant Physicians of Jamaica, in recognition of the 30th anniversary of the UWI's first DM graduate.

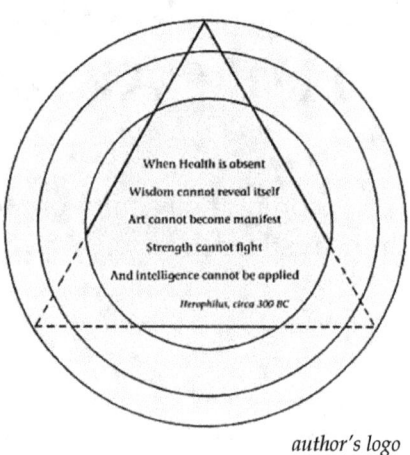

When Health is absent
Wisdom cannot reveal itself
Art cannot become manifest
Strength cannot fight
And Intelligence cannot be applied

Herophilus, circa 300 BC

author's logo

Epigraphs:

"How often had I heard myself dismissed in those years as a dreamer, and the whole scheme as a fantasy, even by eminent colleagues!"   *p. 261*

"...now you must change fantasy to reality...   Michael Manley, PM of Jamaica, 1972

"... don't expect any thanks from colleagues; bear in mind always what satirists say of the stages of a project: Rivals, at first, reject your plan; ignore your successes, until established; then they seize your work and rename it; and then reject and expel you, if possible, to claim all credit!"   *- Professor EK Cruickshank, UWI, 1972*

"I want a generalist, someone who can see me as a whole."
          -Sushruta, Indian Ayurvaidic Physician, 'father of surgery', before 600BCE

"No specialist can be trusted to run this company."   *- General Motors, 1947*

"No man can be a pure specialist, without being in the strict sense an idiot." - GB Shaw

DEDICATION

To my late parents, and to my sister Mahadai, who urged me to study Medicine, and whose unmatched devotion to the welfare of her extended family and community filled me with the love for life and living things, and respect for what has passed away.

To my own family and friends, who enriched my life, and to those who helped me realise the original dream, some named in the text, others unnamed.

To my wife, Mary, who edited, and helped in other ways, and prepared the cover and digital versions of the documents included in the Appendices.

I wish to recognise the original staff of the Medical Faculty, UCWI, most of whom have passed on, the latest Professor Kenneth Stuart, in November 2017. The founders included G. Asprey, E. Cruickshank, G. Escoffery, W. Harper, H. Flint, C. Hassall, S. Martin, G. Bowen, R. Cade, I. F. McKay, N. Millott, K. Hill, G. Ovens, J.L. Stafford, D. Stewart, H. Annamunthodo, G. Bras, J. Golding, L. Grant, T. Hugh-Jones, E. Back, J. Pinkerton, J. Tulloch, W. Levene, S. Patrick, R. Miles, C. Gardner, H. McD Forde, C.P. Douglas, T. Cummins, J. McIver, T. Goreau, R. Cooke, K. Royes, D. Degazon, M. Sugar, L. Marsh, R. Gourlay, K. McNeill, and other staff, including Ms. N. Barrow (later Dame Barrow), and Ms. V. Carby, Nursing; V. Sutherland, Hospital manager; and the students, who showed courage and initiative to inaugurate a new university in an untested environment, who made "oriens ex occidente lux" a reality; and the others who helped to keep the flame glowing in troubled times, and place the UCWI and UCHWI on a sound footing. And to Sirs Thomas Taylor, the first Principal, Philip Sherlock and Hugh Springer, and Dr W.W. Grave, the second Principal, who together set and maintained a worthy standard for those who came after them.

TABLE OF CONTENTS

Acknowledgements		v
Chapter 1	Introduction	1
Chapter 2	A Taste of Medicine	9
Chapter 3	Examinations: the bane of students	19
Chapter 4	An action group, 1969-70	31
Chapter 5	Reforming the curriculum	45
Chapter 6	PGME, the colonial medical service, UCWI	59
Chapter 7	PGME: Brain drain; T&T campus	65
Chapter 8	PGME: UWI chartered; EI heart	71
Chapter 9	PGME CHMC, III, Bermuda	77
Chapter 10	Faculty reforms; Full-time Dean	97
Chapter 11	Other faculty reforms; *IADB committee*	105
Chapter 12	COPMED	113
Chapter 13	Project HOPE, role in PGME	121
Chapter 14	Faculty expansion: IADB Special committee	131
Chapter 15	Jamaica approves	141
Chapter 16	Second term: the dreamer	145
Chapter 17	CHMC IV, Guyana	153
Chapter 18	The eastern Caribbean scheme	163
Chapter 19	Socialism and Specialty Training	171
Chapter 20	CHMC V and VI	179
Chapter 21	Assessing the programs	189
Chapter 22	"Quenching fires"	195
Chapter 23	Campus strike; turmoil in the city, 1973-5	209
Chapter 24	Housing the programs	213
Chapter 25	A crisis meeting	221
Chapter 26	Community Medicine	235
Chapter 27	Swansong	251
Epilogue		261
Maps of Caribbean, 1970		vi-viii
Illustrations, various pages		
Appendices		293
Bibliography		380
Index		383

ACKNOWLEDGMENTS

My late parents and sisters were models of courage as they toiled to achieve success in a difficult land; they were full of ideas, examples, guidance and support, which allowed me to achieve what little I have in this life. They provided seminal assistance and were my best teachers. My wife, Mary, was in their mold.

My children and family were an inspiration. Friends, co-workers, teachers, and students at the UWI in Jamaica and across the Caribbean, in PAFAMS, and others as mentioned in the text, gave critical help.

The late Dr Rabin Sahoy, a key member of COPMED, and one of the pioneers of Cardiothoracic Surgery at the UWI, and later head of Medical Associates, Kingston, gave invaluable support, even after he had left the Department of Surgery; he provided notes and data on events at the UWI, and on Jamaican medicine, society and politics, critiqued my 2004 *Jeffrey Wilson Memorial Lecture*, and urged its expansion and publication.

I thank Prof. R. Wilks, President of the *Association of Consultant Physicians of Jamaica*, Secretary Dr Amza Ali, and their 2004 executive colleagues, for inviting me to honour Dr Wilson, re-live these events, and meet several hundreds of UWI-trained specialists.

My colleagues, some of whom are credited in the text, supported me through harsh times in the bitter days of social turmoil and nascent racial intolerance, which drove many away from the Caribbean, locals and foreigners alike, many not replaced. I received steady support from VCs Philip Sherlock, Roy Marshall and Aston Preston; Registrar Carl Jackman and Bursar Hugh Holness, and their staff; colleagues Karl Smith, Colin Miller, Molly Thorburn, Sir Harry Annamunthodo, David Hoyte, Eric Cruickshank, Rolf Richards, Ken Stuart, Andrew Masson, Ken Standard, Ummul Amin and many others, including Paul Ellis, Hospital Manager.

I could not have done much without the efficient, loyal and patient service of my lean staff: Ann Costa, Dorothy Jung, Norma Rainford, Johanna Young; Dorothy, our unflappable office assistant; and our head photographer, Mr. Brammer, who, with technician Austin, and their small staff, kept Faculty facilities functional, in tough and lean times.

The HOPE team, led by the talented and patient Professor Richard Meltzer, and his wife Amy, came at a time of critical need, and remained when many locals were fleeing the perils of the early seventies; they stayed with the projects and saw them survive and thrive. They and the many unnamed, are the heroes of this tale; some have passed on, others honoured, some not, some forgotten, but their work remains fresh.

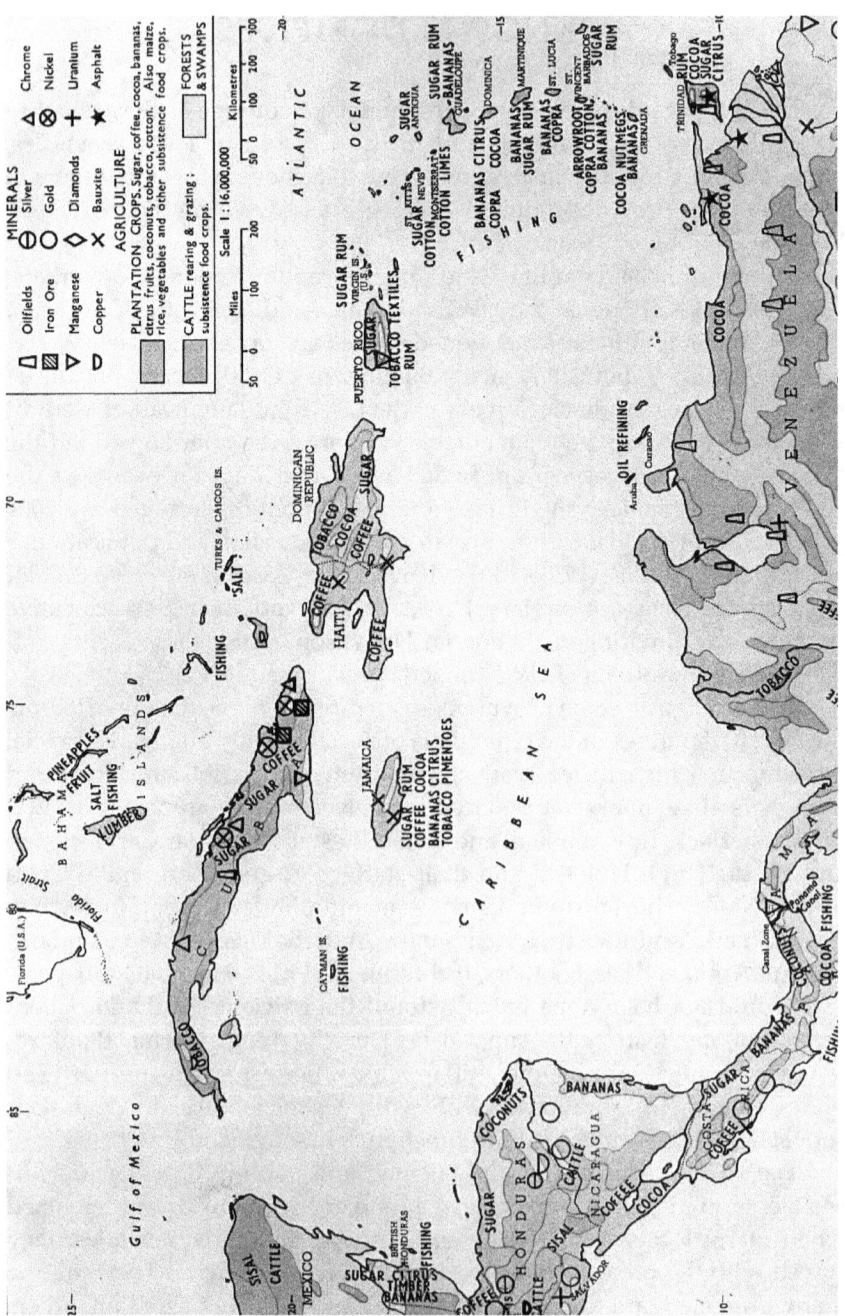

The Caribbean, 1971; Guyana is partly shown at extreme bottom right (in landscape view)

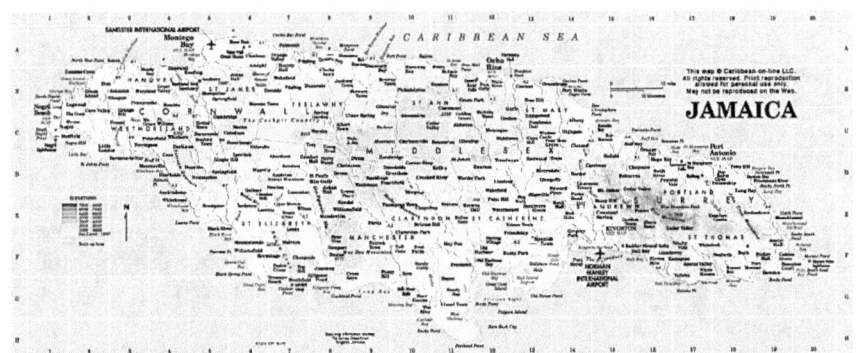

JAMAICA

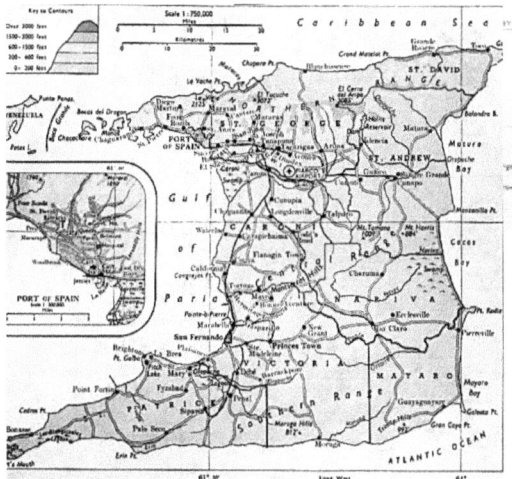

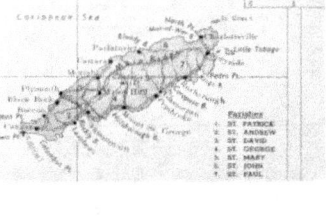

TOBAGO

Trinidad and Tobago, 1971

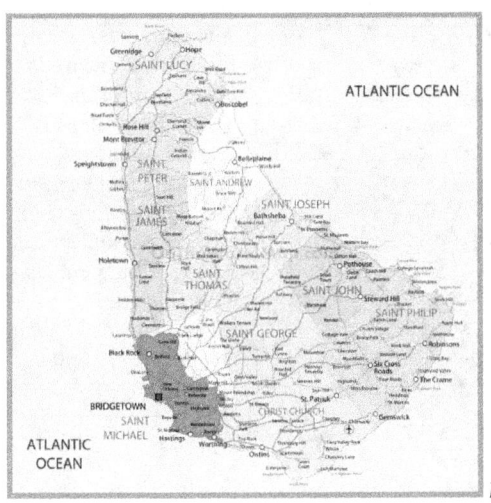

Barbados

.The three islands with campuses today. Jamaica (top), was the original, starting in 1948; Trinidad (middle), and Barbados (left), began with clinical programs in 1968, and developed full campuses in 1989 and 2008 respectively, the latter growing from a clinical school started a decade or more earlier.

All maps are credited to Collins Clear-type Press, London, Caribbean School Atlas.

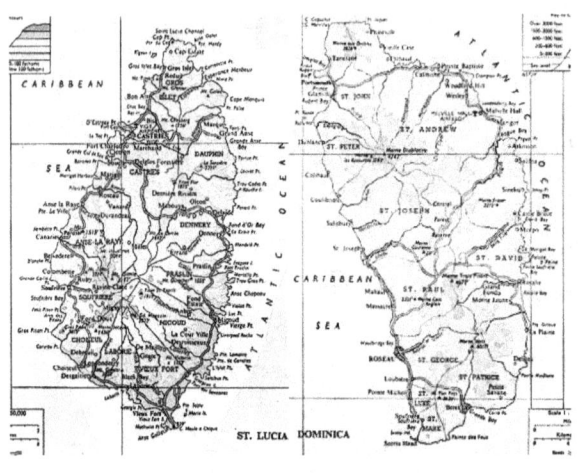

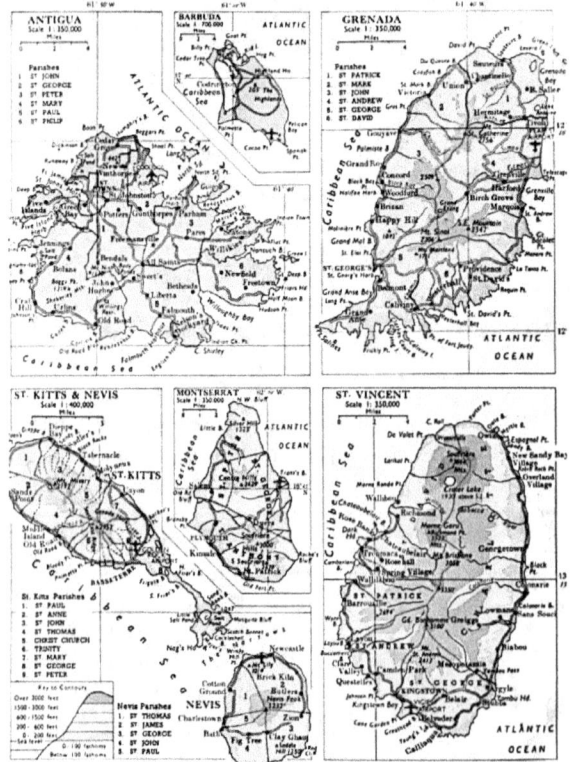

"The UWI serves 16 Commonwealth Caribbean countries and has faculty and students from over 40 countries". (UWI)

Maps show some of the Antilles, which make up the open campus, plus others listed below; clockwise from top left:
St. Lucia, Dominica, Grenada, St. Vincent & Grenadines, St. Kitts/Nevis, Montserrat, Antigua& Barbuda

Other current supporters are: Anguilla, Belize, The Bahamas, the British Virgin Is., Cayman Islands, Turks and Caicos Is.

"Present enrollment is over 39,000 students in all Faculties and about 5,800 students graduate annually, from undergraduate, graduate and diploma programs." (UWI)

PART 1: The Narrative

"Whatever you do, don't tamper with the Curriculum." London University.

Chapter 1: Introduction

In the book, *The Indelible Red Stain* (Bibliography), I had touched on the deprived conditions of British colonies before World War II, with criticisms for London's excessive concentration on law, order and repressive government, while neglecting to provide jobs, education, justice, financial and other infrastructural support for colonial peoples, especially the underprivileged. There were gross deficiencies in, or absence of social services, such as housing, public health and sickness care, labour relations, and social welfare; there was no office or organisation to provide social support. The conditions were grim in town and country and by the 1930s had led to labour unrest throughout the Caribbean. The Colonial Office in London had responded to the turmoil by creating a Social Services Department in 1937, and in the following year, appointing a Major Orde Browne as Labour Advisor.

They also commissioned various enquiries, chief among them the West India Royal Commission, headed by Lord Moyne, with a mandate to identify causes and make recommendations. He reported in 1938-9, and recommended improvements in education, including higher education. The later Irvine Commission recommended the founding of a University College of the West Indies (UCWI) as a College of London University. The Moyne Report was withheld for the duration of WWII, lest its findings stir pro-Nazi reactions among disgruntled colonials, infuriated by the obvious neglect of their wellbeing.

On July 17, 1940, the British Government passed the *Colonial Development and Welfare Act*, providing the sum of £5,000,000 pounds annually for approved schemes throughout the Caribbean, as Lord Moyne had recommended, plus £500,000 pounds for research. These funds were administered by the Secretary of State, and a Comptroller of Development and Welfare was appointed; Sir Frank Stockdale was the first incumbent. The Jamaica Government offered the recently-vacated

Gibraltar Camp and facilities at Mona, with a spectacular view of the Blue Mountains, as the campus for the proposed College.

Thus, in 1948, the University College of the West Indies began as a Medical Faculty at Mona, Jamaica, with 33 students. It admitted its first General Arts and Science students in September, 1949. From 1947, the Caribbean press and radio had given heavy publicity to the new College, and extra-mural tutors had begun work in BG (Guyana), Trinidad and Barbados. The BG tutor was a Jamaican, Adrian Thompson, who spoke

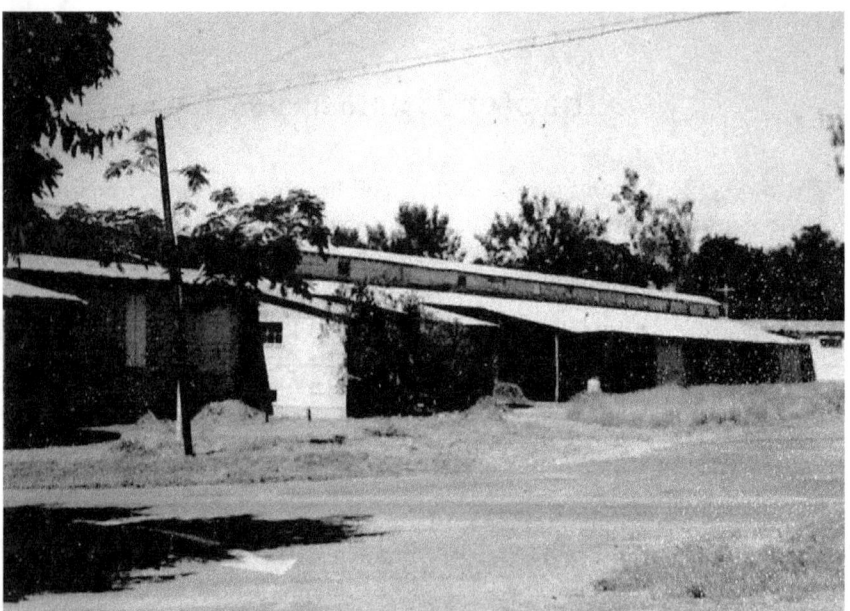

Fig1-1: UCWI, Gibraltar Camp, 1951: The Science complex, where the Pre-Medical Biology classes were held until permanent buildings were ready in 1952. New glass and concrete buildings would replace most of these buildings over the next thirty years.

highly of the beautiful Mona grounds and pleasant climate, illustrated by photographs. (A similar College was founded in Ibadan, Nigeria, which, interestingly, some British experts felt would be enough for their West African colonies; three decades later, there were nine in that region!)

The Mona site was an abandoned sugar estate, set on a low plateau between Long Mountain, on the northern edge of Kingston, and the foothills of the Blue Mountains further north. To the east ran the seasonal Hope River from the foothills of the main range to empty in the sea just east of the city at a place called Yallahs. The site was indeed pleasing, and occupied then by nearly a hundred wooden huts and a dozen or so official residences that had housed the Gibraltar Internment Camp in WWII, so named as it held many individuals transferred from Gibraltar. For the College, these huts became the assembly and lecture halls, offices, laboratories, student residencies, common and dining rooms, library and theatre. The homes of the camp commandant and other officers became staff residencies, greatly cherished by some, including me (between 1969 and 1975), for comfort, space and coolness.

The College prospered, expanded, and sprouted new permanent buildings of concrete, aluminum and glass, and became the UWI in 1962, having absorbed the Imperial College of Tropical Agriculture, at St. Augustine, Trinidad, which formed the nidus of the second campus in the Eastern Caribbean, while a third was planned for BG (Guyana since 1966). But BG withdrew from the University in 1962, and the third campus was developed at Cave Hill, Barbados (see Bibliography, *Indelible Red Stain Book 2,* , for details of the deciding events). Later, a fourth, the open campus, was started, using the techniques of distance education. Today, all have thrived and trained some 40,000 students in all faculties. The University has survived many trials and surmounted obstacles, and achieved many successes; its graduates are versatile, have roamed the world, and succeeded wherever they went.

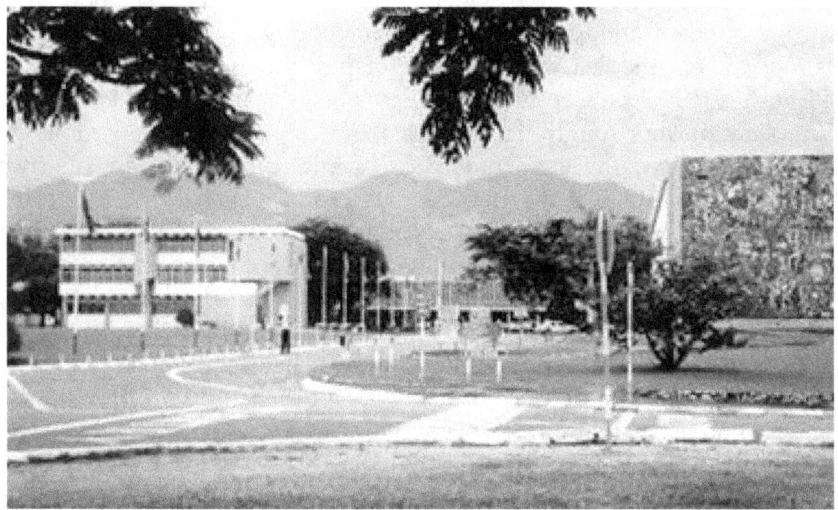

Fig 1-2: UWI: Main Entrance, Mona Campus, Administration Buildings, 1998

Much has been written about the West Indies, the collection of small mountainous and scenic islands lying mostly in the Caribbean Sea, a western arm of the central Atlantic Ocean, and contained within a semicircle that curves to the west and south from Florida to Mexico, Central and South America, which separate it from the Pacific Ocean. The islands form a wide arc that starts just south of the Gulf of Mexico, from Cuba, Cayman Islands and Jamaica in the northwest, runs east to Hispaniola (Dominican Republic and Haiti}, the Virgin Islands, Puerto Rico, St Kitts, Nevis, and Antigua, then curves south to form the Lesser

Antilles down to Grenada, and lastly Trinidad and Tobago. Barbados is in the Atlantic, east of St Vincent, and not included in the Lesser Antilles. The Bahamas, and Turks and Caicos Islands are north of Haiti, in the Atlantic, and are coral islands, like Barbados, while the Antilles are volcanic. The "West Indies, " a misnomer, usually refers to the islands, but the region is politically better known as "The Caribbean," and the states include all lands with a Caribbean shoreline. By convention, Guyana, although not on the Caribbean, is included, by virtue of its political and economic ties to the islands and to its neighbour, Venezuela.

Today, the islands are known mainly for tourism, sugar, rum, faltering agriculture, and off-shore banks, which shelter the funds of the rich, and contaminate the islanders. Jamaica has bauxite and there are oil and gas in Trinidad, offshore Guyana, and in the Gulf of Mexico, which is dotted with Mexican and American oil wells, which at times spill crude oil, contaminating the waters, spoiling the shores, and killing sea life; the last major one was British Petroleum's *Deepwater Horizons* spill in 2010, the world's largest, nearly 5 million barrels in 5 months.

But there was a time when agriculture thrived, seafood was uncontaminated and plentiful, and brought great wealth to European nations, when the Sea was the scene of piracy and naval battles, from skirmishes to Nelson's best against Napoleon. For three sordid centuries European powers fought to possess them, to develop plantations of sugar and tobacco, the slave trade, and bases for piracy. Island properties became some of the world's most desirable and expensive.

Historically, the islands have changed hands among squabbling European powers, following Columbus's journeys, which had begun in 1492. Before that, they were populated by several aboriginal peoples, among whom the Taino and Caribs dominated, until the latter defeated and decimated the others, several centuries ago, and those left were killed off by European germs, to which they had had no prior exposure, therefore no natural immunity, even to the viruses of the common cold.

In 2004, Professor R. Wilks of the UWI Epidemiological Research Unit, and President of the *Association of Consultant Physicians of Jamaica*, invited me to give their annual *Jeffrey Wilson Memorial Lecture* in celebration of the 30th anniversary of the first medical specialist to graduate from the UWI postgraduate program. The lecture honoured the late Chief Medical Officer of Jamaica, a key Government supporter, from 1970, of the Faculty of Medicine's program for specialty training.

At the time, I doubted that Dr Wilks or anyone at UWI knew of the close working relationship between Dr Wilson and me, and I thought the invitation a hoax — as my name had been dropped from the UWI lexicon since the late 1970s — until verified by Dr Rabin Sahoy, my friend, at

Kingston's Medical Associates Hospital. Prof. Wilks kindly left me the choice of topic. I recalled that Dr Wilson was the first physician to study the rarer infectious diseases and Sickle Cell Anaemia in Jamaica, so my first thought was to present samples from a series in my files that I called *"Curiosa et Exotica,* involving people from many lands, including the Caribbean, who had suffered the afflictions he had studied. Other possibilities: nutrition, ageing, and disease incidence in a rodent population; first reports from Guyana of an excess of heart disease in East Indians (today's *metabolic syndrome*); South American aboriginal use of herbs in prevention and cure of disease; our concept of "Community Medicine," as endorsed by Drs Wilson, Comissiong, Smith, PAFAMS and others, but discarded by my successors; or perhaps another topic.

After reading an exchange of emails among the event planners which Prof. Wilks shared with me, I was astonished to note that barely a generation after the seventies, none of these academics—all specialty graduates of the UWI—had any knowledge of the origin of postgraduate medical education (PGME) at their university. They had heard vaguely of "COPMED," mainly because Dr Deanna Ashley, one of the planners, had served briefly on it. I thereupon suggested to Prof Wilks a talk on the origins of PGME, as Dr Wilson had played a crucial hand in it.

This change suited me, as I was assembling material for this book, to document the reforms made and others started at the UWI, between 1965 and 1975. That period included my service to the Faculty of Medicine as Coordinator of PGME and Associate Dean, Student Affairs and Medical Education (1969-71), then as the first full-time Dean, and Director of Community Medicine (1971-75). I also wished to supply information that was apparently missing from Faculty documents since 1976.

I had left Jamaica in July1975 on two years no-pay leave, to study medical systems, and insurance-based universal health care, a topic of great interest to Caribbean Health Ministers, but I was forced into exile by events and personalities at the UWI, ostracised by my successors, for reasons that seemed fuzzy, in the season of "Black Power," as related contextually in this book. At the end of my leave, when UWI declined an extension, I accepted an offer from the Chedoke Hospitals, a teaching complex affiliated with McMaster University (McMU), Hamilton, where I stayed for 19 years, including two as visiting professor in Saudi Arabia. My work as a medical educator at McMaster included development of a model in Community Medicine for Chedoke Hospitals; continuing medical education for the Medical Faculty; development of a tool to assess clinical competence of physicians for the College of Physicians and Surgeons of Ontario (CPSO), the provincial licensing body; and the maintenance of competence program for specialists (Fellows) of the Royal College of Physicians and Surgeons of Canada.

In 1994, as a nominee to the Council of the RCPSC and Chair of its ad hoc *"International Role Committee,"* I proposed the development of mutually helpful links with universities that conducted specialty training: in the Caribbean, especially the UWI, Latin America, and eastern Europe, after the fall of the USSR; and to help to develop specialty education in Saudi Arabia, and elsewhere, as contacts and enquiries were made. We had met with several groups to put flesh to the various ideas, hoping to pilot one project in the following year.

Dr Dilip Raje, then Dean of the UWI Medical Faculty, was prompted to contact me after reading an excerpt of a presentation I had made on this. Thus, on behalf of the RCPSC, I invited him to the 1995 meeting of the College in Halifax, where he described the *"UWI's unique specialist training program, started in 1970 by Professor Ragbeer, when I was a Senior Registrar in Surgery...The university served fourteen small countries then, each as independent-thinking as you are here, and he and colleagues got them to agree to this and to other new programs."* He then discussed ways in which the UWI and the RCPSC could collaborate, suggesting various activities, from specialty seminars, workshops and educational conferences to an exchange of residents, elective or regular, in selected specialties.

An International Role for The Royal College of Physicians and Surgeons of Canada

. . . . . .

Mohan S. Ragbeer MD, FSMT(Hons), FRCPC; John Augustine MD, FRCPC*

Introduction

A few years ago, the Office of Fellowship Affairs (OFA) of The Royal College of Physicians and Surgeons of Canada (RCPSC) invited a small group to inform it about an international role for the RCPSC, and recommend action. The group came to no clear conclusion. OFA raised the issue at subsequent meetings of its Regional Advisory Committees (RAC). At the Ontario meeting (RAC 3), there was general support for the idea. In May 1994, RAC 3 discussion of a position paper prepared by Dr. Mohan Ragbeer led to a resolution requesting the RCPSC to become involved internationally. Many of the points raised in the paper and discussions are presented here. Proponents of the initiative recalled that RAC 3 had played seminal roles in several RCPSC endeavors, the most recent being the Maintenance of Competence Program (MOCOMP®) and resolutions on community electives for residents.

Torstar Corporation of Toronto, presented a paper[1] and Drs. John Ruedy and John Parboosingh provided information on RCPSC activities.

Bases of Involvement in International Health

Individual Fellows confront the problems of other nations in various ways[2,3,4] including:

- professional contact with people from other nations and cultures in their activities as academics, teachers and care-givers
- service with local organizations - governmental and non-governmental, research and educational institutions, foundations, service clubs, religious organizations
- working in health services in other countries
- reports in the lay and medical literature
- other media reports

Fig 1-3: Introduction to article describing the basis for the RCPSC participation in international projects in specialty education, printed in Annals RCPSC 29:266-269, 1996

Our Committee followed up by proposing a joint venture with the UWI, the RCPSC offering advanced training for senior residents in areas chosen by the Faculty at UWI, while they would offer expanded clinical experiences for Canadian residents, e.g., for senior residents or fellows: studies in Sickle Cell Haemoglobinopathy, Tropical Diseases, Nutrition, HIV, Emergency Medicine and so on. These would be offered initially as 3-6-month electives, later, as a regular part of residencies. Another model was the use of expert teams to teach, on site, specific procedures for which a Caribbean country was ready but lacked expertise e.g. certain emergency procedures, minimally-invasive, robotic and distance surgery; complex investigations; distance education, among others. Other projects could be specialist exchanges to teach short courses, and related ideas as identified by the partners, refined, and implemented, if adopted, such as Quality Management, Continuing Education and Maintenance of Competence.

Sadly, Dr Raje became ill, and left the UWI. He was succeeded by Professor Nigel Gibbs, a colleague from our student days, and later a fellow member of staff in the Pathology Department at UWI, and of the *Action Group* in 1970 (Ch. 4). Dean Gibbs had been fully informed of the initiative and continued the interest. He agreed that the UWI could use help with training in certain subspecialties, in research, and other techniques, including information technology. The UWI had a reliable base and the machinery to spread education electronically, which we thought could easily extend to the less developed islands as well.

At this stage—with images of bright, warm Caribbean beaches in their heads—institutional predators with University affiliations and backing, and College clout—emerged from their special interest dens, as they always seem to do in my life, and began to make commercial pillage of the initiative, without fully understanding what we had in mind or how we had thought to proceed. This coincided with a change of leadership at the RCPSC that brought in a profit-oriented President who, with others of like mind, decided that international activities should generate income for the College, or at least be revenue-neutral. They went so far as to adopt a business model for it, guided by a business consultancy, changed existing administrative titles from academic to business ones, and even began to use stereotypical business language and methods in organisation and communications. Those of us who opposed the change in RCPSC to a business, were sidelined.

In 1998, Dean Gibbs invited me to collaborate on a 50th anniversary project and write the history of the Medical Faculty, particularly the evolution of PGME in the Caribbean, and other reforms and innovations in that restless and eventful decade of 1965-75, which he would publish as a series in the *West Indies Medical Journal* (WIMJ), of which he was editor. The first was published as *The Faculty of Medical Sciences, Notes of a Personal Odyssey*, in WIMJ, 1998,47:5-9. This was an introductory and somewhat nostalgic paper, to be followed by others on the reforms of that decade. The first draft of the second article was hardly on his desk than he sadly and unexpectedly passed away. That project remained in draft, awaiting word from the new Dean, in vain, until I received Professor Wilks' invitation to give the *Jeffrey Wilson Memorial Lecture* in 2004, the 30th anniversary of the first DM graduate, Dr Clarence Bankay.

In my 2004 Wilson Memorial Lecture, I said, "*I think that Dr Wilson – and our friends Carlyle Burton and Len Comissiong – would have welcomed the Ragbeer-Raje-Gibbs educational partnership, and the community focus, which was sure to add value to both, or all, partners while preserving their basic programs and individual controls, a principle we had held dear, and promoted in the most troubled of times and through difficult, and at times fractious negotiations at Mona and in the Eastern Caribbean.*"

On a recent visit to the UWI, I was welcomed by the outgoing Dean, Professor Horace Fletcher, met his successor, Dr Tomlin Paul, Vice Deans J. Branday and T. McCartney, a classroom of current students, and Professor A. McDonald, Campus Principal. Dean Fletcher gave me a tour of the new Basic Sciences building (cover), and its many functions. It was impressive. I thank him sincerely. Thanks also to Mrs. A. Spence of the Alumnus office and Mrs. S. Francis–Brown, UWI Museum Curator.

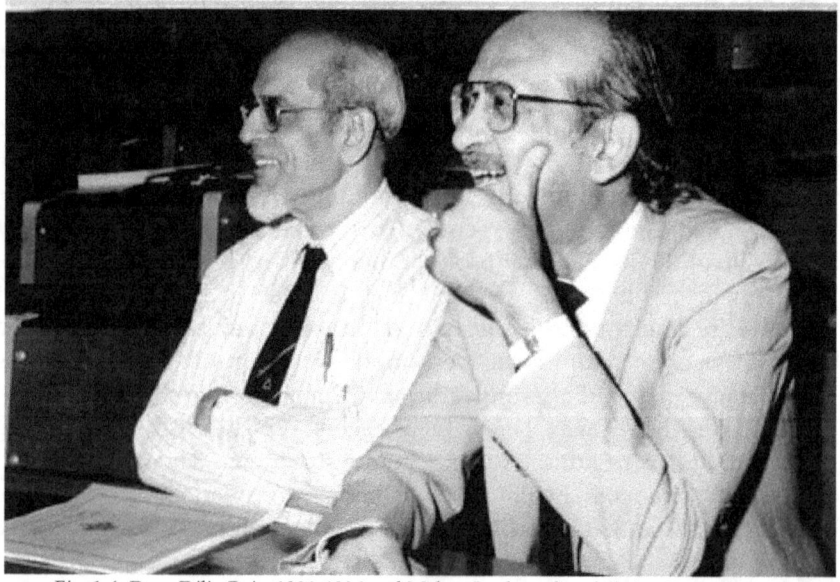

Fig. 1-4: Dean Dilip Raje, 1991-1996;and Mohan Ragbeer, first full-time Dean,1971-5
(Photo: UWI Seminar in Medical Research, 1995)

Sat, vipra bahadha vadanti (from Sanskrit)
One truth; people describe it in different ways

CHAPTER 2
A taste of Medicine; an unlikely medical student

I had been awarded a CDW full scholarship on generous terms to study Geology at a university of my choice in the UK, to start in October 1950, on the basis of my performance in Geography at the 1949 London Higher Schools examination (Arts section), with exemption from the Intermediate BA examination. Capt. Nobbs, the Principal of Queen's College, had asked Mr. Rawlings, my Geography mentor, to file my papers with the British Council by the end of April that year, since they had to be completed in his office and taken in by him or one of his staff. Mr. Rawlings forgot, and the scholarship went to someone in Malaya. The CDC informed the school that I would receive a new scholarship in 1952. I started a temporary job as a personnel officer in the colonial Government's Health Department, to wait out the time.

After about eight months in the Civil Service, despite having ample time to study, play cricket and to socialise, I felt restless, and when I learned of UCWI entrance examinations for 1951 and that a team will follow to interview those who passed, to give final offers, I applied and was accepted into the Arts Faculty to study languages. The interviews had been conducted by Philip Sherlock (Vice-Principal, Arts), Cedric Hassall (Professor, Chemistry) and Eric Cruickshank, (Dean, Medicine); I had mentioned my delayed Geology scholarship and my wish to resume formal intra-mural academic studies, having started second year study as an external student towards a London BA degree. I would lose nothing, if I had to transfer later, and meanwhile would gain a year of languages. Sherlock was encouraging; I was surprised that he had read some poems I had written (now sadly lost) and said he was impressed with their maturity and would encourage me to continue.

Friends and relations questioned my situation and my sanity, one comparing the value of a British Geology degree—and the worldwide vistas that it would open for me—with the common Arts degree, despite my option for higher studies and a diplomatic career. For BG, this would mean toeing an uncertain and thin line, judging from the unsettling militancy and bewildering ultra-left polemics of the first political party to be formed there, the Peoples Progressive Party, headed by Dr CB Jagan, an Indian, my family dentist and close friend, and Mr. LFS Burnham, a Black lawyer, who liked the whisky my brother-in-law served whenever Jagan brought him over for political talk. I was finally persuaded by the UCWI motto, *Oriens ex occidente lux,* and thought that contributing to institution building from the ground up, and to helping the new light shine brighter, should be more challenging than to follow a model already cast in stone. So I chose the UCWI.

Early in the first term, I had applied for exemption from first year as I already had a valid Intermediate Arts Certificate from the University of London. My teachers and the Principal, Sir Thomas Taylor, were sympathetic and encouraging, but my application was denied because of a residency technicality, even though I had offered to complete that at the end of the BA program — the principle of sufferance — while working towards a postgraduate degree. That was not a novel situation, as two or more science students had already done that, but London was unwilling to start it among Arts students. I appealed, but the rejection stood.

The only effect of that decision was to gain me more sympathy when I applied for a transfer to Medicine, prompted by a chance vacancy in the pre-medical class by the decision of a Trinidadian friend to accept a late offer from Montreal, where he had done a BSc. I knew that this would present me with tough new challenges: four science subjects I had not studied before. But a career in Medicine was what my late father had predicted for me, and what my sponsoring sister wished me to do. Despite the slim chance of success without a science background, both with the application and the course, I was surprised to get approval for the transfer, on condition of "satisfactory progress."

I started pre-medical classes four weeks before the end of the first term, failed all the terminal examinations, one or two with the lowest marks in the history of science examinations, received the expected warning from Principal Taylor, but with a reprieve because of the late start. From then on, I worked and played my way to graduate on time, near the top of the class. Because my entire science education was at the UCWI, I had a unique perspective of the school, the educational methods, the Faculty, the curriculum and my colleagues, seeing things and questioning others that my classmates had taken for granted.

I assessed teachers according to the speed with which I had learned their subject, which reflected the way they taught, and how well they distilled a complex set of ideas or information into an easily absorbed one for the novice. The bright teacher who really knew his subject was so much easier for me than the plodder who crammed his points the night before a session and couldn't really get down to the sub-basic level of real familiarity that I needed. I also gained insight into examinations and examiners, from the rare excellent and shrewd one, to the average fellow who was best when he had to check off facts, and was not so good when dealing with arguments, differences of opinion and the relative weights of different points. But I survived and actually did well, to the consternation of several of my classmates, a few of whom had been cool to my entry and had regarded me as an intruder or a spoiler.

When I passed the MBBS 1 (first MB or Pre-Med) examination in June, I got clear passes in Physics, Chemistry and Botany (Professors Bowen, Hassall and Asprey), with first place in Physical Chemistry (Martin), near first in Organic Chemistry and high marks in Physics; but Professor Millott failed me in Zoology by a scant 3/240 marks, and my pal, Otto Sylvester, with 238, a degree of precision that few can justify, and for which an oral by a skilled examiner could have saved months of heartache. But we were allowed to proceed, subject to passing a Zoology examination in December that year. Otto had brought me the news while we were on holiday in Georgetown; perhaps Millott was also punishing him for being my friend and co-worker! Dr Taylor was however quite pleased and said as much to me at the start of the new academic year, October 1952, suggesting that several critics had been stilled, and later expressed his pleasure that both Otto and I had passed the December Zoology test. I had ascribed his unusual frankness to his love of cricket, and support for the College team, on which I played, even near exams.

My outlook on medical education was shaped in part by experience as a personnel officer in the colonial Medical Department, BG, where I also reviewed files and prepared summaries for the Director of Medical Services, Dr LG Eddey. This allowed me to learn something of the structure of the Colonial Medical Service, and Colonial Development and Welfare (CDW) plans for the Caribbean. My training in languages provided me with a broad coverage of literature on a multitude of topics, most dealing with human nature at particular times, places and conditions — social, cultural, healthy, unhealthy etc. — and its mental and physical responses, in order to survive and prosper. For example, I still recall the vivid description of the clinical features of ectopic pregnancy in a French textbook, the chapter titled, *"La Grosseuse ectopique."*

Geography, with its large component of demography, economics, ecology and social studies — eugenics, religions, and what are today referred to as medical or health geography, and medical and social anthropology[1] — blended with history to create for me a perfect prelude to medical education. They fitted especially nicely with epidemiology and socio-biology. Medical education thus expanded my previous interests by adding scientific principles and facts that explained human make-up, function, vulnerabilities and adaptations in the biosphere.

---

[1]"Medicine is an applied or specialised social science," I had argued to the Board for Higher Degrees 17 years later in defending new items of study that should be included but were not usual in the purely medical model that we were following, although Dr Gourlay (Public Health, in my time as a student), would have disagreed and cited the number of topics in his lectures and discussions that overlapped with social sciences.

Thus it differed from what seemed a constituted battle, with arcane medical terms and complex disquisitions, to which it could so easily descend, as some students suggested. A few were justifiably baffled by scientific writing that was not always friendly or readable! Many, chiefly those who had studied in the USA, with no basis in Latin and/or Greek, and victims of "freedom" in education, as in life, found the terminology cumbersome and hard to memorise, as students do today, and marvel at the simplicity of the terms once shown their roots.

Financial need and an early marriage added to my burdens and curtailed, but did not stop the somewhat deeper explorations into ancestral languages that medical studies had provoked, to explore the myths or truths of Sushruta and his Ayurvaidic school of Medicine, which Hippocrates might have explored over 500 years before Christ. My post-graduation completion of residency rotations for General Practice, Surgery, Paediatrics, Pathology and Microbiology and two turbulent years in the teeth of severe political and social unrest in BG—which could have ended my life[2]—were followed by a year and a half of relative tranquillity in Britain and the USA, to conclude specialisation in General and Anatomic Pathology. With no response from the BG government, for months, to either the Commonwealth Office or to me re the job for which I had prepared, I went to New York and received a fabulous offer, in December 1964, from a Columbia University affiliate, but had to leave the USA to await a visa. Later, I would confirm that the racial policies of the Burnham government had denied me a position in Georgetown, just as Idi Amin would do to Ugandan Indians in 1973.

I went to Jamaica, my wife's homeland, to await my visa, and worked temporarily at the UWI, where familiarity, friendships and fine weather, my teachers, Professor Bras and others, and the unique Mona campus, sustained me during the months of waiting. The CIA had just ousted communist Dr Jagan from BG leadership, and as an Indian, I was included in the Indian quota, then 7,500, not Guianese, so I was in a long queue and merited close scrutiny. Ultimately, my wife's debilitation by a prolonged bout of dengue fever persuaded me to accept a UWI contract.

I enjoyed the challenges of life and work in Jamaica, until the mis-direction of the economy, social upheavals and violence during Michael Manley's administration in the 1970s, a period of close alliance with Guyanese dictator Forbes Burnham and Cuba's Fidel Castro—colloquially referred to as the era of "heavy manners" or "heads will roll"—exiled many, including my family, members of which were threatened with lethal harm. My three oldest children were assaulted for being fair-skinned, and twice I had felt the cold steel of a revolver

---

[2] Bibliography: *The Indelible Red Stain*, Books 1 and 2, second edition, 2016

pressed to my temple, for taking a principled position in an illegal strike by certain campus workers in 1973.

But none of this was foreseen a decade earlier, in the relative calm of the 1950s-1960s, except in BG. It is thus useful to evoke a little of the tempo and spirit of the fifties and sixties. The UCWI was barely started when US President Harry Truman—recoiling slowly from his nuclear annihilation of two large Japanese cities and slaughter of their citizens, to ponder, one hoped, what a dastardly, if not criminal thing he had done, as two of our history teachers had accused—thankfully denied his bellicose Pacific commander, Douglas McArthur, the use of nuclear arms to clear Korea of Communists, forcing an armistice in the hot war, as China moved in to support North Korea and beat off the Americans.

Japanese business was reviving, under US strictures, and had begun to make copycat American and German products, while using their unique oriental approach to life, to carve out increasing segments of heavy industry, including motor vehicles, consumer electronics, optics and precision instruments for professional and recreational use. They also made a variety of ordinary items, from office and school supplies to trinkets, toys and kitchenware, which had reached the Caribbean and South America. One I remembered vividly, a fountain pen, which I had bought for ten cents from a friend, whose uncle had become a distributor of Japanese "petty" goods. It was an exact copy of a Parker pen that sold for $10-20, and marked "Made in Usa." There is an old town by that name in Kyushu Island, which the Japanese probably used to fool unwary buyers outside the USA that the product was American-made. It taught me the meaning of "cheap Japanese copy" so that I avoided Japanese goods, until 1960, when I bought the revolutionary Canonflex SLR camera, and learned a lesson in avoiding hasty judgements.

The UK was floundering economically and had to devalue the pound. The effect on the Caribbean was succinctly and plaintively stated in *Dollar and the Pound* by a Trinidad calypsonian, Lord Beginner, who sang *"Devaluation give me a blow/ When de pound that went down so low/The cost of living gone up so high/Dey got de goods, but Ah cannot buy..."* etc. It was a time of rising Calypso stars who were finally being recognised as artists and composers, even though they wrote in local dialects about the earthy and ribald side of life, vividly enough that some of their lines brought a blush to the Victorian aunts that thrived in the Caribbean.

But they were always, or nearly always, good-natured in their teasing, funny, with lilting melodies that evoked a jaunty mood at each recall. Lord Kitchener (Aldwyn Roberts) had already made a name by war's end and had spent six months in Jamaica, just when 33 young and not so young men and women began to study Medicine and begin their own economic rise. Kitchener's *Kitch* was common at parties, and

Trinidadians did not allow anyone to forget him. Nor indeed Lord Beginner (Egbert Moore), who endeared with his *"Two little pals of mine, Ramadhin and Valentine"* (11 and 8 wickets respectively), when the West Indies defeated England in 1950 for the first time at Lords ground in London. Eastern Caribbean cricket fans debated the qualities of the "three Ws" — Worrel, Weekes and Walcott — while Jamaicans sang the praises of centurion Allan Rae. All West Indians could relate to *Hill and Gully Ride / Mandeville Road* by Lord Composer (Roger Ramirez), while Mighty Sparrow's *Jean and Dinah*, Harold Richardson's *Healin' in de Balm Yard*, The Lion's *Mary Ann*, Lord Melody's *Mama look a booboo dey*, George Symonette's *Don't Touch Me Tomato* etc. were catchy and popular at student parties. Count Owen's *Island In The Sun* was more sedate, and pilfered by Americans, as was Lord Invader's lively *Rum and Coca Cola*.

Besides pilfering others' work, Americans began violent crusades against "socialism" everywhere, funding right-wing extremists, attacking anything that smelled of communism, executing the Rosenbergs, cousin to Mrs. Jagan, who was briefly an elected member of the British Guiana assembly, with her husband as premier, and ending at the instigation of the six-year old CIA. The Cold War between the USA and the USSR was firmly entrenched, the US invading Viet Nam, ostensibly to assist the French to hold that colony. The CIA arranged the ouster of popular elected presidents of Guatemala and Iran, the former for bananas (United Fruit), the latter for oil (Aramco). Caribbean societies were peaceful, and even Jamaica was calm, despite a background of violent protest and a penchant for scrapping. In Trinidad, Albert Gomes, the top politician, was confronted by an economist, Dr Eric Williams, who would lead the colony to independence.

One by one, the Anglophone colonies became independent, starting in the sixties: Jamaica on Aug 6, 1962; T&T August 31, 1962; Guyana 26 May, 1966; and Barbados 30 Nov, 1966.[3] Earlier, in Africa, Ghana had become independent on 6 March, 1957; Nigeria on 1 October, 1960; Kenya 12 December, 1963; and Tanganyika and Zanzibar (Tanzania) on 26 April, 1964. The Central African Federation had collapsed and Ian Smith had declared Southern Rhodesia independent from Britain in 1962. Since it was a white take-over, Britain did nothing, and allowed Smith to thumb his nose at the Secretary of State for the Colonies!

The University College at Mona slowly and steadily took shape, with new buildings in white or cream concrete replacing the old weathered

[3] Bahamas gained independence on 10 July, 1973; Grenada, 7 Feb 1974; Dominica 3 Nov., 1978; St Lucia 22 Feb, 1979; St Vincent 27 October, 1979; Belize Sept 21, 1981; Antigua 1 Nov, 1981; St Kitts, Nevis September 19, 1983; and so on. Most of the Lesser Antilles had passed through a decade or more of "associate statehood'" with Britain.

"huts" that had given such good service, as if under camouflage. The Hospital should have been ready to take its first student in October, 1951, but was not ready until 1952, and for a year the Kingston Hospital substituted, and revealed the changes it needed for prolonged use as a teaching hospital.

The College had its first Arts and Sciences graduates (BA and BSc) in 1952, a momentous event that we celebrated, and its first medical graduates (MB,BS) in 1954. Thirteen of the original 33 who had launched

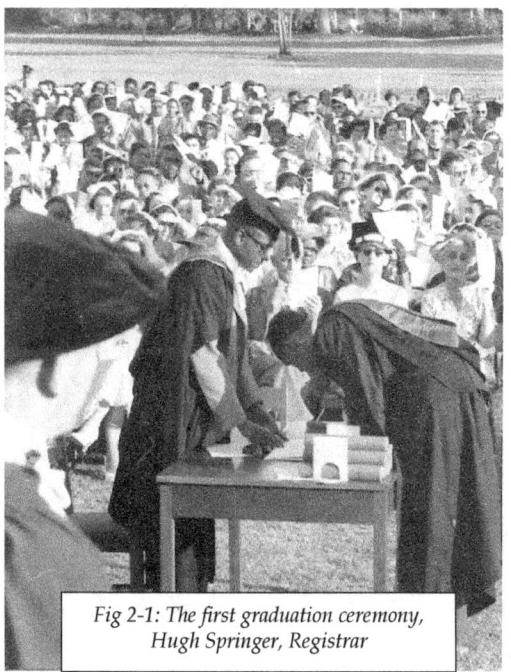

Fig 2-1: The first graduation ceremony, Hugh Springer, Registrar

the College in 1948 passed; the final percentage (42), completing on time, signalled that the six-year course to produce general practitioners, with a proud London MBBS degree, was uphill all the way. We, the students looking on, wondered if these thirteen, —who had inspired such awe—and we, later on, would be given the same recognition as foreign graduates. But the external examiners had commended them and their teachers for *"exceptional preparation,"* and the College praised for the high quality of its first graduates from all Faculties.

It was therefore somewhat excessive to have it complete a solid decade of "successful apprenticeship" before taking on full University status. In 1962, the UWI received its Charter, in the same year that Jamaica and Trinidad, the major contributors, became independent.

For students, independence was no illusion, even to the non-historian; it evoked a great emotion: concrete fears of insolvency, squelched by an almost irrational ecstasy, as only the young can feel. Expectations were great, fuelled by the lavish claims and promises of politicians to launch a grand new age. But the bravado was empty, the claims feeble, and funds for education had to be squeezed out of fragile island economies. Long gone were the "glory days" of King Sugar, when Barbados was a preferred investment to New York, New Hampshire exchanged for one of the Lesser Antilles and Caribbean landlords built elegant homes and lifestyles in Britain, arrogantly commanded *rotten boroughs,* and ruled the Houses of Parliament!

In the USA, the *Beat Generation* had stirred a literary revolt, and the *San Francisco renaissance* had become well-known as a result of writings on social revolt, drugs, aberrant sex, and eastern culture by a variety of writers, including Donald Allen and Jack Kerouac. The trends influenced the Beatles, the "flower" people, and the general cultists of degradation, spawned by the abuse of mind-altering drugs that the US army and others had tested as possible weapons in WWII. Their movement spread to the "chic crowd" in Jamaica, among whom were some University students, who quickly mastered the rhythms and language, though only a few copied the drug and other behaviours. Young members of the privileged set aped American behaviour in detail, a trait more common among Jamaicans and Bahamians than other West Indians. Castro's take-over in Cuba was generally lauded. Criticism for Duvalier and Trujillo was muted but the latter's overthrow in 1962 was welcomed, as much as the US invasion, a few years later, was condemned.

Cuba, relieved of Battista, had foiled the USA and switched to communism and alliance with the Soviet Union, creating tensions in the Caribbean and Latin America, especially after the failed Bay of Pigs invasion. John Kennedy was uniformly popular; I had "campaigned" briefly for him in the June 1960 presidential primaries in New York. His murder was widely mourned. Johnson greeted it with some scepticism, which dissipated with his Civil Rights actions, although the invasion of the Dominican Republic in 1964-5 was regarded as high-handed, and solely in the USA's interest, a case of the giant swatting a fly, as was the CIA overthrow of overtly-Marxist Jagan in British Guiana in favour of covertly-Marxist Burnham, who exploited US fears of "another Cuba," and gained campaign funding from them, support for independence in 1966, and the establishment of a dictatorship through rigged elections. Social unrest, job scarcity among the poorly educated, led to poverty and malnutrition, especially in Jamaica; the poorer enclaves of all cities were shantytowns, overpopulated, underserved, in want, and violent.

The islands were never encouraged by colonisers to be self-reliant, being almost exclusively commercial farms for European companies, which gave little space and no time or effort to food production. Even in independence, they depended heavily on imports for every need, even basic food supplies, a continuation of colonial business practices that flogged "mother-country" goods, and nurtured its cuisine, which had become *de rigueur* even among the poor. Thus, canned pears and peaches, which tasted like blotting paper dipped in syrup were more classy than fresh mangoes, and canned pineapple from Hawaii sold better than fresh ones at the local market, or which you could grow yourself on a few feet of suitable backyard soil. Mango, guava, sapodilla (naseberry), star apple, cashew, sidyam, jamoon, guinep, golden apple, awara etc., were widely available and far more nutritious, but not cultivated for the market; they grew "wild" but, as treats and choice desserts, they paled before expensive "ice" apples, dates, walnuts, figs, and canned pears and peaches in thick syrup, which the rich flaunted and made them fat, while the poor longed in slender envy.

This perversion of tastes and culture was everywhere, except among the Indians of *rural* Trinidad and British Guiana (Guyana), who, from need, preserved their cuisine and grew their own food. Similarly, the rural Blacks of Jamaica grew food crops for themselves, sold the excess, and some prospered. Food scarcity and import dependence were firstly an urban condition that combined, in inner-cities, with under-education, joblessness, social neglect and early pregnancy, to maintain and increase the problems of poverty. The latter slowly leaked into the country towns.

Malnutrition—with or without gastroenteritis or pneumonia—was the foremost cause of paediatric admissions and deaths in hospitals in Jamaica, and provided steady work for local and itinerant researchers into the biochemistry of human need for solids and liquids. A steady stream of Britishers flowed through the University College Hospital of the West Indies (UCHWI), Medical Research Council's Tropical Metabolism Research Unit (TMRU), the Caribbean Food and Nutrition Institute (CFNI, and regular clinical departments, to collect some data, perhaps share a few pearls and enjoy the lovely climate, especially the amenities, which the imperial authorities had carefully fashioned to cater almost exclusively to their own. People like me were tolerated, or dismissed as humbug, more so after WWII, and the really snooty places, like Frenchman's Cove in Portland, Jamaica – then owned by Canadian race supremacists and imperialists, the Westons, with Garfield the chief at the Cove—would in 1964, in defiance of Jamaica's independence, refuse entry to extempore visitor, British PM Hugh Gaitskell, even to the grounds. What would they have done to a coloured person?

The assassination of John Kennedy was followed by the Civil Rights movement under Johnson, and the rise of Black power. Jack Kerouac had yielded to Elvis Presley, Malcolm X and Martin Luther King—who mesmerised the UWI campus when he visited in 1965 and shared his dream of a peaceful and united world. In the USA and Europe, student protests grew, by 1968, into a mass action against the Viet Nam war. Some students opted out, literally and metaphorically, with or without the help of drugs, fuelling an expanding and violent trade in various mind-altering substances, which have grown to threaten modern life, but cruelly maintained as a source of immense wealth to drug lords, like opium to British and American imperialists, since the 19th century. The

Black American, Stokely Carmichael, stressed this by telling Trinidadians and Guianese, *"When I say Black, I don't mean Indians."* Trinidad expelled him but Burnham shielded him in Guyana for weeks, allowing him to spread his message of hate and division, in every town and village in the country. These messages infiltrated and poisoned UWI campuses in Jamaica and Barbados, with their majority black or coloured students. But in Trinidad, it stoked divisions between the large Indian and Black student groups, already fired into rivalry by PM Eric Williams, whose enfeebled governance was criticised by sociologist Lloyd Best and his Tapia group, raising it by 1973 to a political party, *Tapia National.*

In the medical school, we were, by 1967, questioning the *aims* of medical education, after five years of avoiding the issue. But the questions were coming more from the new ranks of Caribbean staff. In 1973, Kamaluddin Mohammed, Minister of Health, T&T, at CHMC V *(Caribbean Health Ministers Conference)*, in Dominica, reminisced, *"The achievement of nationhood was followed by a period of hectic activity in the provision of jobs, social services and physical facilities to satisfy the demands of a population, suddenly awakened to its new rights and privileges, and filled with rising aspirations, which understandably saw independence as the gateway to everything they had been denied previously."*

But it was an expectation preached loudly since 1950 by Cheddi Jagan and Forbes Burnham in British Guiana (Guyana); its failure to materialise there surprised people when the magical transformation turned out to be for the worse! But not all were surprised. The insightful, the well-read, the critical, the silenced, had long seen that the promises were hollow, and they had begun to migrate, one by one, and steadily, to Britain, where they had a right of entry as British citizens and could get jobs as clerks and technicians, by virtue of their "English education," and in various trades, in the re-building of cities and towns laid waste by war; and their children could complete their education, seamlessly.

Nowhere was this phenomenon, this draining of talent, more dramatic than in Guyana, the one among all regional colonies that had the potential of enriching its *total* working populace, the one forecast before WWII for early independence, based on the maturity of its organisations, exemplified by the centennial resolutions of the *British Guiana East Indian Association (BGEIA)*, 1938. But WWII intervened and delayed progress. The post-war economic slow-down allowed political folly and ideological militancy to usurp good sense and leadership, and elevate two tyros, Jagan and Burnham, as the new leaders, who moved away from the sure path to prosperity that their predecessors had laid, to Burnham's dictatorship, violence and racial paramountcy; these have consumed the country and made it poor and one of the world's most corrupt, wasted its health services, and exiled half the population.

CHAPTER 3
Examinations: the bane of Students

When I became a UWI faculty member in January 1965, I acquired as colleagues many of my former teachers, including a few with whom I had had differences as a student, most unexpressed. I reacted by becoming a student advocate quite early. When advisor roles were voluntary, in the mid-sixties, I was swamped with students, as were some others, similarly motivated, until the Dean, then Professor Bras, formalised the advisor role, assigning each staff person a list of students. Even so, I would get "special requests", and found it difficult to deny anyone who asked for help, or who had a perfunctory adviser, of which there were several, who gradually drifted away to the new medical schools that the sixties had brought to North America.

It was this, plus personal experience that led me to my first major challenge at the UWI, or distraction, really, since the University gave little or no credit for anything but publications; thus time spent in planning, education or administration was of no account, which I would come to know later as the "publish or perish" philosophy.

It had become my lot that each time I complained about something, I got the job of finding a solution. By 1965, students had grumbled often about the conduct and content of some examinations (topic emphasis, the obscure vs. common, reproducing content exactly as taught, examiner biases, complaints re orals, and no effective appeal). It had seemed as if the "subject examination" was the aim of all teaching-learning activities, rather than production of sensitive and competent doctors for small states. But the complaints and calls for reform had fallen on deaf ears.

The examination system had been in place since the Faculty's founding and had followed the London model: MB,BS 1 (Botany, Chemistry, Physics, Zoology), after a pre-medical year; MB,BS 2, after two years pre-clinical studies (Anatomy, Physiology, Biochemistry and Pharmacology); and, 30 months later, MB,BS 3: Final, Part 1 (Pathology and Microbiology), and after six months Parts 2, 3 & 4 (Medicine, Surgery, Obstetrics and Gynaecology). Each consisted of theoretical and practical (or clinical) tests, and oral tests for MB,BS 2 and 3. That continued until the pre-medical class was eliminated in the early 1960s.

A review of the method, and a survey of current and past students raised the suspicion of bias or inexperience in the way questions were chosen, or orals conducted and assessed, especially in pre-clinical sciences — Anatomy excepted — and in Microbiology. For instance, the pharmacologist, Dr Feng, was cited for often wanting answers in the same words used in his lectures, and acceptable paraphrases were often assessed as wrong. Instances of examiners not putting candidates at ease, or rushing answers, or giving upsetting cues to nervous candidates, were more common; and a few examples were given of non-expert external examiners, who were unable to act as referee for the student.

The problem had been known for a decade. As graduates became teachers, the desire for change increased. This resulted in one of the first modifications to examinations, whereby orals were given less weight, or discounted for those who had clearly passed theory and practical (or clinical) papers, and retained largely for honours, borderline or fail level performances. Central to any reform, however, would be a curricular statement of the final aim of medical studies e.g., to produce a graduate able to meet primary care needs of Caribbean populations, or to engage in further learning to provide specialist care. Thus, the elements needed to achieve the learning aims determined the inputs from each discipline, rather than the subject-based model, where each discipline delivered a comprehensive sample of its content, in enough depth that the student could readily proceed to a degree in each; it was questioned whether this depth was required, or whether the material was retained in its entirety, even by the best students. Instructional approach should apply adult learning principles, content based on terminal aims, and the examination plan follow an agreed blueprint.[4]

Confining teaching to essentials for medical practice could result in a reduction in time devoted to basic studies, permit completion of the undergraduate program in less than five years, and provide time for elements missing in the current curriculum. For example, did students need to learn and be examined on therapeutics in advance of studying illnesses and their management? Must they know how to smoke a drum, or cannulate a jugular vein—taught using dogs—when they would not be expected to do so in ordinary clinical practice; or, as a general physician, to recognise specific cancers histologically? Yet we taught those, and students had been held back for "failing" them.

I had started—as agreed by department heads and with the cooperation of teachers—by reviewing examinations for Final Pathology

---

[4]M.S. Ragbeer: (i) Objective Examinations in Medicine, a critique of eight types in common use in North America, and (ii) *Comparison of Objective (MCQ's) and essay examinations for Part I (Pathology and Microbiology) of the Final MBBS Examination,* UWI. Medical Examinations Board, 1966, 1967.
M.S. Ragbeer and P. Jutsum: *Computer-assisted analyses of multiple choice questions,* UWI, Department of Pathology Examinations Committee, 1967.
M.S. Ragbeer: *Performance characteristics of 3300 multiple choice questions tested for Part I Final MBBS Examination,* UWI, Faculty of Medicine Examinations Board, 1968.

and Microbiology, probing the scope of test topics, the validity of essays as a test of factual knowledge; examiner reliability in rating essays; precision among examiners, etc. Examinations demanded much staff time: a class of 60 students produced 480-600 essays in an examination (two papers of four or five answers each). Four examiners, all senior staff, each marked 15 students (120-150 essays); the marks were listed in rank order, and added to those from the practical and oral, thus giving them equal value (a doubtful conclusion), and the total determined pass or fail, and for those passing, whether an honours level was reached. Percentiles and "z" scores were not given, and letter grades not used. No one checked marking consistency or accuracy at any stage of the process, nor inter-rater reliability. The orals were personal chats between the student and the most senior examiners (two or rarely three, plus the external examiner). The session might be a formality, or more searching to confirm a failure or excellence; oral marks were arbitrary and subjective, and hopefully matched performance. The only objective marks were those of some essays and the practical tests, since the latter were mostly factual, except for any part that required comment.

Essays, however, exposed students to gain or loss from the extent of inter-rater and intra-rater reliability. It had been rare for examiners to meet beforehand to agree on a minimum pass answer to each question. For example, if a 100% answer should cover ten points in answering a "describe" question, of which four were crucial, the pass student should have at least three crucial and five or more total; those with all crucial and 8 or more total would qualify for honours. A student fails with 0-2 crucial, regardless of how many others were correct; an oral would give this student a chance at corrections and a pass rating.

A "discuss" question was more woolly and qualitative; it asked for a critique of the issue: pros and cons; good and bad; positive and negative; worthy and unworthy; comparing its value with others in the topic class etc. It would help examiners to have the framer of the question provide an "ideal" answer, but this rarely happened, if ever. Thus, variations in marking were common due to differences in examiners' judgements.

To test inter-rater reliability, I chose the same essay by an honours student (82); five average students with a 20-point spread in marks (54-74); one borderline (48) and three weak students, with almost identical marks (40, 39, 41). The rankings were based on 80 and over, honours; 50-79, pass; 46-49, borderline; 45 and below, fail. Those between 75 and 79 and borderline would have orals, to gauge qualification for honours, or pass/fail respectively. Failed students usually received an oral.

The ten essays (staff time restricted us to this) were given randomly over a two-month period to four staff, who marked them in rotation, blinded to the identity and source of question. Averaging the four results for each student, I ended with 2 honours (81, 85), 7 passes (50-76) and 1 fail (41). The individual marks were more revealing: one rater was very demanding and had no honours, 5 passes, 2 borderline and 3 failures. One was generous and had no failures, 3 honours, 5 passes and 2 borderline. The other two were in between. Interestingly, nine of the 40 marks deviated by 5 or more from the index mark—the mark given in the real examination—and two by 10 or more.

To test intra-rater reliability, the same teachers marked the essays they had marked two months earlier. None had reproduced the first-round mark; the closest match was a 5% variance; there was as much as 20% difference in nearly a quarter of the items. Interestingly, the better honours student retained his rank with 80 instead of 85 and there were four instead of three failures and two versus one borderline. Allowing for the small sample size, the results did suggest a need for more objective ways of testing performance.

I had had some experience with Multiple Choice Questionnaires and had taken two such examinations for the ECFMG, and had studied the subject from library sources as applied to a variety of university subjects. With input from Kassim Bacchus, Senior Lecturer in the Faculty of Education, I decided to pilot a test, with approval from the chief examiners, Professors Bras, Pathology, and Grant, Microbiology. The late Dr Earl Been helped with the Microbiology items, while Pathology teachers agreed to supply items relating to the courses or lectures they had given. Peter Jutsum, a lecturer in the Physics Department, was pleased to help with computerising and analyses.

I spent months creating MCQs of all types: 5-choice completion; multiple completion; 5- and 4-choice association; case history analysis; excluded term; relationship analysis; quantitative comparison; variation relationship; structure and function matching, and true-false types. I tested batches of each item, hundreds of each type, enrolling 20-50 anonymous student volunteers at each session, and in 1967 had suggested to Ken Standard, head of S&P Medicine, that I could include test items for his courses. Ken was my neighbour and we often had over-the-fence talks on educational issues. In the end, he declined to try the system due to time constraints, though he had agreed that his discipline could be tested as an element of Part I Final, which would be new and would enhance his clerkship.

After each trial, I received feedback from students on overall acceptability, on the clarity of instructions and precision of wording of answer choices. By the end of 1966, we had assembled over 1500 questions with satisfactory reliability, comparability and validity characteristics and student comments. Based on these, we decided to limit the item types to 5-choice completion, multiple completion, and case analysis. We started objective examinations in 1967 with 150 MCQs, and two essays to test organisation, presentation, and writing skills, especially for honours students. By April 1969, we had 3300 validated items in our bank, over 90% prepared by me from topics submitted by teachers. Items were approved by staff and chief examiners for balance and tested in six term examinations, not part of University assessments, but filed in departmental records for use as a form of continuing evaluation, which could help students at Part 1 Finals.

The structure of the Final examinations (Parts 1-4) demanded intense effort by examiners to have the theory and practical (or clinical) marks assembled before the orals. Up to then, all students had an oral, in every subject, thus four for Basic Sciences, and four for Finals. These orals were seen by some older faculty as a replacement for the system of term reviews called "Collections," which the early UCWI had practised.

I include this commentary for historical and other interest, and to illustrate the value of testing based on pre-set goals (Dr Taylor's remark, underlined p. 24). Collections were held in the early years of the College, when class size was small. In a letter home to a literary friend, I wrote, at Christmas 1951 (while listening to the third Test Cricket match, Australia vs West Indies at Adelaide, which WI won, the only one of five):

"All teachers involved in that term assembled like a French revolutionary tribunal examining the guilty next to the guillotine. They sat, teeth bared, at a long menacing table, with the Principal at the Centre and his deputies on either side. They dissected the performance of each student in turn, diagnosed his/her ills and offered a prognosis. Every class had teacher favourites who usually sailed through "Collections," while heaven help the unpopular or outsider, unless the Principal was unduly alert or prescient to spot unfair or insensitive treatment. My first experience was an example; I was dismissed as a singularity and aberration by Bowen of Physics, micro-analysed by Martin of Chemistry, whose reaction was somewhat acidic, and dissected, skinned and pinned out in display by Millott of Zoology. Principal Taylor listened patiently. Pre-medical Collections were scheduled for three hours. There were 33 students, allowing about five minutes each and time for a wrap-up by the team.

"It was a beautiful end-of March Saturday morning, and our cricket season was in its third week. I was on the team and that day we were playing an exhibition match (pre-season), starting at 12.30 p.m., against the Kensington Cricket Club, captained by Colin Bonitto, whose brother, Neville, would later play for Jamaica.

"Taylor knew about the match. He was a keen backer of our team and would usually be seen watching 'net' practice and a game; he knew each player in the twenty-four man squad who qualified to represent the College, and had become familiar with all the first year additions, which included Bud (Wallace) Lee and me from our class. Bud was an accomplished science student and had sailed through the Collections process 20 minutes earlier. So had Bunny Lowachee and

Jim Munroe, QC colleagues and Glenn Nymm of Trinidad; all had completed sixth form science and would make any teacher proud. Now here was I, a plain anomaly, an imposter, with only fourteen weeks of the "Sciences" in all my life, and just finishing and failing, with low scores, the same examinations that my friends had "hit for six." I was grist for the mill, slop for the pigs, ready to be tarred and feathered, guillotined, and so on. I had failed my first term exam, after spending four weeks in the class, having transferred from Arts with no science worth a scientist's scorn even. I was given at that time hardly any marks in Zoology, Chemistry and Physics, not even a token for attendance, though I did get 30% in Physics Practical, a huge achievement.

"Millott did not like me, on sight, and had accused me, as I joined his class, of wanting to join the wealthy, who lived in Stony Hill (at the time I knew little about this Hill, stony or not, didn't take to the description, and resented his characterisation). Our dislike had become mutual, but I did admire his ambidexterity at the blackboard, his clear drawings and almost copybook style of lettering with either hand, at times incredibly together. I think I exaggerate, but he was good at the blackboard, the greatest showman 'who ever got chalk on his coat,' as Tom Lehrer might have said. But he saw nothing good in me, and would often pick on me to answer questions, just to hear me say, 'I don't know,' allowing him to insult me. At the end of the second term, I had passed his Zoology Theory but failed the Practical — because my drawings were "art, not scientific diagrams". My tapeworm was every bit what I saw in the display, my drawing almost a photograph, my labels in the right places. But Millott wanted massive and stylised schematics, not copies! I passed two others, but failed Martin's chemistry and almost passed Physics Theory. But Millott was unsympathetic and chose to expose me as an impostor unveiled.

"But he didn't reckon with Dr Taylor, who, looking at this and last term's marks, cut him short, as he was sprinkling salt on me, <u>'Come, come, Millott, the man's done what we asked of him.'</u> And he abruptly changed the subject, asking me, 'Are you playing today?' I hesitated momentarily at the sudden switch and peremptory swatting of Millott off my back. 'Yes,' I said, near gleefully. 'How's the pitch? Didn't have a chance to see you all yesterday. Who's visiting?' I told him. 'What time do you start?' 12.30. He looked at his watch. 11.35. 'Hurry on then,' he finished, glancing balefully at the discomfited Millott, who would give me the same look of hate for the rest of our enforced association.

"In less than a second I was gone, my sweat fanned dry by his comforting termination of the session; I had been before them for over twenty minutes, and considered the session as an enactment of the comments section that each teacher is asked to complete on a school report card. The hoopla was all theatre: the format, the assembly and student parade, the costumes, their finery, our imitations, but we did look as good in our own white suits and flowing red gowns, clean-shaven, with bushy hair nicely combed. The girls looked as if they were all virgins getting married, so immaculate in elegant white dresses, it was hard to believe they were students, and half the time on their backs, or wishing

to be! Those "Collections" did not last; they were, though, a grand exemplar of plain sadism, the exhibitionism buried in every teacher, and especially developed in the British, the desire to perform without fear of public ridicule, even if the show bombed, which it hardly did, with a captive audience of one!"

But a compulsory oral examination *(viva voce)*, for students who had already passed the two major parts, the theory and practical (or clinical) easily comprising 90% of the whole test, was not only a humbug, but a waste of time and money. A hundred students (the increase by 1968) would require 20 intimidating hours or 2½ days of 3 examiners (two internal, one external), or 7½ man-days per subject. There had been rare instances of a student passing the Theory and Practical Papers, yet failing at the Oral. This had occurred, notoriously, in Pharmacology, the students blaming Dr Feng, the acerbic chief examiner, for "punishing" them by this device, simply by asking abstruse or clinical questions.[5] Those instances were not probed in the days of the College, though word of this had reached the Dean. But there was little he could do in the absence of a formal complaint, which students declined to do, fearing staff reluctance to criticise colleagues or fellow foreigners.

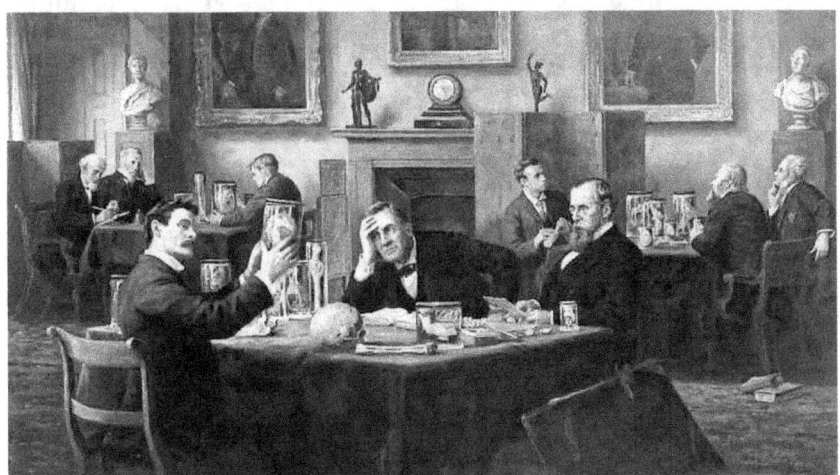

Fig 3-1: The VIVA: Royal College of Surgeons, Court of Examiners (1894) by Henry Jamyn Brooks - http://www.bbc.co.uk/arts/yourpaintings/paintings/the-viva, RCSEng Public Domain.

---

[5] Dr Marryat, radiologist at the UCHWI in the fifties and a minor British aristocrat by birth, tells of the short O&G examiner at Finals posing him a difficult term delivery problem happening to a young primigravida, in the middle of the desolate Derbyshire moors. The full clinical picture was given, and he was asked, "How would you handle this?" Marryat, a 30+ year-old student, and a veteran of WWII, had had enough of "blood and guts," and had stiffened his stance with each detail; he stood erect to his full six feet, stared at the examiner, and answered, pausing hardly at all, head high, "What, my dear man, would *I* be doing in the middle of the Derbyshire moors?" He failed.

Thus, anyone having the temerity to complain might face repercussions by spiteful teachers, according to an informal classification by students. I had therefore argued, with evidence, for changes, which were adopted for Part 1 Finals (Pathology and Microbiology), and suggested for the others, at least partially e.g. two essays and 150 MCQs, in lieu of each 3-hour 5-question paper, thus resulting in 200 essays to be marked, versus 500, while the computer—even the slow minicomputer we had then, an IBM 1164—could mark, rate and analyse the MCQs in a few hours. Examiners accepted the argument for selective use of the "oral" for failing, borderline and honours level performances. We started this in 1967, and by March 1968, had assembled enough data to limit the types of item to 5-choice completion, case studies, and a few multiple completion items for special topics, as noted above. This decision settled some of the semantic and "framing" issues of other types, especially as careful wording allowed most of the others to be adapted to the 5-choice method. I had a chance to discuss these points while in Chicago in 1968.

At that time, global tensions had become increasingly threatening, flowing from unrest in the USA and USSR. My trip to Chicago from Europe had been delayed two days by the Chicago Police riots during the Democratic National Convention to select a candidate for President, with damage to the Hilton hotel, where I was booked to stay for the short time it would take me to find lodgings near to the Michael Reese Hospital. Earlier, on August 21st, Warsaw pact troops had moved into Prague, ousting Alexander Dubcek's government and ending the "Prague Spring" reform movement, on the very day my train to Prague was turned back to Vienna. The invasion sparked anti-Soviet rallies in many countries. But in the USA, it was the Vietnam war. 1968 was the year of global riots among students, workers, the *Youth International Party* members *(Yippies),* Blacks and draftees, wanting to end the War and railing against the *Tet offensive.* They wished peace, civil rights and freedoms for minorities and women. Americans had discovered sex and drugs, and the *hippie* movement had swelled. Hordes of young people filled the streets, airports, train and bus stations, with bulging backpacks, running from the draft, mingling with saffron-robed *Hare Krishna* followers, cymbals jangling, as they chanted *mantras* on peace.

The murder of Martin Luther King on April 4th, 1968, and the slow progress of Black civil rights had aggravated tensions. Student uprisings upset Paris, France; New York, USA; Berlin, Germany; Sweden, London, and several cities in Yugoslavia. A rise of Black Power in the USA and calls for improving rights and social justice spread everywhere. Black sprinters protested at the podium during the Olympics in Mexico City in October. At the UWI, Jamaica, students had protested the banning of leftist Walter Rodney by the JLP government of Hugh Shearer, leading to riots and the death of five. Earlier, on Oct 2, in Tlatelolco, Mexico, Police had killed between 30-300 students and other civilians. In Trinidad, Black Consciousness and the New Left movements had spilled over from South Africa, and influenced the mutiny by army officers in Trinidad (p. 266). The UWI campuses seethed with dissatisfaction among social scientists and students. In Chicago, I shared in the state of alert.

However, I visited with the Christine McGuire school of evaluators, looking at their use of case-based analyses or "patient management problems,"(PMPs), as they called them—with new stylings for old concepts, at which American educators and psychologists excel. But I liked their approach to the "clinical" examination—even though it did not test the diagnostic process at the bedside with live patients, as we did, nor with live simulated patients as some Canadians were beginning to do. Their approach handled some of the criticisms of the "long case," the lynch-pin of Final Examinations in British schools, by placing more emphasis on accurate and thorough histories, which were seldom, if ever, directly observed by our examiners, who *inferred* competence in history-taking from the results examinees presented, whether their procedures were well-performed or not. Nor did we review behavioural aspects of a student-patient encounter: greetings, manners, interview styles, rapport, putting patient at ease, speaking style, particularly avoidance of jargon, obtaining permission for physicals, ending the interview politely, and so on. American examining boards avoided real clinical tests, believing that students would not get MDs from their school unless they had passed such tests.

The "long case" in itself was a defensible clinical test for the case type used, and satisfactory performance was generalised from it, knowing that students were exposed to a wide variety of clinical cases and would likely perform consistently in encounters with them. They knew that doctors must be equally competent over the wide spectrum of disease found in the environment. The long case fell short in that it was a single encounter, and the case was different for each student, and presented more often than not a single diagnostic problem, whose elucidation and management often differed from other system problems, even though the process might be the same. Thus one's performance could not strictly be compared with another's, for rating purposes, e.g. prizes, honours etc. In a sense, at UWI, this was defensible, as every student up to then, was supervised by his seniors and reports on performance and abilities given to the department heads, so that they knew the weak, the average and the strong. Quite often, it seemed that the "long case" was more for the benefit of the external examiner, and to show off the UWI.

Our use of short cases came closer to the PMPs of the McGuire team; it was cheaper for us to assemble a variety of these than they could in Chicago, to test, interactively, many aspects of the clinical process, even principles of health promotion and disease prevention. They envied our advantage and ability to cover a wide range of clinical states, live, which mimicked the clinic situation, and was worth emulating.

I also discussed these issues in 1970 at a meeting of the *Association of Caribbean Universities and Research Institutes* (ACURI) in Cali, Colombia, where, with Dr Karl Smith, S&P Medicine, I met several Latin American educators who were struggling with the Hubbard system of MCQs, in their typical verbatim copying of Americana. Dr Smith and I spent a "free" session discussing our findings with an appreciative group. The shorter examination time in our model was student-friendly and fiscally smart. However, the long and critical preparation time for objective tests and the lengthy instructions for some types were inhibitory; but the change in student response from ambivalence to acceptance, the elimination of inter-rater disagreement, the improved reliability of the tests, the quick identification of poor items, the time saved marking by computer, and the addition of test items with each examination, were powerful arguments in favour of objective tests of proficiency at various stages of the course, and justified the high initial cost in faculty time.

We discussed in Chicago, in Cali, as at UWI, with the Dean's group, the growing role of continuous assessment, which was used at the new school at McMaster University, Ontario, and was a main part of their small-group tutorial-based program, arranged in units of ten weeks, where peer and tutor assessments were done at the end of *each* tutorial, and a formal summary written by tutor and students at the end of each unit, with ratings for all students and *tutor*. The method was sound in theory, and worked fairly well with the mature students (Honours BSc, MSc or PhD) studying medicine there, and accustomed to hearing frank, or even harsh evaluations that might, if done improperly, create ill-feeling or anxiety among younger peers. But it was staff-intensive, considering that each group was no more than 6 students, average 5, and that the school had *hundreds* of tutors; many coordinators; ample clerical staff; numerous meeting rooms, centrally registered, and booked in advance; and a plethora of library and audio-visual resources! Contrast the UWI, with larger student numbers; little money; less than 100 staff and dwindling; few AV resources; a small library; and few tutorial or lecture rooms. It was thus easy for our Examinations Committee to decide on exploring less costly ways to achieve learning and evaluation.

The Dean's Group deferred consideration, pending study of cost, staff commitment, value gained, and implications for the current system of examinations. The Group was not convinced that a financially strapped school could embark on a scheme with dubious merit, however much "the rich educational psychologists in North America might want to flog it here, and justify a winter holiday," as one department head cynically remarked. One significant difference between the UWI and North American schools was that our pass qualified the holder for a licence, whereas the North American could graduate and yet fail the licensing examination[6].

The Board of Examinations for the Faculty was fully briefed on the issues, but in general, the clinical departments of Medicine (Part II), Surgery (Part III), and Obstetrics and Gynaecology (Part IV), deferred any changes, "pending further study," adversely swayed by the time demands of preparation and verification I had described. Some defended essays as requiring students to rely on their own resources, not written cues, and dismissed the "American method" that rewarded guesswork! Few of them realised that "True/False" questionnaires were hardly ever used in Final Medical or licensing examinations. Some even questioned the wisdom of changing a system (essays) "so tried and true!"

The final argument against significant change was that it must await improvement in staffing and technology to afford time for the refinement of new techniques. The fact that Pathology and Microbiology were able to effect changes in just two years with one staff in each dedicating time to it, largely as an add-on to, not instead of regular duties, supported by contributions from all teachers, was not seen as a model to be copied, although it was offered, and papers distributed to all staff. The pre-clinical departments were more interested, and some teachers had used limited objective tests in term examinations. They undertook to explore further use, after a workshop for staff, conducted by Dr Jutsum and me, attended by Dean Bras and about twenty staff, one at least from each department involved in examinations, as the Dean had requested. We showed examples of each type of MCQ described by Hubbard, explained their attributes, and student reactions to each type. We agreed with students and avoided types with lengthy instructions, settling, as noted, on the 5-choice completion, case studies, and fewer multiple completion types, which should test both content and performance processes.

---

[6]By an unusual irony, I ended up as a professor at McMaster University in 1977, saw the system up close, and joined with others to trim its fat, which became an imperative as the bravado of the 1965-75 period gave way to fiscal reality and budgetary constraints. Mc Master had no examinations, merely cumulative unit evaluations; the lack of exposure to exams was a source of student anxiety. Change was pushed when reviews of licensing examinations failures showed McMaster University graduates at the head of the list; I saw how easy it was to pass the unit evaluations, when I failed a student who had passed two previous units, with no useful knowledge of elementary sciences, e.g. he couldn't define pH or electrolyte. I introduced my students to MCQs unofficially, as exams were anathema.

Clinical departments reported to the Dean and declined to participate. But each had sent at least one person to the seminar, and conceded that they might revisit the issue when staffing improved. That still left the issue of testing components of health promotion, disease prevention, and public health, whose omission might make students feel that these were not important. By comparison, in the Canadian Licentiate examination (LMCC), the MCQs routinely included several items on these topics and also on basic Biometrics. No one involved in Parts 1-4 Finals claimed these topics as "theirs," since only S&P Medicine taught them specifically, but did not test students in the Finals, nor in any way that mattered for their practice, beyond course assessment; those results, though reported, hardly ever influenced any candidate's ranking.

Professor Standard was a member of the Dean's Group and, like Dr Smith, his colleague, agreed to include Biometrics, which they could test by MCQs or "short answer" questions, including calculations from a batch of data, to show mastery of terms and procedures used in medical statistics. An essay was not an efficient way to test such knowledge, and, in any case, no one wanted to "waste" even one of the ten precious essays required for each subject (or Part) on anything other than diseases. Ironically, UWI students paid attention to public health and medical statistics only because they were tested in the American ECFMG, and Canadian LMCC!

This illustrates an advantage of MCQs in expanding the range of topics tested. As it was, each department regularly had to decide what final ten essays would be chosen from among the dozens submitted by the various lecturers. When I enquired into this process, I calculated from information given by Professors Stuart and Cruickshank that the department of Medicine regularly spent as much faculty time each year on examinations as we in Pathology had spent amassing our tested bank of 3,500 items! But they consistently resisted the argument and declined to construct a trial batch of MCQs, with or without help. When I asked for an explanation, Professor Cruickshank simply noted, with tongue in cheek, that their majority British or British-trained staff could not relate intellectually to MCQs, an American "invention!"

In later years, changes in examinations had to be made in line with curricular changes, the aims of medical education, and demand for training relevant to types of practice, to replace the training of all as toti-potential doctors for comprehensive care or solo practice in underserved and isolated areas of colonies, outside the populated, attractive, comfortable and remunerative cities, where colonial leaders tended to congregate, in clubs. It would have been better to have fashioned a curriculum to produce primary and community care physicians, not hospital-ready operatives for the UK and North American markets!

CHAPTER 4
The Action Group, 1969-70, *a necessary distraction*

In the years following completion of my reviews of the examination system, and the reform the Board of Examinations had authorised in 1967-9 for pre-clinical subjects, Pathology and Microbiology, I took courses in Education, with the advice of Kassim Bacchus at Mona, and in Management, guided by Marshall Hall of Management Studies. I had also begun research on several problems in oncology, hoping to apply immunological reactions both for diagnosis and treatment of disease.

About the same time I had a long serendipitous discussion on immunotherapy with Denise Thwaites, a GP, one of UCWI's first graduates and wife of my classmate and good friend, David Thwaites, an O&G specialist. I had met her at the Hope Institute, a Jamaica Cancer Society palliative care centre for terminal patients, tucked away on a hill slope on the road leading from the University to the Hope River bed. She had been visiting a patient and had read an article on immunotherapy and other treatments practised entrepreneurially in the US; one of these touted an enzyme called *Laetrile*, whose inventors were claiming many "cures" of advanced cancer; could we not get some?

But Laetrile was a hoax, and banned from the USA by the FDA; its base then moved to Tijuana, Mexico. In the mid-sixties, Bill Brooks had loaned me a paperback triumphantly called, *Laetrile, the Conquest of Cancer*, describing it as a wondrous hope, but lacking data to support it. We discussed the plethora of bogus cures in the USA and the extent that faith, hope, entrepreneurship, and *laissez-faire* allowed them to flourish. But immunotherapy was different; its base was sound. She had a busy practice, mainly children, but would find some time to do any therapy if it came to that. The issue was in line with my own research interests.

I had begun with the standard literature search on aspects of lymphomas and breast cancers, of which I had quite a collection: the first phase of work I had hoped to do for a PhD on the behaviour and properties of these groups of malignant cells. The literature search itself was tedious and the library often had a delay in getting reprints (photocopying as we now know it was several years in the future). I had also agreed to review the drafts that Eric DePass of the Government's Kingston Laboratory had produced on *Cancer of the Oesophagus* for an MD thesis, and to double-check his slides, with Bill Brooks. I consulted Professor CV Harrison, a former teacher, and head of Histopathology at RPGMS (p. 60), who had visited as external examiner. He reviewed my material and the suggested further work; he agreed that for a London PhD, I should go beyond morphology, and use the electron microscope and immunocytochemistry, such as Professor AGE Pearse, one of my former teachers, was doing at Hammersmith, to probe cell behaviours. He offered to discuss this with Dr Pearse on his return to London.

But the course of work outlined required equipment we did not have, except for an electron microscope; Paul Keane, Clinical Chemist, was then trying to procure some of the others. The tools required skilled technicians and a sizeable grant for the equipment and supplies that neither Paul nor I had. So when Bras asked me to assist Alex Talerman, a newcomer, with a research project, I turned over my "Lymphoma material" to him, especially as a morphological and serological work-up was enough for an MD at Sheffield, Talerman's University.

One day, Bras gave me a slide and asked what I thought it showed. I could see several stained tissues and after studying them suggested they were a small animal, rat likely, with a small cell benign tumour completely replacing a gland which I concluded was endocrine. He said it was a pituitary adenoma in a Sprague–Dawley (SD) rat, and how would I like to join him and his NIH grantee, Dr Morris Ross, a biochemist, in a more substantial study of *"Nutrition, Longevity and Disease Incidence"* in rats of the Sprague-Dawley strain?

I saw his solicitude as perhaps in remorse for denying me my rightful position as an author of the *Lancet* report, two years earlier, of the discovery of Burkitt's lymphoma in a canine in Jamaica, the first report of the virus-induced lymphoma outside East Africa. I had made the diagnosis over the doubts of everyone else, including Bras, written the paper and given him the draft. But in submitting the paper, he had replaced my name with that of Selwyn Murray, then nearing the end of his contract, to "compensate for his fruitless search" for Burkitt's in the department's ten-year files. The publication would be a "nice send-off" for Selwyn, who apologised that he knew nothing of the switch, and had in fact drafted an article reporting his negative finding! I had responded stoically, and instead of grumbling, had concentrated on the education and examinations challenges, which eventually stalled other research.

The rodent study was quite interesting and matched my interests in nutrition, neglected so far, but which I had nursed since studying its biochemistry, and seen its ravages in malnourished children during a six-month internship in Paediatrics.[7] I gratefully accepted his offer to

---

[7] But we also saw the miracles that kept us going. One of mine was Maxine, 2½ y.o., 7½ lbs on admission, mere skin and bones, with gastroenteritis and bronchopneumonia, and barely responsive, even to a "cut-down" procedure. Her outlook was so bleak I was given permission by her mother and the chief paediatrician, Eric Back, to do whatever I thought would help her. Though moribund for a long time, she refused to die, surviving my various

enrol me as co-researcher in the NIH-sponsored project based in Newark, Delaware, to serve as the pathologist "blinded" to the identity of the animals, whose autopsy tissues I would get, already prepared as stained slides, for review and histological evaluation. For those reports I got a small fee, approved by the University, and welcomed, as by then my commitments had extended to the hosting of my younger brother for his Bachelor's degree in Education, and my oldest fraternal niece through a 4-year Diploma program in Medical Technology.

Bras had made another gesture of appeasement in 1967, recognising the work I had done on Examinations, when he recommended my promotion by three additional salary increments; the University awarded two, noting that three were very rare.

The first result of the NIH assignment was a paper on the influence of diet on the incidence of pituitary tumours in the study population, published in *Journal of Nutrition*. We then analysed longevity outcomes with various diets, and the ultrastructure of the peculiar nephrosis that occurred in SD rats fed standard Purina "lab chow" or a high protein diet. The work was progressing well by 1973, and we had assembled much data on diet-related disease and longevity, when the US government abruptly ended the grant, in the wake of the OPEC oil price "crisis" — citing their decision to terminate nutrition grants, since *"the United States of America was the world's best-nourished nation!"* This ignored the rising incidence of obesity, cancer and immune dysfunctions in a population gorging on high-calorie processed food, low in fruits and vegetables, and high in calories, hormones, antibiotics and pesticides!

In January 1968, I was re-appointed in my position for three years and promoted to Senior Lecturer. But the promotion was not plain sailing, as the Promotions Committee emphasised "scientific research" as measured by published papers in peer-reviewed journals. I was criticised

---

parenteral invasions, and with excellent nursing care, under Sister Wells, gradually became viable. Her colour, pale grey on entry, changed to a dark tan, Six months later, she went home, able to walk and weighing over 15 pounds. Prognosis for learning was poor, and for life, guarded, although her resistance and tenacity had impressed us. That was 1958. I saw her thrice thereafter on OP visits, even though I had left Paediatrics; her mother, proud of her progress, wanted me to see her. I lost touch when I left Jamaica in 1961, and ten years later, reminiscing, wondered what had happened to her. One day, Colin Miller, who was SHO and part of the team in 1958, now Senior Lecturer in Paediatrics called me to his OPD, where he introduced a pretty, slim and shapely early teen-ager, with smooth tan skin, the picture of health. When it was clear that I didn't know who she was, her mother emerged from behind a mobile screen, and greeted me, "Is Maxine, doc; you no remember Maxine? She just finishing school; she do a'right!" The girl looked at me, quizzically, then glancing briefly at her mother, wrapped her arms around my neck and gave me the warmest hug and kiss. It was a wonderful reunion, another that made all labour worthwhile.

for having only seven such publications in three years, which certain science and one influential medical member of the Committee thought "too few." Had Bras not pinched my Burkitt's lymphoma paper, or failed to mention my two substantial handbooks for students on *Chronic Inflammation* and *Basic Immunology,* and included three papers presented in 1967 in Guyana, it would have been easier to account for my time.

Teaching activities and my work with students counted, but the papers resulting from these — though they had led to changes in teaching and examinations — had been internal, and had not been published in a "Medical Education" journal. On our joint European trip in summer 1968 preceding my study leave in the USA (Chicago and New York, to learn new procedures in electron microscopy), I had discussed my work with Kassim Bacchus, then finishing his own PhD thesis for London University, which was conferred on him at the end of August, 1968.

I gave him details of what I had done, the subjects covered, how and with what results, particularly on learning theory and examinations, and the implications for curricular reform. He asked many questions, then agreed that with formal composition and presentation, he was sure that the work would qualify for at least his Faculty's M.Ed. degree, especially as I had completed the content of qualifying M.Ed. courses. Professor Ken Stuart had earlier given a similar appraisal, suggesting that I add to it: tables, diagrams, photos and a more detailed critique, such as were later presented to the *Inter-American Development Bank Special Committee on Faculty expansion/ duplication,* and register for a London Ph.D. With Professors Bras and Cruickshank's strong support, I did get the promotion, and did register for a London higher academic degree.

Perhaps for this and my work on animals, curriculum and ongoing work to develop the Faculty's proposals to the Academic Board and the CHMC for Postgraduate Medical Education, Bras financed me in 1970 through a two-month evening course in *Cybernetics and Leadership Training,* a unique exploration of refined management techniques, conducted for a mixed group of professionals and business folk, by the Society of Jesus of Kingston, and eloquently led by Fr Alexander, SJ.

I had earlier been helped in my Faculty efforts by a chance meeting with VC Roy Marshall and Dr Karl Smith at a conference of the *Association of Caribbean Universities and Research Institutes* (ACURI) in Cali, Colombia in early 1970, where I had presented a paper on *Educational research for curriculum planning.* I described hindrances to curriculum reform new programs at UWI, which had led to an ear-bending session with the VC, who said he had been assured that all was well in the Faculty of Medicine, but he would follow-up our assertions re staff and student discontent, which were "new and quite troubling".

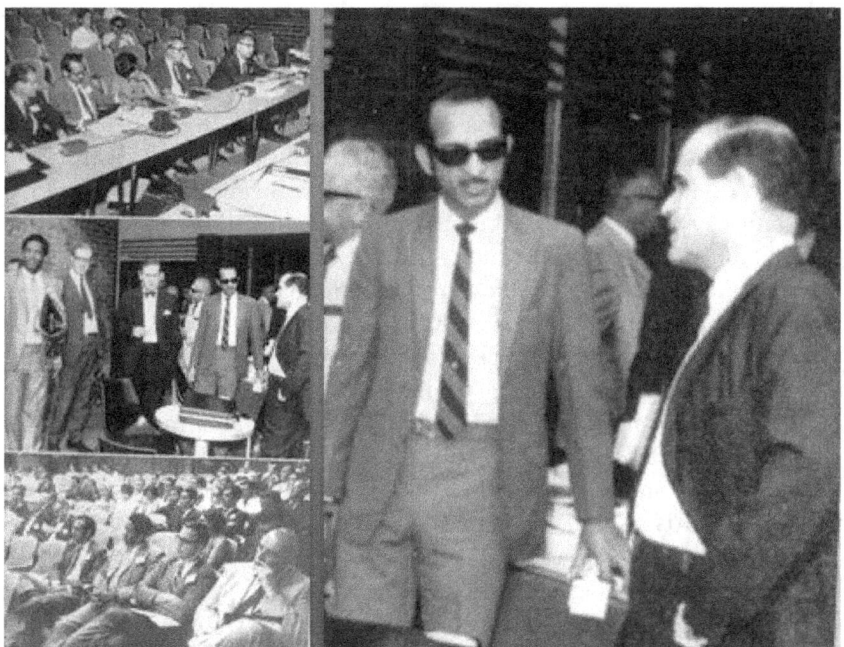

Fig 4-1: Cali Colombia, 1970: L: top, education session; middle, Karl Smith, S&P Med., UWI, Bob Hill, CFNI, Sandy Robertson, P Millbank Fndn., MSR and VC Roy Marshall, UWI; bottom, plenary session. R: enlargement of self and VC Marshall discussing "problems" at UWI.

He was as good as his word, but Dean Stuart's report (Professor Stuart had succeeded Eric Cruickshank in the yearly rotational part-time deanship) had allayed fears and promised action on the staff issues: research funding; teaching loads of junior staff; high student:staff, patient:staff and student:patient ratios, and slow progress on the Eastern Caribbean scheme (p. 163). This last measure had been planned to show EC governments that training could take place there, as they had wished. At the same time, it would relieve pressure on clinical staff at Mona by distributing clinical students to Trinidad and Barbados.

The VC's acceptance of the Dean's assurances — who, meanwhile, had told the Faculty Board that delays were due to University inaction — had halted University investigation of our position. We responded with the formation of an "Action Group," which I chaired. It wasn't a "strike," more a meeting of like minds, finally discovering one another. My prior service as Vice Chairman of the Hospital's Medical Staff Committee (Chair, Andrew Masson), and Chair of the Records Committee had informed me of the workings of the Hospital Administration (I attended Board meetings with Andrew) as well as our monthly staff meetings, which were poorly attended, thus, most staff were ill-informed on Hospital affairs; in those days, when everything was in short supply or labour intensive, a newsletter was beyond our reach.

Prominent members of the Action Group were staff members Rolf Richards, Malcolm Adam, Karl Smith, Errol Walrond, Nigel Gibbs, Molly Thorburn, Colin Miller, Bob Gray, Paul Milner, Winston Chen, Viv Brooks, Reg Carpenter, Marie Campbell, Mike Woo Ming, Andy Joaquin, Val Young, and Brian Sharpe, plus Rabin Sahoy, Gene Burkett, Paul Arscott and Fred Hickling (Junior Staff). Dawn Swaby ('70), L. Matadial ('71) and P. Figueroa ('72), were among the many students. The Report covered all Faculty activities and was presented to VC Marshall, PVCs A. Preston (Finance) and L. Robinson (Planning); C. Jackman, Registrar; H. Holness, Bursar; and R. Augier, Chair, Board for Higher Degrees.

Some residents had surprised me by staying away from the issues, although they had held strong positions for or against, e.g. Herbert Ho Ping Kong (65) and Keith Prendergast (68), both Jamaicans, who were among those seen as future Faculty members. The non-Jamaicans who took an active interest were those who wished to stay at UHWI, e.g. Sahoy, Richards, Adam; or were married to Jamaicans e.g. Woo Ming, Gibbs, Thorburn, and Bankay. Abstainers included Bill Brooks and Vasil Persaud from Pathology; Don Christian, Pam Rodgers and James Ling and their residents from Medicine; Dave Picou and George Alleyne from TMRU, Hal Dyer from the Health Centre, though he sympathised with many of our views, but felt that we were somewhat quixotic, and biting off more than we could chew; and a few others.

They were informed, like all members of the Faculty Board and Committees, and were aware of, if not interested in events, but didn't show any appreciation of the detective work needed to ferret out some of the "confidential information" that underpinned our recommendations; some medical researchers would regard manpower and education studies as "non-medical," and stuff for social scientists, not proper medical men! (See Alleyne, p. 370-1.)[8] There were others on the sidelines, mainly expatriates, and some West Indians, neutral, and willing to listen to any sound proposal, e.g. Andrew Masson, John Golding and Dave Atkinson (Surgery); Bill Whimster, Harold Chan, Herbert McDonald and Joan Summerell (Pathology). Others were not willing to show their hand,

---

[8]Some would a few years later show the result of their aloofness by their ignorance of the ground we had covered, when as Senior Faculty in the late 1970s, under Dean Sam Wray, they groped for a way forward, repeated some and ignored most of the self-reliant work done and progress made in the early 1970s to create a "Caribbean doctor", plagiarising my papers of that period, and latching on to the coat-tails of the new McMaster Medical school, which had begun to publicise itself globally, powered by lavish grants from the Ontario government, and a University President and founding Dean of Medicine with family connections to one of Canada's largest banks. Several seminars on curriculum were held, involved PAHO, under its new Director, Hector Acuña, with US and Canadian participants; they adopted a McMaster style study plan at the Trinidad campus when it opened in 1989, after lying idle for four years after completion (*vide infra*).

mostly for personal reasons, or career concerns. The latter included UN Pathak, Mavis Anderson, H. Wynter, and S. Singh (a registrar), from O&G; Ted Belle and Dorothy King from Microbiology; John Hayes, F. Cole, A. Talerman, E. Ahern, and several residents: Shirley Amin, Pam Da Camara, and Olive Williams, from Pathology; O. Minott, S&P Medicine; O. Morgan and O. Barrow, Medicine; Eve Palomino, Paediatrics, and others. But we had bright minds in support, and momentum, with detailed facts on the issues, and enough sympathisers.

The Action Group presented its report on Sept. 25, 1970 at a special forum with Vice-chancellor Roy Marshall, and teams from the University and the Hospital administration. It covered the following:

Hospital Affairs: The administration; medical staff; number of interns, residents (house officers and registrars), and consultants (dermatology, ENT and other special surgery e.g. ophthalmology, plastic surgery); space needs: inadequacy of beds, offices, housing etc. created an unproductive milieu; the telephone services were poor, both internally and nationally; the wait for a home phone could be up to six months, even with the priority given to physicians and emergency workers; maintenance and security were unreliable and underprovided.

Faculty & University matters: these centred on the mission of the Faculty: what kind of doctor should it produce? At the time, we graduated a "multi-mini-specialist," which sounded like what small nations needed, a jack of all trades, but many graduates tended to find this overwhelming in practice and chose to pursue single specialties instead, which only the largest populations could absorb, and even so, only in small numbers. Meanwhile, the CHMC was telling us that primary and community services were inadequate. Should we then modify our product? Examinations reforms had begun following my work re Part 1 Finals, which had been accepted by the Faculty Board and in use since 1968, while changes to other parts were promised.

The group focussed also on new programs, urgently needed to address outstanding concerns re health care in contributing territories. These included Postgraduate education, Community Medicine and Family Practice. The hurdles included staff unrest, insufficient research time (not enough SHOs and registrars for service work), a flawed promotions process, based on criteria copied from an affluent British model, with half the work-load and twice the staff; residents did little research in training; besides we had scant or no resources for this. A prominent complaint was that staff were poorly informed on Faculty matters and had no voice in governance of either Faculty or Hospital. The Dean's Office was under the hegemony of Department Heads, some of whom controlled resources as if they were personal property, and often had no factual knowledge of the basis of financial management, a situation similar to one afflicting certain officers of government.

These raised questions concerning the poor political relations among governments that had led to the collapse of the WI Federation (in any case a poorly-considered act of an imperialist eager to shed colonies, and blind to the corrosive divisions created by its former colonial policies). The emerging nations, educated in a cloud of British fables and fantasies, suddenly were exposed to economic and social realities of independence, and to demands that swiftly exhausted their purses; and when the mists began to clear—and far too slowly, stalled as they were by class, colour and race—those who could see, realised that most governments were almost broke. The economic and social adjustments they had chosen, from Trinidad's racially-biased oligarchy to Burnham's communist dictatorship, were often capricious, and fractured relations, uprooting many of the best talent, leaving the new nations weaker than before.

The relationship between governments and University was that of ownership by the former and aloofness by the latter, nurtured by the culture of exclusivity of higher education and the "higher educated" in the British Empire. This "town versus gown" mentality was perhaps acceptable in private universities, such as the American Ivy league, which some of their acolytes on the UWI staff touted as models, without reference to their nature, mission or wealth. The Colonial Office did not study the effects of this attitude on the viability or survival of the UCWI as a multi-national institution, and might not have properly anticipated the storms through which it had to pass to survive. That it did is thanks to a succession of dedicated and almost sacrificial leaders from its inception.

Faculty finance, administration and governance were inadequate to the demands of a high student intake, and it was soon obvious that intake exceeded both facilities and academic capacity. The specialties of Anaesthesia and Radiology should have become full academic departments by 1966, or the departmental structure, with its overlaps, territorialism, and possibly waste, should have given way to groupings of departments into "divisions." The new areas of Family Medicine and Community Medicine could develop academically as a Division, with Psychiatry, Social and Preventive Medicine, and Public Health. But the matter remained to be debated by the Faculty Board, and was unlikely to be debated as long as that body remained a cabal of department heads.

Staff workloads *(Fig 25-4, p. 226)* had increased as intake increased, with the common complaint that appointments and promotions were often contentious, focussing heavily on research and publications, while staff had little or no funds or support for research, while fully occupied with teaching and service.

Government criticisms of UWI and its products mounted, as graduates increasingly failed to return to serve their homelands. This was straining relationships with the University, which could hardly be expected to control the movements of graduates, but governments could, if they routinely bonded physicians — whose education they had financed — for a set period of service after graduation. Governments pressed instead for a curricular change to reflect their needs, and wanted their voices heard. Yet neither would guarantee retention of graduates.

Many heads balked as they were "sceptical of a non-academic's ability to grapple with learning issues." Should there be a committee of CHMC and the Medical Faculty on curriculum? Could one expect any major input from a gaggle of politicians beyond motherhood political statements and views on the type of product they wish to finance? As Chairman of the Curriculum Committee, I had issued a standing invitation for a CMO representative to attend meetings. I believed that Governments and providers of care should have a voice in our councils. We needed to know their needs and how well our graduates performed in meeting those needs. Comments made at Council meetings often failed to reach the Medical Faculty. Later, at a CHMC meeting, we suggested, and CHMC welcomed a permanent joint forum to discuss issues on education for the health services.

The CMOs of CHMC members constituted a technical committee, which met before each annual meeting to prepare the agenda and prime the Ministers. In 1970, I had attended one of their sessions in Barbados and discussed the curricular issues, among others. They suggested that it was enough that we considered their views on the final product and would not be concerned with details. If any was of crucial importance, they could communicate by writing or by personal attendance on our invitation. Dean Stuart had agreed, and so it was left.

The Action Group Report had included data on performance in teaching, service and research that surprisingly exceeded expectations and confirmed the hard work done by staff at all levels, and that quality was maintained. The Group recommended an external review of the issue of workloads, which might not be such a great impediment to research output, if adequate *support* were available, e.g. more audiovisual and stenographic and other support, in a pool available to all researchers, with time for research protected. External examiners of high calibre visited twice each year, and could constitute such a review panel.

The Report was signed by *"Drs M. Ragbeer, M. Woo Ming, E. Walrond, A. Joaquin, and R. Sahoy,"* and later endorsed by C. Miller, K Smith, M. Thorburn, N. Gibbs, P. Milner, D. Carpenter, H. McDonald and several others. Added and unexpected support came from members of the central administration who had become increasingly critical of the Medical Faculty's sloth in carrying out reforms, and its reliance on the same nucleus of influential voices, the academic heads, to convey Faculty views to University Committees, giving the impression that the Faculty had a single voice, and that everyone was conceited and content. This was inevitable since the pool from which selections were made was limited to the Faculty Board, then excluding junior and middle-grade staff. I was an anomaly, a non-voter, there by virtue of my role as Associate Dean for Education. I remember how surprised members of the University Board for Higher Degrees were, when I became the Faculty nominee to the Board.

OUTLINE OF RECOMMENDATIONS, ACTION GROUP, 1970

A.   HOSPITAL AFFAIRS
    (1)   Strict limitation of Clinic size.
    (2)   Replacement of General Practice type "Casualty" practice
        by an Emergency and Accident Service only.
    (3)   Government to strengthen its Hospital Outpatient Departments
        and CLINICS by
            (a) adequate staffing
            (b) adequate medicines
    (4)   Increase UHWI links with other Corporate area hospitals;
    (5)   Definition of hospital areas of responsibility for patient care,
        geographic and special services.
    (6)   Change Staff Structure of Hospital and Teaching Staff:
            (a) "Separation" of Academic from Routine Services
            (b) Increase part-time staff in major specialties
                (load, teaching)
            (c) Increase junior and middle grade hospital staff
                (service load and postgraduate study);
    (7)   Careful definition of Conditions of Service and Contracts,
        including work in sub-specialties;
    (8)   Reorganise Hospital Administration, especially its Financial
        section and reform its management:
            (a) Budget on an Annual basis
            (b) Create Contingency Fund
            (c) Appoint a fully trained Hospital Administrator
            (d) Obtain services of a "top class" Financial Director
    (9)   Establish Adequate Public Relations;
    (10) Expand Hospital & Increase Sources of Hospital Revenue:
            (a) Establish Private Block
            (b) Develop Specialties

       (c)   Encourage development of endowments, e.g. Heart Foundation.

B   FACULTY AFFAIRS

    (1)   Strengthen Administration

       (a) Full-time Dean/Medical Educator vice volunteers
       (b) Trained Administrator for Dean's Office
       (c) Change structure of Faculty Board
       (d) Reorganise curriculum planning

    (2)   Departmental Development

       (a) Change hierarchical status; have separate academic and clinical heads.
       (b) Improve management of departmental affairs, e.g. policy-making, service and teaching duties by adopting democratic methods.
       (c) Encourage development of specialties.
       (d) Involve a larger number of part-time staff.

    (3)   Improve Conditions of Service for Academic Staff:

       (a) Reduce routine service load
       (b) Provide adequate research facilities
       (c) Improve remuneration urgently
       (d) Reform Rules re Promotions and Appointments

    (4)   Improve Conditions of Study for Students:

       (a) Amenities
       (b) Library
       (c) More effective teaching at all levels
       (d) Streamline processes of assessment
       (e) Reorganise courses
       (f) Create "Dean of Students"
       (g) Increase staff:student ratio and improve relationships.

    (5)   Organise postgraduate teaching (specialty development is essential for this)

    (6)   Improve Medical Communication & Faculty Public Relations, through media such as W.I.M.J., which should expand its scope to include sections with discussion papers, letters, and other communication.

C. UNIVERSITY AFFAIRS

(1) Insist on Maintenance of high academic standards by Faculty.

(2) Reduce student intake (until imbalances remedied).

(3) Relations with Hospital:
    a) Insist on reforms in Hospital administration and fiscal arrangements (planning, budgeting, etc.)
    b) Urge construction of private block, and development of subspecialties

(4) Wider recognition of specialties for University appointment

(5) Revise attitudes towards the Medical Faculty in view of its essential differences and unique position within the University.

(6) Urge extension of basic clinical training to Hospitals outside Mona.

(7) Establish a new Medical School in the Eastern Caribbean
– Action Group Recommendations, end.

The University team listened with care, some disbelief, and surprise that the giant had awakened. At the end, VC Marshall listed those reforms that could be done within the Faculty: Board structure and membership; research time; workloads etc.; and those that required University action. The latter included aspects of Faculty restructure; finance; staffing; communication; and a full time Dean, to which the University had already agreed in principle, and was awaiting action and a recommendation from the Board of the Faculty of Medicine! That was a surprise and caught Dean Stuart and other senior Board Members off-guard, as they had not informed us of this, nor had Department heads been open with *all* their staff, tending to take a few senior or favourite ones into confidence and ignoring others, on the principle that "Father knows best; trust us." One department head was enraged enough to announce to us, "You can have my job!" He settled down soon after, when he recalled that he too had had to rebel to get ahead.

Financing of extra posts was another matter, but the VC advised that we must first try to fill all vacancies, of which there were several. We suggested that money for unfilled posts should be deposited into a Faculty research and development fund, instead of simple reversion to the general purse of the University. That was resisted by PVC Finance as contrary to the rules of the Finance and General Purposes Committee! We responded with the view that a Faculty budget should be under that Faculty's control, and rules should permit a Faculty Finance Committee to move unused funds to areas of pressing need. Faculty members were far more qualified to assess this than any central University group, however bright or well-meaning. To facilitate such actions, we opted for a divisional structure to share budgets, space, equipment, time-tables, staff and so on, to reduce administrative costs and facilitate curriculum planning and implementation. The Faculty itself could eventually develop into a self-governing "school" within the University, and be responsible for its own financing.

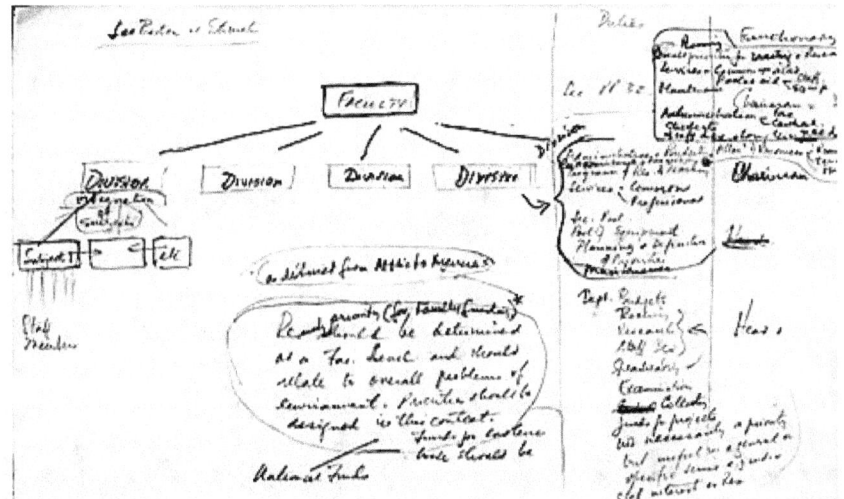

Fig 4-2: Original draft of Divisional Structure as scribbled during discussions with VC Marshall in 1971, and later revived with VC Preston for Faculty or School of Health Sciences,

This displeased some Faculty administrators, as it seemed the British system had held sacred the silos of departments that could directly plead with the Centre and bypass the more critical eyes of their Faculty peers. The shifting of the sort we were suggesting, from one pocket to another by the person wearing the garment, was anathema! This became a source of contention as evidence suggested that the Faculty of Medicine was subsidising other departments or Faculties, and filling of positions had frequently been delayed to accrue "savings", which were not all channelled to the appropriate Faculty, and seemed to be used as a slush fund to reward "favourites." As expected, the argument was vehemently rejected by PVC Finance and colleagues, who deflected discussions to what the Faculty could do within the rules, and defer those that would require a debate in Council and Charter change. Its leaders were free to bring matters to the appropriate University committees, especially Planning and the Joint Committee of Council and Senate (JCCS).

We noted that since becoming VC, Professor Marshall had made useful change to the senior administration by appointment of PVCs for Finance (Preston), and Planning (Robinson), while he and the two PVC's in the EC—Lloyd Braithwaite, T&T, and Sydney Martin, Cave Hill— would continue to perform the duties of campus principals. We hoped that he would next consider our plan for Faculty organisation. By this time students had gained representation on University committees, but at Mona, they had protested the exclusion of sociologist Dr Clive Thomas from Jamaica in 1969, and in T&T against the visit by Canadian Governor General Roland Michener because of expulsion of rioting students from Ottawa's Sir George Williams University. In 1970, the same students protested service to the Chancellor, Princess Alice, and joined Black power groups, while further unrest plagued the Mona campus (Ch. 25).

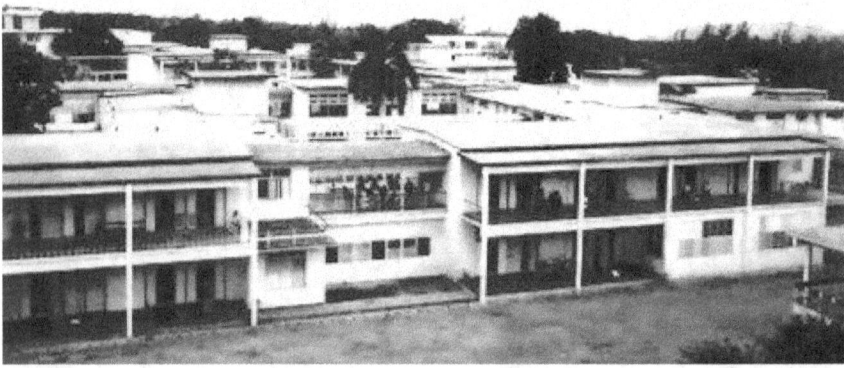

Fig 4-3: UHWI, showing Wards 3 and 7, upper floor and 1 and 5 below, part of the original structure; Wards 4 and 8, and 2 and 6, mirror these in the middle distance; central supply and ORs are at middle right. A later addition of specialty units is shown in background.

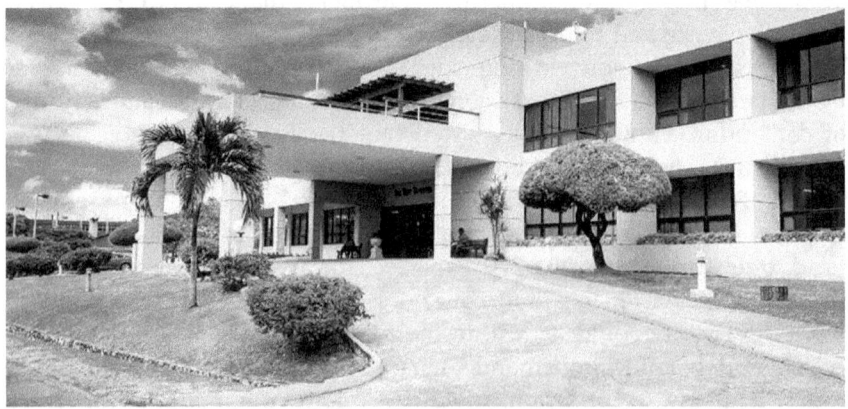

Fig 4-4: UHWI: Façade of the Tony Thwaites Private wing on Ring Road, UHWI (http://ttwing.com/wp-content/themes/ttw/images/ttw_home_2.jpg)

CHAPTER 5
Reforming the Curriculum

Caribbean communities supporting the UWI were all islands, except for Belize, and as deprived of scientific medical services as communities in African and Asian colonies. A look at the belated and desultory development of medical schools in British colonies post-WWII showed a singular pattern, whether Makerere in Uganda, Ibadan in Nigeria, U. Malaysia in Kuala Lumpur, or UWI in the Caribbean. All were wards of a major British University, all following that University's aim of producing enough doctors to work in communities in their native districts, to which they would all dutifully return. The added benefit of diverting colonials from British schools was appreciated. Each of these schools was planned to serve an entire region, e.g. UCWI, the British West Indies; Ibadan, Nigeria; Makerere, British East Africa, and so on. It wasn't long after that all of these places founded several universities.

How late universities came to non-white colonies could be realised by recalling that white Puritan settlers in America had started Harvard in 1636, just a few decades after the Massachusetts Bay colony had been founded; it had started as a private religious college, headed by a priest, and grew from that base to today's prime Ivy League University. No such motivation existed in the non-white slave colonies until the British Raj found it necessary to educate a local colonial civil service.[9]

Colonial universities were established as Colleges and academic copies of their parent universities, as wards of their governments and subject to Government policies, but protected from political change by their charters. Thus, in each medical faculty, pre-medical preparation preceded a detailed study of pre-clinical subjects, leading to a thorough coverage of nearly all aspects of clinical medicine and surgery. These included radiology; anaesthesia; ENT; dermatology; forensic medicine; and public health. The last included site visits—after survey lectures—to an abattoir; restaurant kitchen; sewage treatment and water purification plants; dairy; milk pasteurisation plant; cement and clothing factories; and clinics for VDs, leprosy, and others. The UCWI curriculum included a course in dentistry, where one learned oral hygiene and performed extractions. In Pathology, each student had to assist in at least nine autopsies, fully charted and marked; and, for O&G, complete 20 ante-natal cases and supervised deliveries, some domiciliary, when that new

---

[9] See my book *India, under siege, the enemy within,* Bibliography, where this is discussed.

Year	Oct – Dec	Jan – Mar	Apr – June	July–Sept
1	Anatomy (A) Physiology (P)	Anatomy Physiology	Anatomy Physiology Biochemistry (B)	VACATION
2	Anatomy Physiology Biochemistry	Anatomy/ Physiology & Biochemistry Pharmacology	Anatomy/ Physiology Pharmacology (p) **Exams A,B,P,p**	VACATION
3	Introductory Course	Junior Med. Casualty	Junior Surg. + 1 month Anaesthesia	Surgery
4	Medicine Eyes Casualty	Paediatrics V.Ds. Prev. Medicine	Pathology Skins Prev. Medicine Forensic Medicine	Obst & Gynae Prev. Medicine
5	Obst & Gynae Prev. Medicine	Medicine Ante natal Mental Dentistry **Part I Final Exams** in **Path/Micro,** mid-April)	Surgery E.N.T.	Free **Final Exams: Parts II ,III, IV** in early October

TABLE 5-1: "Program of Work" – Faculty of Medicine, U.C.W.I.,1949–1965.

This UCHWI "London Curriculum" emphasised sciences in medicine and was successful in producing a medical scientist, competent in all clinical disciplines, although in practice the "minor" disciplines suffered as students increased and teachers did not. This curriculum was widespread, but neglected to require mastery of behavioural and community aspects of health and disease, thus branding doctors generally as insensitive, dogmatic, and arrogant, despite those who have risen above this stereotype.

service began in 1956. Indeed, I was honoured to be assigned its first patient and do her home care and delivery. Students were rotated on call through Casualty, did all the uncomplicated suturing and whatever care the physician delegated. No stage of training was lightly passed over. An index of this rigour is seen in the fact that only 13 of the original 33 entrants completed their training on time six years later. Thus, after the icing provided by an internship, most graduates could take on anything that came their way in their own city hospitals. But colonial governments were too poorly financed to offer them employment, so were ill-prepared for them, except to fill vacancies, or set up practice in places deemed unsuited to British doctors! Many found this daunting and stayed away.

Medical services in every colony were part of the general civil service, even though many of their demands: personnel services, hours of work, worker training, other conditions of service, organisation, management, and so on, were better served independently, as I had concluded in my time as a personnel officer in BG's Medical Department. When the colonies became independent, however, they stuck to colonial ways: customs, laws, procedures, structures, attitudes, which were strong deterrents to returning graduates (see *The Indelible Red Stain, Bk 1*, Bibliography). With the shortage of specialists generally, and their exalted positions in the Civil Service hierarchy, it was no wonder that so many pursued specialty education, effectively "wasting" all that "other" knowledge they had acquired in preparing to deliver confident and *comprehensive* sickness care.

The UWI obtained its independent charter in the same year as the major states, Jamaica and Trinidad, became independent, and the WI Federation collapsed. The British had hoped to pass the University to the Federation it had cobbled together, with the same flaws and fate as those in central Africa and Malaysia. Soon after, questions began to be asked about the aims of medical education, and focussed on the curriculum.

Subdued colonial society had given way to restless independence and ambitious politicians, who quickly carved out sectors of popular support, and clung to them by ideology and/or personality. In Jamaica, Alexander Bustamante bought his support with charisma, salt fish and ackee! But Government funding was tight; Britain was still crawling out of near bankruptcy, and when even an islet claimed self-rule, was quite delighted to grant it, however irresponsible the decision. The islands soon felt the weight of financial obligations, and in time began to consult one another to find solutions. By 1967, five years after UWI, and the breakaway of Guyana from it, the Commonwealth Caribbean Health Ministers got together, targetted joint property, such as the UWI, which most saw as a liability forced on them by Britain, and started to pen resolutions. The UWI was in fact the only tangible joint asset left, beside the cricket team, after the Federation fell in 1962.

It had not suited the imperialists to have their colonies talk amicably or get to know one another, to forestall any union that could blossom into a revolt. So the UCWI was a brave, some say foolhardy experiment, by politically naive British academics. But the students had taken it seriously, made friends, intermarried and worked in each other's territory. Jamaica was the main beneficiary, and Barbados, when Guyana withdrew. Trinidad was troubled by a racial problem that Eric Williams fostered rather than squelched. But his bias was cast in stone and he held to it and created, as did Burnham in Guyana, a racial rift that would fester, become chronic, infect their successors and spoil society for good.

The UWI at its birth had acquired important Trinidad resources, the chief being the *Imperial College of Tropical Agriculture*, a reputable school at St. Augustine, which became the Faculties of Engineering and Agriculture, to which new ones of Arts, Sciences, Education and Sociology were added. This second campus brought rivals Trinidad and Jamaica into closer association, not without friction.

When Guyana quit in 1962, the third campus went to Barbados, a community with probably the highest proportion of people with secondary education. Barbados became independent in 1966, despite white "apartheid". But under Premier Errol Barrow, it steered a sensible economic course, avoiding clashes with whites, and the ideological adventurism that tended to scare away highly-trained people, like doctors, who, by then, were finding positions in North America, and fleeing restless regimes in Jamaica, Guyana, Trinidad, and others.

Nearly half of the 1969 class interned elsewhere; Jamaica's losses were relieved in part by retention of graduates from Guyana and the EC islands. This degree of brain drain, internal and external, prompted a greater demand for its end, or at least reduction. The causes were complex, but repeated surveys of migrants and would-be migrants identified curricular compatibility with those in Britain, recognition by GMC, UK, and availability of specialty training in the US as major pulls.

Year of graduation	% outside of Commonwealth Caribbean in Sept 1970
1965	30
1966	45
1967	59
1968	42
1969	40

Table 5-2: The Brain Drain

At their first meeting in 1967, Caribbean Health Ministers demanded that they needed to "taste, not just see a piece of the doctor pie," as one said. They had paid for medical education for nearly two decades, and were still waiting for the promised "adequate and well-trained staff." Instead, the only beneficiary seemed to be Jamaica, and, to a lesser extent, Trinidad and Barbados. But that did not mean that all graduates were satisfactory. Though generally competent in urban hospitals, they were quite uncomfortable in clinics, especially in rural areas, and in dealing with behavioural, family and community issues. The matter was referred to the Curriculum Committee.

Curriculum reform began slowly, struggling against the entrenched positions of departments, especially pre-clinical ones, which commanded two years of training of nine academic months each. The two three-month holidays were welcomed by students who tried to get a job to help with tuition and living expenses. But there was a significant opinion that at least half of those months could be used to shorten the period of medical training. The mood of the school at that time was to move away from rigid structures or programs, and develop flexible systems that would facilitate amendments or expansion, and to make training in the Eastern Caribbean viable and attractive. Already the number of beds at UHWI (500) was insufficient to provide 200+ clinical students with a consistent exposure to clinical work (*see Fig 25-4, p. 226*). This pressure had convinced even the most resistant Faculty member of the necessity to find more clinical space or partners. The Eastern Caribbean islands, especially Trinidad and Barbados, were developed enough for clinical students; expansion would please their people and governments, and stem criticism of the University for failing to "return graduates" to them.

By 1967, we had drafted, and by 1968 started the scheme to develop clinical training in Trinidad and Barbados. We learned that the Trinidad Government had obtained funds for a maternity Hospital at Mount Hope, near St Augustine. At that time, the Government of Jamaica had agreed to build regional hospitals, one of about 400 beds — the Cornwall Regional Hospital — on the outskirts of Montego Bay, and another, 300 beds, in May Pen, at the centre of the island. These, the Queen Elizabeth Hospital, Barbados, and the planned Mount Hope Hospital, Trinidad, held promise as learning centres, although as yet no Faculty member had been involved in their planning. Trinidad had involved University engineers as structural consultants, but no one from Medicine, except informally. At Mona, few knew anything about these developments, but we would have a chance to get solid information when we met the CHMC in 1971 to present our plans for specialty training.

Most of the troubles we had in this, as in other contemporary projects, were rooted in the undergraduate curriculum, then virtually written in stone. When I reported to Professor Cruickshank that I could not rationally proceed with educational planning because of curricular hurdles, which I partially explored in an article for the student magazine, *The Stethoscope*,[10] he appointed me, with Professor Bras's agreement, to the Curriculum Committee, to make my case there. At that time, the

---

[10]The Undergraduate Curriculum, Medical Faculty, UWI - an opinion, 1970, *Stethoscope* 6,8

Committee had no agreed statement of aim for medical education at the UWI, or for the Caribbean—now called *'mission'*, replacing a military term with an evangelical one! The Committee consisted of subject agents who met to bargain for "teaching hours," and thus resources, in the model common to all London Colleges: to cover the syllabus and produce an informed graduate. Community skills, including behaviour, attitudes, communications etc., were not emphasised, thus not tested.

After exploratory discussions, I reported to the Dean and Prof. Bras that we could not decide how, what, or how much to teach, without knowing what kind of doctor(s) we were expected to produce, in terms of competences and behaviours. It was by then plain that the classic UK model of a toti-potential doctor, a "multi-mini-specialist," trained in hospital medicine for all sickness needs, was out-dated. However, the Chair of the Curriculum Committee, Professor Louis Grant, advised that that was not an issue for his group, but for the Faculty Board, which then consisted of all Heads of Departments, all Professors and Readers, three Senior Lecturers and two Lecturers, the last five all appointed.

We had also questioned specific aspects of the curriculum, where the knowledge learned was mistimed — generally too early and forgotten by the time it was needed, or non-contributory, or useful insights had been withheld.[11]. This criticism was shared by several members, who had passively sought to retain departmental hours and had simply haggled for them, without too much consideration of the education issues. Professor Grant had not faced the issue, and had carried on what London had begun, assuming that given the time, the learning will follow.

Facing arguments for reform, he deferred discussion to the next meeting. Reporting to the Faculty Board, he suggested that as Associate Dean, I should handle the matter. Having no wish to argue it, and preferring the status quo for his department, Grant resigned as Chair, saying it was time someone else took over. Dean Cruickshank agreed, as did Bras and Ken Stuart, the Dean-designate for 1970-71. So much for complaining! Despite protesting re lost research time, I ended up with the issue in my lap, on the argument that it was *educational* research!

I had, at the start, made a motion, seconded by Paul Milner, head of Haematology, that the Curriculum Committee should urgently consider making a statement of the aims of medical education at the UWI, a

---

[11]The rebuttal to this was that issues were easier to revise than to learn fresh, and it was doubted that the good student would totally forget learned knowledge, even if it was not immediately applied. Advocates of problem-based learning and Carl Roger's learning theory, however, argued that new knowledge gained in relation to problem-solving tended to be retained better as the problem was likely to occur in another patient and solutions thereby reinforced. By the same token, if one relied on problems to stimulate learning, new knowledge is not gained for its own sake, and much basic information could be missed.

matter then seething among undergraduates, graduates and junior faculty, who were brimming with ideas and teaching plans. The CHMC had also begun to ask for *"a doctor more suited to the region than for the corridors of US hospitals!"* I thus viewed the appointment to the Chair of the Curriculum Committee as a penalty for causing trouble; it added to my already overflowing files as Coordinator of Postgraduate Education (PGME), which Professor Cruickshank had labelled me in 1968-9.

Satisfying Caribbean realities called for a changed approach, aimed at competence in Primary Care, Community Medicine (Ch. 26), and a range of specialties. The Faculty also had a key role in training ancillaries (aides, assistants etc.), and Continuing Education for all cadres *(See Fig 5-1, p. 56)*. Clearly, the Faculty may not directly train ancillary staff, but must know how they were trained and what they did in the continuum of care, as part of health teams, whatever the task, simple or complex; it could contribute to staff development of supervisory skills. Departments could define the work for specific aides, and regroup as "Divisions," to facilitate this, which might require a Charter amendment. Training of ancillaries could be coordinated by the proposed Division of Community Medicine, with inputs from Governments. While the UWI must be vigilant to keep *politicians* out of daily routines, the states that supported it were too small to afford town-gown schisms at the level of policy and planning. (*Ragbeer and Burton*, CHMC IV, 1972, Bibliography).

In 1969, I took to the Curriculum Committee a paper on principles for a new curriculum, which Professor David Hoyte and I had drafted, based on the aims stated in a 1968 revision of the model by Case Western Reserve University, Cleveland, Ohio, which I had reviewed while in the USA. It was flexible, with goals that reflected ours: to teach students about health and disease, their natural history and what can change that; to treat patients as persons and members of a community, integrating teaching of basic sciences and clinical disciplines, promoting self-directed and life-long learning, and research to integrate new knowledge in the clinical problem-solving matrix, under critical eyes of teachers, to enable them to deliver holistic health care as defined by Ministries. Learning would expand from hospital wards, to emergency rooms, laboratories, clinics, occupational and public health units, rehabilitation centres (e.g., polio), to prevent disease, promote health, and give efficient service.

The Committee agreed that we *had* to teach facts on human biology and clinical medicine, and prepare students for community practice. Ideally, an integration of studies could begin by exposing students early to clinical cases as a reason and basis for structure and function studies, but staffing and the error of planting pre-clinical buildings a mile from the hospital precluded that, and its correction became our *cause célèbre*.

Chief Medical Officers gave *provider* opinions on medical education at each meeting of the CHMC, starting in 1969. That year, the Dean had invited Dr Sam Street, CMO, Jamaica, to a Faculty meeting, at which he shared Government's outlook for the services. The Committee of CMOs had agreed on the holistic nature of a doctor's function, from promotion of physical and mental health and disease prevention, to sickness care and rehabilitation. Thus, although education in human biology was a major part of the cake, other less tasty layers or visible ingredients influenced health and illness: human behaviour, socio-economics, ecology, education, sanitation, agriculture, food, politics, jobs, personal choices and habits, government, health care organisation and administration, etc. Doctors must learn their roles and combined impact.

After several consultations and discussions with Carlyle Burton, their ad hoc Chair, and Head of the Barbados Civil Service, at the 1970 CHMC meeting in Barbados, I received this summary: "*All medical practitioners should have a core of knowledge: basic facts of normal anatomy, physiology, biochemistry, or cell biology, or whatever name is fashionable or most appealing; pathologic processes, basic and as affected by environmental circumstances, social and cultural phenomena, diet, economics, religious practices, climate, geography, etc., and include an understanding of health care organisation and facilities in the various territories. The fare must be adequately balanced and examples drawn from local experience primarily, and supplemented or amplified by extraneous ones that have a high impact on local health e.g. jobs, travel, tourism, international business, agencies and similar contacts. The remainder of the formal education period should concentrate, through required and elective opportunities, on exposure to the whole spectrum of health disciplines, including needs, organisation, delivery, etc., and give the student a period for elective studies of his/her choice.*"

The statement was inclusive and in line with our ideas, which had been tested at previous CHMC meetings. We stressed for our Committee a few epidemiological facts in health care and how resources were affected. Of 100 persons in a community needing care, over 75 or more would have common ailments like cuts and bruises, rashes, benign coughs and temporary colds, upset stomachs or bowels, children to be immunised, pregnancy, and routine ante-natal or similar primary care that could be managed at home, after some specific attention by a doctor or other primary care-giver. Another 15-20 may have ongoing chronic conditions and at risk for sudden complications, therefore needing more focussed or special care, mostly ambulatory, but at times institutional. Five to ten will need special care in and out of hospitals; one or two will need intensive hospital care, from accident or disease, or for certain types of treatment. The diagram below (*Table 5-3*) shows this distribution.

Table 5-3; see also Fig 5-2, p.57		
Primary Care >75% 1		
Secondary Care 15-20%	2	
Tertiary (Hospital) Care 5%		3

Our training plan exposes students to Groups 2 and 3, that is, 20% or so of the population at risk and in need. The other 80% are barely seen by students, except in casualty and outpatient clinics or as part of field work in Social & Preventive Medicine, and by the few on general practice electives.

"We should be training our doctors," I argued, *"to care for this sector of the population as diligently as we do for those in hospitals. Their needs are more varied and at times more complex, however simpler they may appear technically or biologically; but they often require more mastery than we teach of human behaviour, environmental and social realities, occupational and domestic relations, and of nutrition and education, as they affect health. Too often, hospital care is neglected primary care."*

The literature from the WHO has already begun to address specifics of this. On our part, we had not done enough to add to our curriculum human behaviour, social studies, health promotion, disease prevention, community practices, health care organisation, and the importance of research. The Pathology Department had started to give students data on disease incidence and longevity in animals fed various diets from nutritional experiments on rodents, in which Professor Bras and I were involved; choice of diet could prolong the healthy active life of animals by 2-3 times. Jamaica and the Caribbean have long had a problem of malnourished and undernourished children, their complications providing daily work for regional hospitals, the resulting learning disability retarding their chances in society.[12]

Most of this illness is very expensive and preventable. Yet the medical curriculum had no emphasis on nutrition in the basic sciences, other than the biochemistry of metabolism, and clinically only at ward rounds on malnourished children in the Paediatrics clerkship, despite dedicated metabolism and nutrition research units on campus. Doctors should be major advocates of good nutrition. We hoped to stress this in the syllabus for Community Medicine, a major aspect of the reforms, and by inviting the TMRU, ERU and CFNI to join with other disciplines to make Nutrition a strong feature of the curriculum. Thus, we would stimulate research into the properties and value of local foods common to the majority, including any medicinal use, and more and more the harmful effects of processed foods, heavily marketed by the USA.

---

[12] See Bibliography, under Ross et al, Richardson et al., Waterlow at al. See Fn. 7, p. 32

Year	Oct. Nov Dec	Jan	Feb Mar.	Apr	May June	Ju Aug Sep
1	Basic Sciences: Organic Chemistry,	V	Anatomy,	V	Physiology	V
2	and Biochemistry + Behavioural & Social Sciences		Ex abp	V	Pharm; Intro. Path/Micro Intro. Clin Med &.Surg. 3/12	Jnr. Clerk in Med.& Surg. 3/12
3	Pharma Med/Surg Path/Micro Intro. Psych.	E v Ex Ph₁ / V	Med/Surg Path/Micro Intro. Psych. / Ex m pa (1)	V	Apr-Sept: Paed. 10/52 Clin. Path Micro + VDs 10/52 / O&G. 5/52	Ex Mp a (2)
4	Psych. 5/52	Orth 5/52 Anaes. 5/52 + Part- time in Ophthal. for 5/52	Social & Prev. Medicine 5/52 +"Special" subjects 5/52 e.g. ENT, Dermatology, Radiology, Dentistry		Senior Medicine * 12/52	Senior Surgery * 12/52
5	Obst & 12/52	Gynae*	Elective* 12/52	Rev 6/52	Exam F May	

Table 5-4: First Revised Curriculum, Faculty of Medicine, UWI, 1969

*These periods may be spent in Trinidad, Barbados or Jamaica; electives anywhere approved by program

Ex= Examination (1) = first attempt (2) = second attempt. V = vacation

abp = anatomy, biochemistry, physiology, organic chemistry ph = pharmacology; mpa = basic microbiology and pathology F = final examination in clinical pathology, medicine, surgery, obstetrics & gynaecology.

Governments had no coordinated national food policy beyond public health handouts, and the work of international bureaucracies like the UNFAO and UNICEF. There was no encouragement for food research; the CFNI (PAHO) was committed to this subject, but staffed mainly by expatriates, and not directed by the nation's welfare; but they did address as many of the issues as budgets or staff interests allowed. A focus on nutrition should add to the current emphasis on other measures such as immunisation, public health, sanitation, vector biology and control etc. to promote health and prevent disease.

But while accepting the intent of the 1969 curriculum (Table 5-4), many members declined it for want of resources, and the physical gulf between basic sciences and clinical facilities; we were mindful too of GMC rigidities and settled for conjoint teaching of such disciplines as could be readily merged, e.g. structure and function studies in the basic sciences, and providing for overlap with clinical studies. The draft of the revised curriculum was completed, and the first phase of implementation agreed for the 1971-2 academic year, providing one year's notice. But it was delayed for three years, ostensibly by the need for GMC approval, and lack of staff to teach behavioural sciences — despite positive reaction in informal talks with social scientists. PAHO funded a 2-week seminar for medical staff, in December, 1971, on the teaching of behavioral sciences.

The Faculty Board assigned authority in all curricular matters to the Dean's office. The first drafts of the new curriculum were not well received by several of the senior staff, pre-clinical and clinical, based on apparent loss of teaching hours, rather than on aims, concept and design. These settled, once assurances were given that through regular review we could identify and correct problems, and that the Dean had undertaken to attend straightway to such problems.

In a subsequent review, a preferred model was adopted (Table 5-5, p. 58) and the overall design of medical studies Fig 5-1, p. 56). Students, ironically, objected to the very section their forerunners on the Curriculum Committee had welcomed: that dealing with Community Medicine, and delayed its formal launch as a requirement in the clinical plan. The Faculty Board had, after *four* years of debate, approved the Community Medicine changes in 1974, to start in 1975, under my directorship. The changes had shortened the pre-clinical period by one term and applied the time saved to introduce human behaviour, demographics, sociology, the environment, epidemiology and society, and an elective. Pharmacology was stretched out to overlap preclinical and clinical programs, allowing more integration with clinical studies and pathobiology. Community Medicine was added to the existing clerkships plus lectures in the second clinical year. Examinations would be re-arranged, to include the new topics, but the formats maintained. For the GMC, nothing was lost; instead, essential topics were added.

We had, by early 1970, cleared the academic hurdles for specialty training, whose initiation would help to retain at least the number of approved residents. Professor Stuart took over from Prof. Cruickshank as Dean for 1970-71, and renewed my appointments as Associate Dean and Coordinator of PGME, to concentrate on completing the detailed specialty plans, and arrange for financial estimates by Mr. Preston, PVC Finance; these he would put to the CHMC in mid-1970, in Barbados.

The early seventies had begun as a difficult time for staff, more leaving than joining, even Jamaicans, rattled by the political unrest and violence that had in a short time spread from its primary cauldron in west Kingston into many areas of the city, with bank and shop robberies common. The violence had reached the campus and nearby suburbs, with devastating effects on staff and families, physically and mentally. Several were assaulted, including wives, and others, including several of our secretaries and assistants. I was twice threatened at gunpoint, as recorded elsewhere, by Union enforcers. There was great fear that the violence might torpedo the HOPE program, even as it delayed curricular reform and contributions to PGME from the Eastern Caribbean.

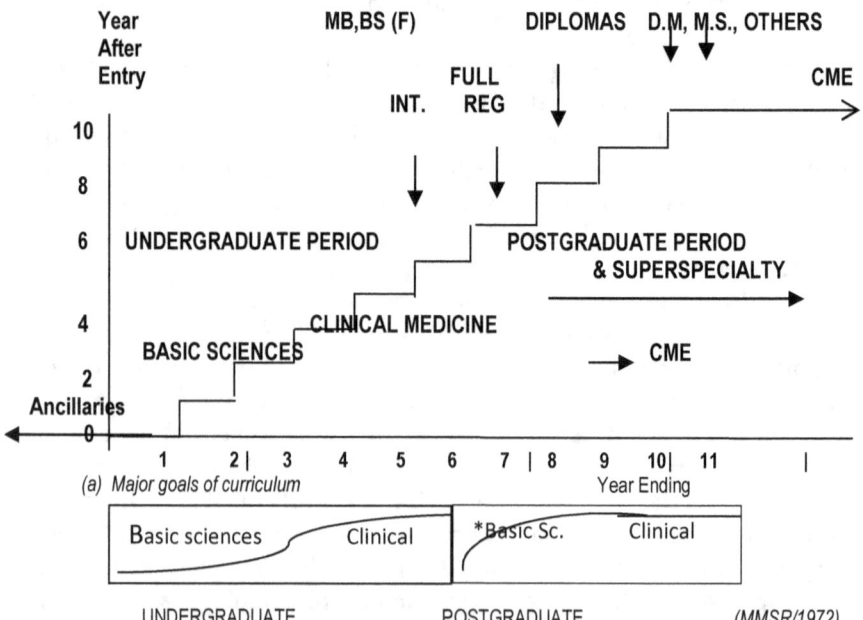

(a) Major goals of curriculum

(b) Approximate Allotment of Time for Basic Sciences and Clinical Practice in Curriculum. This will change as Community Medicine is included, and if the total undergraduate period is reduced to 4½ years.

Fig 5-1 is a simplified scheme showing the various levels of training needed in a health service, and the continuity from the least to the most complex level of training; University responsibility would begin at the medical undergraduate level, but its departments or divisions would, as now, be aware of the full range of expertise needed, and involve university students in their roles, and even in the training of non-medical cadres, of which the aide would require the shortest training and more technical groups a university degree or equivalent. The IADB Report lists 23 groups of "paramedical" or "ancillary" or "allied health" workers, several of which are trained in UWI or UHWI departments for their own use or in affiliated schools e.g. nursing, laboratory technology and radiography, and others, ad hoc. EC campuses would include these; see also p. 180.

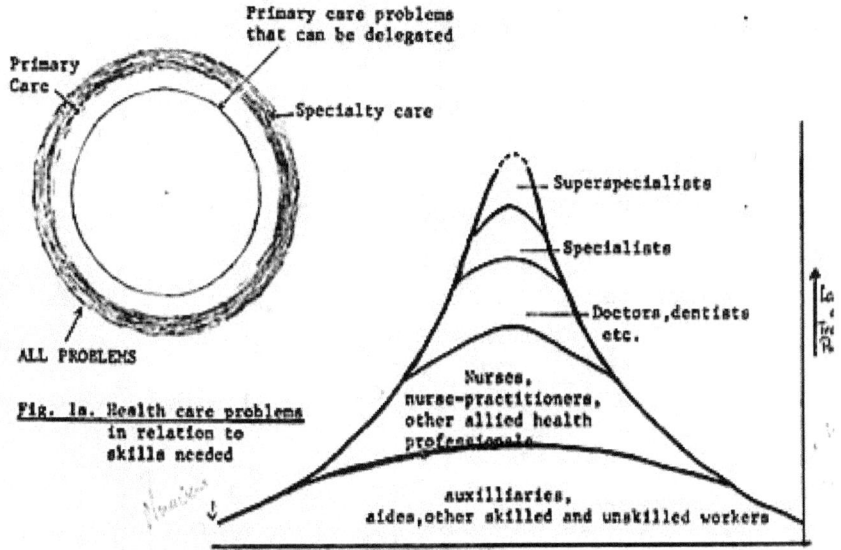

Fig 5-2, (L): a diagram of health care problems, not to scale, showing a core of primary care (up to 90% of circle) and specialty care (black) 10-20% (p 53);
Fig 5-3 (R) shows the required manpower pyramid; note the major component of ancillaries and non-medicals. This figure was used in the talk given to the Association of Commonwealth Universities, Sussex, UK, 1973 (pp 150, 239); see below Fig 5-4.

THE ROLE OF NEW UNIVERSITIES
IN THE TRAINING OF MEDICAL ANCILLARIES

PAPER BY PROFESSOR M. S. RAGBEER

Introduction

The Medical Ancillary

The dictionaries which I have consulted for the meaning of *'ancillary'* g words such as 'subservient', 'subordinate', 'aiding', 'auxiliary', thus indicati that the medical ancillary should be someone who has a *support* role in health services, and could include all such personnel whether in health servi planning, organization, management, clinical practice, community medici public health or in any other health discipline. The ancillary is not then by t definition a 'prime mover' in any particular situation, though he may be only trained person in a particular role at a particular place at a particular tir
    There are at least two approaches to defining who belongs to the group
medical ancillary. The first is to look at the tasks performed by a particu

---

Fig 5-4: First paragraph of paper read to Commonwealth Foundation, Seminar on New Universities, Role in Development, Sussex University, Sept.1973

	Oct	Dec	Apr	July			
PHASE 1, Yr. 1	Introduction to Social Sciences as Studies 2/52, with evaluation Organic Chemistry is B A S I C ←		and Behavioural basic to Medical Educ. by MCQs. mandatory in 1st term SCI ENCES+ →		Elective 4/52 Holiday 6/52	33 + Vac Xmas & Easter, 2/52 each	
Yr. 2 / PHASE 1	12/52 BASIC	12/52	12/52 SCIENCES Pharmacology	2/52 Exam	PHASE 2 Epidem. & C.Med. 4/52	8/52	8
Yr. 3 / PHASE 2	12/52 Medicine Thera-peutics	12/52 Paed	12/52 Surgery 8/52 Trauma 4/52		4/52 Anaes.	8/52 O&G	8
Yr. 4 / PHASE 2	8/52 Psych.	8/52 Comm. Med.	8/52 Pathology & Microbiol.	EXAM; V 4/52	PHASE 3, Part 1: 12/52 Elective, plus 3 of 7 clinical areas as listed below (also in caption)	12/52 rotation	8
Yr. 5 / PHASE 3	12/52 Phase 3 Part 1...	12/52 O&G, Psych	12/52 chosen from Medicine, Surgery, Paediatrics, Community Medicine, Emergency Medicine; 4 additional weeks are given each to Forensic Medicine and Revision		Final Exam	V 252	Internship 12
Yr. 6 / PHASE 3	one year	PHASE 3, Pt. 2 (Internship in up to four disciplines	12/52 periods			Full Reg.	PGME, CME

Table 5-5 Agreed Phased Curriculum (time in weeks), 1972, Curriculum Committee
+ Basic Sciences are Anatomy, Physiology, Biochemistry; exams as on p. 54
Phase 1 ("Stage" in University Calendar) includes a 2/52 course in social and behavioural aspects of medicine, the health care team; the roles of a doctor: scholar, teacher, health promoter; professional. It gives orientation to medical studies and introduces common terms, to supplement the handbook. The rest of the Phase will cover the scientific basis of Medicine, and end with an examination on all content covered. Those who pass will go on to **Phase 2,** which deals with Health, its maintenance and promotion in various environments, the conditions that impair it, the body's responses to challenges, the physical and behavioural changes produced in individuals, their families and community, and ways to detect and alleviate illnesses and prevent recurrence or spread. An examination ends the phase. Success leads to **Phase 3:** eight periods of 12/52 over a 2-year period, each in clinical disciplines to give a broad experience in clinical problem-solving and to delve further into mechanisms of disease, its effects, treatment, and prevention, in specific settings, and divisions: age, gender, location, condition, e.g. Paediatrics, Obstetrics, Emergency etc. in hospital, central, or district, and community clinics.

CHAPTER 6
PGME: before UWI, the Colonial medical Service

W hy spend so much time and money on specialty training? A basic question asked by many, for practical reasons. If one follows logically from the premise that promoting healthy living, practising primary prevention, and treating minor illnesses and accidents would take care of 85% or more of conditions that require a doctor, then proportionately more public money should be spent on these *(see diagrams pp. 53 & 57)*. Instead, health care spending goes to episodic curative and special care for the 5% who have acute illnesses, incurred through neglect or misfortune. Logically, Governments should not be responsible for preventable illnesses, or those due to life-style choices, such as smoking-related emphysema, alcoholic cirrhosis or syphilitic dementia. This may sound harsh and discriminatory, but a Government should be prudent and disciplined in its behaviour, for itself and its citizens. Unfortunately, it is unlikely that a modern "democratic" government would survive such a policy, as each citizen claims equality of treatment, despite blatant inequality of behaviours.

Yet, specialisation is the acme of medical practice, expanding as the more profligate and epicurean in society have become the power-brokers and set the demand at high levels for various services. Although the percentage of population needing specialists is small (some people actually have lived well and long without them), science has made such strides in understanding molecular behaviour, especially genetic, and human organ repair and replacement, that many individuals have come to benefit from their application. As scientific knowledge exploded in the past century, it has become impossible for any one doctor to master more than a small segment of this knowledge; thus, its application requires new experts as each new field is opened, or new diagnostic machine invented and introduced. Training in each is thus needed to ensure high quality and competence, and to protect consumers.

But the training of specialists has not always been a Government responsibility, except in socialist countries, where medical care is centrally planned and state-delivered. Most western countries now have organised specialty training and accreditation schemes, and license doctors for general or special practice.

Britain did not have an organised PGME program until 1930, when the Postgraduate Medical School was set up at the Hammersmith Hospital, London, as recommended by the Athlone Committee, appointed, in 1921, by the Ministry of Health *"to investigate the need for medical practitioners and other graduates for further education in London."* Hammersmith was chosen because it had over 400 beds, was *"centrally located"* and *"not associated with an undergraduate medical school, to distract from focus on PGME and research."* Those were the conditions set by the Committee. Formal PGME began in four specialties: Medicine, Surgery, Obstetrics and Gynaecology, and Pathology, each under a Professor, assisted by *"a reader, four assistants, and a few part-time specialist consultants."* That was just 18 years before the UCWI was started!

Hammersmith Hospital began functioning as the Royal Postgraduate Medical School of London University (RPGMS). At its formal opening in 1935, George V wished for it *"the relief of suffering among my peoples in this country and overseas, and in enabling doctors of all lands to come together in a task where all must be allies and helpers."* This was a time when University teachers were mostly voluntary, at least in the London hospitals. Thus the RPGMS was given an imperial role, trained many Commonwealth physicians and several from UCWI, starting in the early sixties with Eugene Ward, Hugh Wynter and me, contemporaneously, and later, others. Its capacity was limited and has remained so, and has now become part of Imperial College.

Colonial Medical Services, London

Colonial medical Departments, each Headed by Director of medical Services (DMS)

Colonial Medical Department+
(Service, Research, Education)

Hospitals	District Clinics	Rural & Remote Areas
(1*,2*,3* care)	1* care Limited 2* care	1* care
Specialists Generalists Apprentices & Volunteers	Generalist(f/t)	Periodic visits by GP Physician's assistant, where trained
. . . .	. . . .	. . . .

+ Essentially a curative service, with a separate Public Health subdepartment, headed by a Public Health Officer, a GP with Diplomate in Public Health, duties administrative and little or no patient contact. The CMS developed a preventive service after WW2and changed Administrative structure of departments to bring Public Health closer to Curative Services for programming and administration.

Fig 6-1 The Colonial medical Services, as seen from the Caribbean

---

The contributors to the UCWI were all part of the British Colonial Medical Services (CMS) when the College was launched, and fourteen years later, would begin to gain independence one by one, after a failed WI Federation. The CMS was then one of the largest employers of physicians, general and special, distributed mostly in urban colonial areas, with some coverage elsewhere, as shown in Fig. 6-1.

The CMS did not train any level of physician, but did help employees, in an ad hoc manner, to train for particular specialist posts; trainees had to return service for this, a kind of indenture. One of the attractions of the CMS was the chance "to see the world," and employees did roam the world. Some became justly famous for work done, e.g. Patrick Manson, who worked in China and clarified the role of the mosquito, *Culex fatigans* (*quinquefasciatus*) in Filariasis, announced in 1877, and theorised a similar role for a mosquito in Malaria.

Ronald Ross, who worked in India, met and corresponded with Manson for years, and discovered the life cycle of the malarial parasite in birds — avian malaria — which the Frenchman Alphonse Laveran had discovered in Algeria and had called *Oscillaria malariae*, later *Plasmodium*. Ross received the Nobel Prize for Medicine in 1902, but failed to credit Manson, his mentor. Such meanness is all too common in professional competitiveness, and sadly not getting better. Giglioli made advances in study of Malaria in British Guiana, and so had others who had started the British Indian Medical Service in 1800, and the Calcutta school of Tropical Medicine in the 20th century. Laveran won the Nobel Prize in 1907 for his work and donated half the money to the Pasteur Institute.

Manson had founded the College of Medicine, which became Hong Kong University. He persuaded Joseph Chamberlain, the Secretary of State for the Colonies, to set up the *London School of Hygiene and Tropical Medicine* in 1899 at a naval hospital on the lower Thames. He wrote a textbook on *Tropical Diseases* for this and would provide courses and diplomas for those entering the CMS. A similar *School of Tropical Medicine* was established that year in Liverpool, based on strong links with West Africa. Manson later became the head of the Colonial Medical Services.

His book survives to this day and now includes "native" medicine, which had been roundly rejected in his time: Ayurveda in India, and equivalents in Africa, China, Japan and SE Asia, but there are many anecdotes of Europeans of high and low status, who had accepted local medicine and its benefits. Attitudes have changed over the centuries and "alternative medicine" has a chapter now in *Manson's Tropical Diseases*, with a place in most western societies. So also have the many herbal and other remedies of Guianese natives — as related in *The Indelible Red Stain, Bk 1, Ch. 9* — which I had wanted to study, but regrettably could not.

The supporters of the UCWI each inherited a tiny slice of the CMS pie, but lost access to the pastry-maker. The CMS had filled holes in their fabric by episodic training of likely candidates in appropriate British schools, especially those two of *Hygiene and Tropical Medicine*. Candidates were usually required to have given good service over a number of "tours of service", something like a five-year minimum, in general service, with aptitude for the chosen field of study. The CMS had also exploited contacts with the large medical schools and teaching hospitals on an ad hoc basis, to train their specialists, while it grumbled for years over Britain's lack of an organised scheme of PGME.

The Royal Colleges of England, Scotland and Ireland were set on a different track. They were basically membership bodies of single specialties: Medicine, Surgery (including Anaesthesia), Obstetrics and Gynaecology, and, from the early 1960s, General Practice and Pathology. They prescribed conditions for entry to their specialties, including training, approved house officer and registrar positions in various hospitals, organised examinations, and awarded degrees. But they controlled no institutions and largely left it up to the hospitals to attain a standard that would attract graduates wanting to specialise.

CMS employees were career-driven, and none designated as a trainee; in fact there were few formal trainees in colonial hospitals, and education (CME) sessions were held at the whim of section heads, apart from what pearls fell from their lips on ward rounds. Systematic study of error, death reviews, and similar audits of care did not happen, at least not in a mixed (seniors and juniors) audience, or in backwaters, like the remoter colonies, where doctors tended to see their primary role as caring for the local British. Non-white physicians were not encouraged into the system, except in areas of large disfavoured populations, like rural India, the African colonies or the Australian and Canadian hinterlands, where locals could thrive or not, on their own initiative.

In any event, the Colonial Office application process was time-consuming, demanding and expensive. You had to complete a four-page foolscap form (e.g. CSC #CGP&S774/63) in quadruplicate, and account for every living moment of your life, give detailed demographics of your immediate ancestors; provide documentary evidence of every step in your schooling, almost from birth, with certificates, prizes, the lot, each one thus becoming a burden; your professional education; extra-curricular work; wartime and other acivities; and then find ranking non-relatives to write testimonials on each stage of your life, with names, addresses, occupations, and period of your life each would cover. They thereby also became subject of scrutiny, a deterrent. In addition, you had to supply two separate "personal references," with names, addresses and occupations, who could describe your private and public life. And, as if those were not exhaustive enough, you were invited to supply other names and addresses. The one "concession," in the pre-computer or "selectric" typewriter era, was that you had to hand-write the application, (perhaps so that the hand-writing experts could analyse you, if the need arose), but you could type-write the copies! Thus an applicant from a small colony could end up naming the entire literate population! This burdensome practice carried over, with token change in titling, from the Colonial to the "New Nations" Civil Services. This form was still in use in the mid-sixties in BG (now Guyana), until replaced by the PNC membership card when Burnham pronounced the "paramountcy of the Party,"and only card-holders were eligible for civil service positions, which included all doctors.

The colonial UCHWI was spared this imposition, relying on the testimonials of its professors, but fell in with the pattern of specialty education. Its junior staff benefitted from the teaching environment, and thus they, like their counterparts in other colonies, Nigeria, Ghana, Malaysia etc., fared better by landing house officer positions, which were recognised by British examining bodies, but the American Boards were more cautious, and many of those entering that system had to start from first year residency, which made them leave the UWI early.

To facilitate training, prior to WWII, it was not unusual for West Indians, including Guianese, to volunteer, if they wished a position in colonial hospitals, to show their talents, and hopefully impress superiors. "Patience" and "obedience" were rewarded, if matched by ability and diligence. Government promises to those given work, were, of course, not guarantees; and waiting time for specialisation varied from person to person by frustrating years. That was the colonial path travelled by most senior specialists and administrators in the new Ministries of Health that had sprung up, with self-rule, in the fifties and sixties. It explains, at least in part, some of the difficulties—misunderstanding, impatience, and antipathy—that older staff had for student unrest and the calls for change, as these increased in the sixties. When I went to BG in 1961 as a Registrar, I joined at least ten other local doctors in their early thirties waiting in uncertainty to get a rare government-sponsored position in the UK to complete specialty examinations. This situation was replicated in all the territories that supported the UCWI.

The first UCWI graduates in 1954, and in the following years, immediately faced this problem, very much on their own, and had hoped that the Faculty would aim at a predictable and dependable system of specialty training, but the Faculty, then part of the colonial system, maintained its original plan to produce "general-duty" medical officers and to satisfy metropolitan standards of professional competence. That ensured their registrability with the UK General Medical Council, and instant acceptance in the Commonwealth of Nations and in the USA.

These were important attractants to students seeking a medical career, especially in the specialties. By the time the UWI was chartered, it was realised that training had to be modified to ensure that graduates were able to solve problems in the wider community for both individuals and for groups, using existing facilities, often quite spare. This required that undergraduates develop keen clinical skills, an analytical approach to problem-solving, and to see disease from multiple perspectives: personal, family, community and national, and today, international (note Cholera, SARS, AIDS, Ebola), in their customary settings.

In the fifties about half of the graduates obtained internship positions at UCHWI, competing with UK graduates. The "best" from each class were given available positions at the UCHWI, and the remainder channelled into internships in the main city hospitals in Kingston, Port of Spain, Bridgetown, Georgetown, and, by the early sixties, Nassau, each hospital having a specified number of internships. Post-internship positions at UCHWI—Senior House officers (SHOs) and Registrars— were largely reserved for UK nationals, though a few UC graduates did, from the fifties, become SHOs and Registrars. This was all in keeping with the perceived UCWI mandate of training general practitioners.

But the mandate was breached from the outset by a curriculum that emphasised special care in hospitals and little outside, despite exposure to Casualty (walk-ins) and Public Health, the latter having none of the glamour of emergency resuscitation or a surgical *tour de force*, as performed by the late Sir Harry Annamunthodo, the most dexterous surgeon I have ever met! By the sixties, graduates had begun to seek specialisation, and increasingly went into North American residencies. Departmental response to this varied, but most department heads did try to obtain new SHO positions and the more limited registrarships, for which local graduates could compete by the end of the 1950s; thus, by 1960, there were several UCWI graduates in SHO positions in the major medical and surgical specialties. With the added recommendation of British external examiners, many of these would secure SHO positions in the UK, to enable completion of specialty training, almost exactly in the fashion of the Colonial Medical services.

As expected, some departments were better at this than others; some provided hardly any. The weak ones whined; the strong forged ahead. For example, Psychiatry was staffed entirely by part timers from the Jamaica government service, and was for many years a subspecialty of Medicine, hence had no unique departmental basis for promotion of graduate training, not that one was necessary, once the program was justified, as Psychiatry clearly was. Similarly, Public Health, Radiology and the "medical" subspecialties were in the Department of Medicine. Anaesthesia, Orthopaedics, Plastics, ENT, Ophthalmology, and other surgical groups were part of the Department of Surgery. In reality, this arrangement was already what was envisaged in an administrative *Division*, lacking only formal rules, rights and procedures.

CHAPTER 7:
PGME; UWI chartered; Brain Drain; T&T campus

When the UWI received its charter in 1962, its increased student intake was not followed by a corresponding rise in UHWI training positions. Medicine had made rapid advances: disease entities had been clarified, prevention defined, the structure of DNA had been revealed; kidney transplants and open heart surgery performed; vaccines for polio introduced (Salk 1955, Sabin 1962); new antibiotics and drugs had been released; immunomodulators proposed; anti-cancer agents introduced; antibiotic resistance unravelled; new dignostic technology introduced, or at the concept stage, and molecular medicine initiated. A severe epidemic of poliomyelitis occurred in BG between November 1962 and January 1963 (p. 72). Nursing was responding to the School's need for more trained educators and administrators. Medical Technology advanced as the Society of Medical Technologists, based in the UCWI Pathology Department, expanded its intake of general and specialty candidates, and encouraged its members to conduct research towards a Fellowship degree, FSMT(WI). A School of Radiography was established at the Hospital department of Radiology.

At UCWI/UWI new conditions had been discovered: Veno-occlusive Disease, Toxic hypoglycaemia, a Neuropathy (?auto-immune), which quickly raised the profile of the new school. It had made inroads into diseases of poverty and life-style. The high prevalence of cancer of the uterine cervix and diseases of the penis, including cancers, suggested a venereal link with an infectious agent. (Later, virology would identify the role of the human papilloma virus in cervical and penile cancer.)

Every Faculty on the Mona campus shared with students in the optimism and enthusiasm with which the University College had started, and which was expressed with each new batch of admissions. Research publications by new graduates and West Indian faculty, outside of the research facilities like TMRU, ERU and CFNI, added to overall prestige and confidence in the College.

By 1968, the *Caribbean Free Trade Area* (CARIFTA) had been formed. The Declaration of Grenada posed the notion of Caribbean economic integration and a new political unity, and a Caribbean Development Bank had been set up with a mandate to help the lesser-developed countries (LDCs) of the Caribbean — essentially the Lesser Antilles — with soft loans in agriculture, "industry" and tourism, snaring them for good into the jaws of international banks. The CHMC repeated its support for PGME and for the training of ancilllaries, including hospital maintenance workers. The CARIFTA HQ in Georgetown, Guyana, opened a Health Desk for coordination of regional activities, and sharing of information.

These events took place in an atmosphere of continent-wide social protest, starting on US campuses against the Vietnam war, one of the USA's many post-war military adventures, which had drafted students. The *Bay of Pigs* debâcle (failed invasion of Cuba) had soured many young Americans, and, adding to many tangible examples of official foreign affairs mis-steps and arbitrary dealings, culminated in campus riots, repudiation of US might, and escapes to Canada to avoid Army drafts.

At this time, immigration laws had changed, new universities were forming, or older ones expanding; hospitals in North America (NA) were increasing residencies; these attracted many UWI graduates who did not get UHWI posts. Others, influenced by Faculty trained in the US, and by older graduates familiar with the "orderly progression" of training in residency schemes in NA, joined with colleagues to push for *residencies* at UHWI, rather than the current casual *apprenticeships*. In other spheres, the Premier of BG, Dr Jagan, had trashed the sedate, non-militant UWI student body and its dissolute "colonial" professors and administrators, and withdrew from the UWI at its founding in 1962, and so the third campus went to Barbados. Jagan founded the University of Guiana in 1963, with Burnham's support.

The UWI 's first Vice Chancellor was Allan Lewis, an economist, who focussed his energies on consolidation, developing the second campus already started on the grounds of the *Imperial College of Tropical Agriculture (ICTA)*, St Augustine, Trinidad, and, failing to change Jagan's mind, starting the third campus in Barbados. The first medical students for a UWI degree were those admitted in 1962, the class of 1967. Until then, UWI would continue to train those admitted as London matriculants. The transition was hardly noticed.

Postgraduate needs had long become evident, but were superseded by the greater need in the services for general practitioners. But the loss to the region of a third or more graduates was worrisome and a great financial cost to poor countries; their desire for specialty training could not be ignored. The Faculty shifted from a passive to a reactive stance and by the end of the decade was fully involved in promoting specialty training under the aegis of the university. Independence from London provided flexibility in curricula, and hospital expansion offered more training posts. The increase in West Indian doctors seeking a teaching career at UWI, especially those who resented having had to comb the world for specialty training, plus the service needs of Governments for specialists, provided added push. The University responded by conducting an internal appraisal in 1970, which prompted it to secure funds from the Inter-American Development Bank for a Committee (*the*

IADB Committee) to study the feasibility of Expansion/Duplication of the Medical Faculty. It reported in 1971.

Clinical teachers had long been sympathetic with graduate demand for specialty training, but the UCWI did not have a mandate to train staff for its own academic needs, nor to meet the demand for primary and community care physicians, coming from Health Ministers. It was clearly unrealistic to expect such competences without focussed training, or that the colonial aim to have UCWI graduates fill general duty positions – while reserving specialty training posts, and jobs, for British graduates – would be tolerated for long. This was a short-sighted, and selfish British move, as Professor Cruickshank, the first Dean, later admitted.

Teachers were generally disappointed at the steady and increasing loss of graduates from each class, some even before internship. One ruefully remarked that he could not reconcile his virtual "working for the Americans with my West Indian salary!" But for most, it was not that, but the wastage of trainees whose service was denied their homelands, cannibalised by the super-rich, like children lured away by Browning's Pied Piper. It was increasingly likely that most of the graduates from UCWI/UWI would be lost in the mass of new and dazzling technology, and promise of new careers that dominated US medicine, the world's most expensive, while Cuba, the US nemesis, would attain the widest coverage at an enviably low cost:benefit ratio.

In Chicago, in 1968, as a visiting Fellow at Michael Reese Hospital's Pathology Department, I had to give a talk on *"Renal disease in the Caribbean"* to about forty residents and staff in Medicine and Pathology, at the regular weekly symposium. For illustrations, I had mined glossy magazines for pictures and cartoons of tropical scenes, personalities, and events, and copied journal titles of work published by UWI doctors. These I projected with an old unused epidiascope, which someone had rescued from storage, to supplement the few slides from my renal course for UWI residents which I had brought to discuss with experts in Chicago, some having direct experience of repeated outbreaks of post-streptococcal glomerulonephritis (PSGN) in Trinidad.

Knowing that I had no other illustrations, my immediate colleagues, all junior faculty and fellows from the US down to Argentina, wondered how I could do the lecture, without slides. But it was a resounding success, with wonder that I had used "scrap" and old equipment to put over a scientific talk. One said, "Few of us would even think of using such stuff; most photos were not even medical!" My microphotos of SLE nephropathy was introduced with a Jamaican beach scene from a travel magazine showing a Miss Jamaica advertising something (which I was able to hide); I had seen biopsies from several young women and wanted to stress the connection; one researcher on immunopathies said, "That was neat! Each time I see a pretty girl in a bikini, I would remember your talk and the EM changes in SLE."

Chicago was my first in-depth experience of the ways of American Medicine. Although everyone complained of "not enough funds," there was plenty, even an over-supply, everywhere, of materials and small equipment, like slide or overhead projectors, microscopes, and of the ordinary things that we could barely afford, and of people to do things. At UHWI, we had two or three employed as photographers in the whole hospital and were thankful that both heads of Pathology so far had been avid amateur photographers, and had created and maintained a good unit, swayed the University to start one, and trained the photographer and his assistants, who doubled as animal house caretakers.

By contrast, the audiovisual unit in the pathology department at Michael Reese had several graphic artists, designers, colour consultants, and three dark rooms for electron microscopy. That plenty was everywhere, yet they spoke of needing more! The support available to complete a paper extended to the array of experts to turn a crude draft into a final version, with tables and figures done and in order, readied for the final review, while the worker focussed on research: more output, more funding! We had none of this at UWI; each paper was entirely the author's, except for the photographer and typist, unless (s)he was department head. For me, preparation of papers took longer than the research itself, which explains the backlog of unpublished work in my archives; the same might be true of others. Chicago would not allow that!

I was offered positions in Chicago, made so tempting that were I not married with children, and attached to my job at UWI, I'm not sure I could have declined, in the atmosphere then of welcome to doctors, and expanding medical schools. Later, at Mount Sinai in New York—where I went for further work on ultrastructural diagnosis, using their library of renal disease, and to refine photographic technique—I was pitied when I told my supervisor the equipment I used. "Can you get anything useful on that thing?" But he and the department staff were impressed by the quality of my micrographs, and surprised that I had taken and developed them myself. "Where did you find the time?" asked one, skeptically. Again, the job offer. It was thus easy to empathise with a fresh graduate wishing a fruitful career, or a chance for fame.

I still recalled the anxiety each student felt at graduation, as I had felt, knowing that there were two or three applicants for each UCHWI internship, and that having to complete it elsewhere, even in a hometown hospital, was like being thrown in the trash. Several who wished to go home after internship, still felt the need for extra training in certain disciplines that were needed in their area, sometimes never available. Earlier graduates had learned that many hospitals could also use individuals with special skills, even at an intermediate level, which would allow coverage of 70% or more of special situations. And that government jobs nearly always involved solo rotations through rural districts, often with no backup nearby, and included mental health, eye, skin and ENT problems, which they had skimped during clerkships. For some, the handling of fractures and other wounds was a calamity, as were dealings with patients' families. Not surprisingly, many left such demanding positions for the relative security of specialised practice.

I had experienced the Guiana medical services, which were typical of the British colonies, with manpower deficits at all levels, and untapped non-medical talent willing to learn and accept delegated responsibilities in a variety of specific medical tasks; how quickly we had trained teenagers to give oral polio vaccine in schools! At the other end of the scale was the technical excellence of the Royal Postgraduate Medical School in London (RPGMS), where I had refined my skills, followed by exposure to special functions at Columbia university and at Mount Sinai Hospital in New York. There I developed ideas on preparing a broad range of manpower to meet health service needs, at all levels.

In *The Indelible Red Stain*, I discussed the successful training of a Pathology assistant, who proved his worth, but was never properly compensated, a failure to innovate of many manpower establishments, even in the USA. The inflexibility and narrow vision of colonial services persisted after independence. I was 19 when I mentioned to my boss, Mr. Joseph, the Chief Personnel Officer of the Health Department that we could improve process "a lot." He smiled, nodded, and said, pointing to his copy of the *Colonial Regulations*, "We can't think outside that book!"

In 1969, after discussing with Dean Cruickshank and Department Heads, at one of their Wednesday morning meetings, the idea of a spectrum of health care workers, noting that we were already training several cadres of technicians, assistants and health aides, Professor Stuart quoted the views of Dr Len Comissiong, Chief Medical Adviser for Grenada, about needs, one of which was for a "lab specialist" to do a competent autopsy and make sure that tests were "properly done." As a result, I was given the task of developing a Diploma program in Clinical Pathology covering a curriculum based on that of the RPGMS. We could train a doctor in two years—six months each in Histopathology, Chemistry, Haematology and Microbiology—to handle most routine diagnoses in clinical laboratories, referring problems to the UHWI.

A similar initiative was begun earlier by Drs John Sandison and Siva in Anaesthesia and UN Pathak, head of Obstetrics and Gynaecology, to train generalist physicians for a year to perform certain procedures in those specialties, at a level to meet the needs of district hospitals. Health

Ministers welcomed the plan for diplomas, and would release DMOs for this. At the same time, PAHO had agreed to fund the Diploma in Public Health at the Department of Social & Preventive Medicine.

Similarly, we favoured the training of nurse-practitioners, beginning with anaesthesia. Colonial hospitals and health ministries had, for a long time, trained nurse practitioners e.g. midwives, public health nurses, health visitors, sicknurse/dispensers, for service in primary care, mostly in colonial health centres, and were in use in other countries. Another level, *aide*, was proposed, similar to the *feldshers of the* USSR, China's *barefoot doctors,* and India's primary care nurses and nurse assistants.

After several meetings, clinical departments agreed to plan for full specialty training in their disciplines. By then, most faculty, graduates, students and the CHMC, were in favour, and eager to participate.

As Associate Dean and Coordinator of Postgraduate Education, I was appointed Faculty representative on the Board for Higher Degrees (BHD), a most intimidating group of Deans, Science, Humanities, Sociology and Education professors clothed in Masters and Doctorate robes, with hardly a foot or toe touching ground, and just one colleague. My appointment came just in time to carry the case for diplomas and explain their functioning to a sceptical BHD, chaired by Dr Roy Augier, historian and Dean of Arts and General Studies, who kept a neutral ground and did not allow detractors to stray into irrelevance.

I completed *Regulations for the Diploma in Clinical Pathology,* which were approved by Professors Bras and Grant, Drs Paul Milner of Haematology and Herb McDonald, Clinical Chemistry, and presented them to Dean Cruickshank. This and the other diploma programs, led to a general Faculty Board initiative to create two levels of graduate specialisation, the diploma and the full specialty, for which departments had begun to draft educational plans. In 1969, the Faculty Board, the University Board for Higher degrees, and the Academic Board (AB), approved the Diploma plans. Soon after, Dr Faye Whitbourne, a 1963 UCWI graduate, registered for Pathology, and two years later, became our first Diplomate in Clinical Pathology.

Throughout the process, Professors Bras and Grant had involved academic and senior technical staff, adopted or modified their inputs, so that no one was overlooked who would be involved in the day-to-day interactions with trainees *(Fig 11-3, p. 112).* John Hayes, senior Anatomic Pathologist, had been in favour, but Bill Brooks, who had taken over when Hayes left, was opposed, and when he became head of Pathology, after Bras left in 1972, declined further applicants. Dr Whitbourne has remained the only Clinical Pathology diplomate trained at UWI.

CHAPTER 8
PGME: The academic plan

By the time the UCWI had become the UWI in 1962, it had acquired a number of talented West Indian Faculty, mostly with British degrees, and perspectives on, and attitudes to medical education, as varied as their institutional philosophies, but they did unite on the need to define the purpose of medical education at UWI. The West Indian Federation had collapsed in 1962, and for the next five years several territories became independent, and began to look critically to the University for solutions to general manpower problems. Many of their senior civil servants, consultants, professionals and politicians were, by then, UWI graduates, and as those from Medicine began to join the Faculty, contact became easier and more direct.

Student intake increased to 110 by 1968, as originally planned, but with no change in facilities. Soon, UWI began to face the difficulty of recruiting specialists for certain academic positions, a situation that developed steadily in the sixties, as new medical schools arose in many countries, and expanding technology created increased opportunities for British and North American graduates in their own and in affluent foreign countries. Indeed, even Britain would by the end of that decade begin to rely on imported physicians to fill junior posts in its NHS.

The Caribbean nations were all basically too poor to compete for the best foreign specialists even though the islands were among the most attractive physically. With help from the Ministry of Overseas Development (MOD, the re-styled Colonial Office), and British Council, they continued to recruit from Britain, whose cost and quality of living still left much to be desired, until political unrest in Jamaica and Trinidad in the 1970s coincided with British economic improvement to reduce that traffic to the level of the more intrepid and curious. In this global setting, the good teacher had no difficulty finding attractive employment.

Perhaps I might digress to show the kind of work that needed to be done in the region. Although Walter Reed was well known, and Patrick Manson's *"Manual of Tropical Diseases"* was in circulation, it was not a prime text for us, since few of our British teachers or external examiners would have had any real knowledge of the topics discussed there. So we learned the biases of European medicine re disease incidence, prevalence, and their presentations, and only later placed them in the context of environment, culture and belief systems found in the West Indies. We got the impression that a select few, the bright ones—local and foreign—would do the basic research, while the rest would concentrate on clinical care, barring occasional adventures into local problems, like malaria and Veno-occlusive Disease (VOD).

I started my unplanned Pathology career in BG, now Guyana, at a time of great social and political turmoil. Soon I teamed up with a family relation—the late gifted paediatric cardiologist, Walter Singh, who had studied Medicine in Halifax, Canada. A severe epidemic of poliomyelitis between November 1962 and February 1963 paralysed 485 people (attack rate 86.5/10^5, mostly children under 5, with the highest attack rate in those under one. Twenty-two died. The event cooled political rhetoric for a few weeks and anti-US premier Jagan was grateful for American iron lungs and a team from the CDC with the new oral Sabin vaccine, which thus underwent another field trial, reaching some 85% of children under five. A clinical feature of the disease was the relatively high percentage of bulbospinal and encephalitic cases. Walter and I were deeply involved in the clinical and immunisation programs, while Dr ES Tikasingh, from the Trinidad Regional Virus Laboratory (TRVL), had been the first microbiologist to arrive and collect samples, which he sent to TRVL for laboratory diagnosis, confirming Polio. The CDC team, which arrived subsequently, took over, and pursued a strict academic and drug trial agenda. They ignored us, were generally curt, and flashed an MOH fiat to seize our data.[13] An epidemic had stricken Laos at the same time.

In mid-1962, we investigated an epidemic of severe congenital heart diseases, with many fatalities, nine of which I autopsied. The abruptness, clustering, the spectrum of lesions and total numbers of cases were unusual and quite baffling. We eventually found that the cases had all come from two locations which had experienced an outbreak of Rubella, and were connected by a single contact. The literature and experts we

---

[13] In 1954, an epidemic of some 1200 cases had occurred in Jamaica, with 94 deaths. The attack rate was 154/100,000. The worst cases were housed at Mona at an old WWII army building, and every medical student participated in rehabilitation. I had four cases, two of whom had been weaned from iron lungs. I worked with them for three months until enough aides were trained; two of my patients were discharged to private care. The Salk vaccine was given to under-fives in a 1957 epidemic reducing attack rate to 71/100,000 and again in 1960. The Sabin vaccine replaced Salk in a 1962 campaign, repeated in 1964; incomplete coverage was followed by sporadic outbreaks. In 1972, Trinidad suffered an outbreak; Jamaica reacted with a vaccination campaign reaching less than half the under-fives. An epidemic occurred in 1982. Deanna Ashley, a COPMED member in 1971-2 (Ch. 12), wrote in 1985, with R. Bernal (Bibliography), that the 1982 epidemic cost the cash-strapped government J$3,889,882. *"Immunisation coverage of children under 5 did not exceed 50% at any time between 1964-82. The expenditure for an adequate immunization program would have been J$72,618, and prevention of the epidemic would have cost J$363,093 for the 5 years, less than 10% of the amount actually spent in 1982."*

could access had never heard of an association between the two, but the finding was inescapable. Prof John Waterlow of the MRC at UWI agreed, included our paper for the April 1963 MRC conference in Port of Spain, and advised sending a letter to the *Lancet*. Although Walter did manage to attend, he found that CMO Nicholson had added his name to the paper and wished to read it; Walter refused; Nicholson withdrew the paper, which was "read" by title only. Walter was so upset that he forgot to mail the abstract as a letter to the *Lancet* from Trinidad, and so avoid the strike in BG that closed all public services. He could not mail the article until the strike was over in July; in late May, the *Lancet* carried an Australian article on an association of Rubella in pregnant women with Congenital Heart Disease in their newborn infants.[14]

About the same time, the Hon. Balram Singh Rai, Minister of Home Affairs, intent on developing a strong Forensic Sciences Unit, had asked me for a report on the causes of medico-legal deaths at the Georgetown Public Hospital. The results for 1961-3 *(Fig. 8-1)* showed an unexpected feature, which had nothing to do with forensic medicine, but it influenced my attitude to, and direction in medical education. The data surprised everyone who saw them, including Drs AP Brahmam, Harold Hamilton, Walter Singh, and John Waterlow, who had accepted the paper for presentation at the Port of Spain Conference.

Main Causes of Disease-related Deaths

Group	CVA	Heart Disease	Other**	TOTAL
East Indians	14	31	8	53
Negroes	28	13	10	51
Others **	8	5	5	18
TOTAL	50	49	23	122

Fig 8-1 This shows the high incidence of Heart Disease in East Indians, ischaemic, due to Atherosclerosis in this series of coroner's cases (sudden or unexplained death). The percentages are specific to this autopsy population, but show the unusually high incidence of cardiac deaths in Indians, and strokes in Blacks. (This graph was copied from a paper presented in Hamilton, Canada at a 1997 Public Health Seminar, using original data. The first WI paper on this condition was from Dr Wattley of Trinidad, published in WIMJ in 1958. Danaraj noted the same in Singapore in 1959. Stroke and its link to hypertension were being studied by Dr Hamilton and others in the Caribbean.)

CMO Nicholson had insisted on being listed as first author, (he had bullied Walter into including him as an author on our Rubella-CHD paper); I had acknowledged him as CMO, with Minister Rai of Home Affairs—who had requested the study, and was satisfied with the acknowledgement—and the late Supt Brian McLeod, head of the

---

[14] Details are given in the book *The Indelible Red Stain, Bk 2*; the conditions mentioned are described on pp. 355 and 503. A brief comment on the Health Services is on pp.345-349.

fledgling Forensic unit, who was killed by rioters in February 1962. When I refused, Nicholson withdrew my paper from John Waterlow's list at the Conference, and barred its publication *(see also p. 183)*.

The turmoil in BG in those terrible years destroyed more than property, businesses and careers; it destroyed the foundations of knowledge, which fled in flocks to kinder climes. We had stumbled on something that we called *"A Peculiar East Indian Heart Disease,"* for want of a better term, which in time would acquire other associations e.g. Diabetes Mellitus, and be known, tentatively, as the *Metabolic Syndrome*. We knew none of this at UCWI, and our British and American textbooks were silent on the problem, which seemed even then to threaten the very ethnic group to which I belonged. My plan to study the condition collapsed when I left BG. In Jamaica, the Indian population was too small and remote for a resumption. But Trinidad and Guyana remained fertile soils for further probing. Singapore had reported the condition, but Indian literature in the sixties had no reference to it. My paper remained unpublished, but by the 1980s, the topic had become a hot one globally, as more diasporal Indian physicians became aware of the condition.

So when I became a UWI teacher, I had hoped to help amassing information on the population we served, and of focussing research on those silent and chronic diseases that quietly eroded their health. I felt it should happen as a matter of planning. But it was a monumental task to get research focussed this way, or any Government to provide funds for research, as Professor Ken Stuart was finding out in his attempts to study hypertension in Barbados. Nevertheless, through efforts at the University and UHWI, plus the TMRU, the ERU, the CFNI, TRVL (later CAREC) and other units, we began to assemble this information.

A specialist who wished to practise in the West Indies must be steeped in WI medicine, at least from the epidemiological and sociological points of view. Also, it was clear that we could not recruit medically-trained anatomists from elsewhere; we had to grow our own. Vidia Persaud, a Guyanese teratologist trained in East Germany, had been given extraordinary incentives to stay, and pampered by Professors Hoyte and Bras, had but left after receiving the first Canadian offer, at a conference to which Hoyte had taken him! Hoyte did not favour non-medical Ph.Ds. as teachers of human anatomy to medical students. We had to find appropriate incentives to attract physicians into pre-clinical teaching careers. For a start, he had already engaged several senior surgical house officers to serve as sessional demonstrators.

By the late sixties, I began to receive from Dean Cruickshank drafts of departmental designs for formal specialty training. My task was to collate and refine these plans, which consisted of position statements, ideas and facts. They differed widely, related sometimes only by the rubric "postgraduate medical education." In my review, I told him that what I had was a veritable hodgepodge of ideas, and the only uniting factor was that training would take place at the UWI! There was little common ground, even among closely related specialities, for example Internal Medicine and Paediatrics, or the latter and Obstetrics.

Some had proposed that training in their specialty be overseen, by a dedicated "College," a club really, as in the UK, which would grant an award of proficiency that the UWI would endorse. Others wished to have specialty Associations confer degrees after UWI training. These were dismissed as unwieldy and unoriginal. Some training programs were planned to take six years after internship, and the one in medicine, eight years! Clearly, few would consider these, when North America was luring graduates into 4-year residencies and current British regulations required a series of rotations, which could be completed in 2-3 years[15]. From this diverse beginning, we reached, in 1969-70, a consensus within the Faculty to support a residency scheme, but not before much wrangling from both pre-clinical and clinical staff.

At the Board for Higher Degrees, non-medical members objected to the "residency scheme," dismissing it as "mere vocational training," not original research, nor academic enough. None of them would accept the argument that Clinical Medicine could not be strictly compared with Physics or Mathematics in content or the way suitable teachers were developed. We needed practical professionals with years of problem-solving experience in managing a wide range of diseases and community issues, which were not learned in a laboratory or by silent contemplation alone, or as a single discipline. Some of the professors I had to convince understood the point better by analogy with their own medical needs; I asked the question: "To whom would you go when you fall ill?" It was often only by this heuristic approach rather than rational argument that our positions were eventually understood and accepted.

After further debate, and emphasis that our proposals constituted a new program, not a substitution for a hospital one, and that most academic medical staff had completed the type of training that we were proposing, the Board approved the regulations for UWI degrees by residency training. I still have the scars from those battles!

---

[15] By the late 1960s UK Colleges were changing conditions for degrees, with a better structure and taking 3-4 years for a basic specialty degree and longer for a subspecialty e.g. cardiology or neurosurgery, as in the US or Canada. In the US, each specialty degree is regulated and granted by a specific Board. In Canada the Royal College grants degrees after examinations set by subject "committees" from member Universities; and training in accredited hospitals. *See Ch. 22, pp. 201-4.*

Meanwhile staff and students grappling with the increased intake to 110 per annum, *(see graph, p 228),* saw it as threatening the quality of clinical education and almost ending research — scant as that had already become — by adding to high staff workloads and lowering ratios of patients to students. Clinical education was the UWI's strongest feature, where it eclipsed most contemporaries, even in highly-developed countries, on both sides of the Atlantic, which habitually enticed UWI graduates into residencies. External examiners never tired of praising our clinical training, even as they lured away our brightest, to the extent that American recruiters set up stations in Kingston, in the late sixties, for enrolling graduating nurses and doctors.

When political and societal turmoil of the 1970s made campus life in Jamaica dangerous, staff recruitment for the UWI became difficult, as both local and foreign members of the existing staff began to leave. Replacements were doubly difficult as medical education was expanding in North America, the UK and elsewhere, and the number of residency positions in the US was increasing, soon after US and Canadian immigration rules for Indians had relaxed, finally placing them in the quota of their birth countries, rather than ethnicity. The recruitment difficulty and the huge losses of graduates that took place in the sixties starkly exposed the short-sightedness of overlooking the need for specialists, and excluding formal PGME from the initial mission of the Faculty[16].

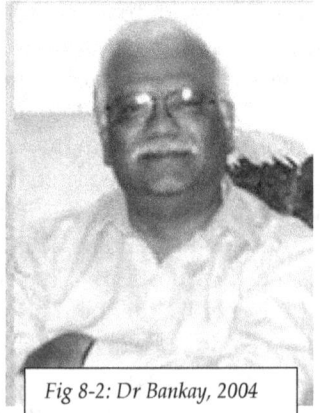

Fortunately, several young men and women had kept faith with our efforts to have PGME recognised, and once approved, had registered, so that when the programs were officially started in 1972, they were credited with up to two years of prior training, that is, to the date the Regulations came into force, enabling a small group to gain specialty degrees in

Fig 8-2: Dr Bankay, 2004

1974, starting with Clarence Bankay, a Guianese, in Internal Medicine, and so qualify for specialist appointments. Dr Bankay was also the first person to pass the UK MRCP Part 1, by examination, held at the UWI, and done at the same time as it was held in London, in a pilot project, for which I was accredited as supervisor by the Royal College of Physicians of England.

---

[16]EK Cruickshank, first Dean of Medical Faculty, UWI and professor of Medicine, p. 69 and Ch. 16; also DB Stewart, on UWI, in *Medical Schools for the Developing World.*

CHAPTER 9:
CHMC III, 1971, Bermuda, the PGME debate
who, what, why, when, where, how

Academic proposals were taken to the February 1971 meeting of the CHMC, held in Bermuda. To start, we needed the agreement of at least one major contributor, hopefully two, and a few of the Lesser Antilles, to show graduates that forward steps were underway for training at the UWI, still a controversial issue that had generated scepticism and adverse comment from a few financial observers and commentators, as at the 1970 meeting in Barbados. Foreign detractors had been unusually free with criticism, which was based purely on North American social values and concepts of medical education; they seemed unwilling to admit any individuality or comprehension by West Indians of what it took to run a program of learning.

Addressing the meeting, Dean Stuart said, following the script we had prepared, "Mr. Chairman, ladies and Gentlemen, I am grateful for this opportunity to present further material on our case for graduate training, which we have been preparing for the past few years, coordinated by our Associate Dean for Education, Dr Ragbeer, who will take you through the documents. The University Appraisals Committee had pondered this matter and realised the practical need for medical specialties, but is limited by having provisions, including rules and regulations for academic degrees, Masters and PhDs, but not the professional ones that the practice of medicine entails—and by medicine, I mean all subdivisions, medical, surgical, paediatric, obstetric, psychiatric, preventive and curative etc.

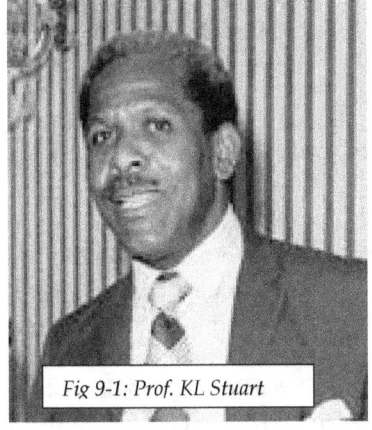

Fig 9-1: Prof. KL Stuart

We had therefore to overcome this hurdle, by first getting our University Board for Higher Degrees to accept this conceptual change, or rather addition, to our Faculty's offerings. In this, our biggest challenges came from within the Faculty, where the academic scientists tended not to want contamination by those who are simply highly skilled, versus learned by empiricism and original thinking. We took this challenge, and prevailed, with the results before you, from which we could start, without much delay. So we began by focussing on needs and how to meet them; we came to an agreed range of training or levels of specialisation, some unique to our circumstances, and devised regulations to govern them. These are among your papers.

"Why do we need programs in Postgraduate Medical Education (PGME)? Our MBBS graduate is entering a regulated profession with various levels of knowledge and skill, and subject to licensing and specific qualification appropriate to the practice. I would encapsulate our aim as follows:

A. *To train and educate*
   i) interns;
   ii) those between interns and consultants in rank and experience in hospitals, styled residents, or house officers and registrars;
   iii) the general practitioner;
   iv) scholars – local and peripatetic;
   v) academics;
   vi) researchers;
   vii) consultants
   viii) others, as identified.

B. *To prevent medical and economic 'brain drain'*

"There is a shortage of health professionals in the world today, in the most economically advanced countries as in the economically deprived, and unevenly distributed. We in these territories, most of which are still colonies, have traditionally depended on the imperial "mothers" of Europe or on our "uncles" from North America for professional training, and in fact for most of our professional people, until the UWI began. These obligatory supports have been slowly withdrawn as independence replaced colonialism, and by the shortages I've mentioned.

"The Faculty has long recognised that the provision of postgraduate training is vital for medical doctors, if we are to keep current medical graduates in the Caribbean, in the face of their increasing drain to the US and Canada. In fact, these two, and to a decreasing but still significant extent, Britain, benefit more than we do from our efforts. In one year, recently, almost the entire graduating class ended up in North America.

"This Conference made a specific request to the UWI last year to provide it with plans for specialty training. In its turn, the UWI has been concerned with the problem, officially since 1961, a year before its independence. It has tried to implement what plans it could, with time and energy squeezed from the altruism and dedication of its staff. One of its earliest efforts has been to date one of its most successful, and that is the sponsoring by the Pathology Department of the Society of Medical

Technologists (WI), and the training of technologists in all laboratory disciplines, now conducted by a mature Society for all territories. We are proud of this success, a most cost-effective one. In the same way, the UHWI contributes to training of radiographers and nurse-practitioners.

"But with the resources we have, it has not been possible to do much formal postgraduate medical training, despite the need. But even before the decision of this Conference last year, we had obtained approval of academic regulations for degrees and diplomas, and prepared detailed proposals for postgraduate training programs in all the common specialties. These plans have been refined by many passages through specialty committees and by consulting with external colleagues in medical education; they are distilled in these pages and approximate costs provided. The price, as you see, is high.

"Lest you feel that this price tag is too steep, I wish you to consider the following facts and implications:

"British influence has dominated life in the member countries that founded this Conference, the primary members, especially in education. British economics dictated our ability to finance projects. We rose and fell with the pound, as the calypsonian, Lord Beginner so vividly sang of the effects of the first big devaluation two decades ago. As new countries grapple with the financial cost of independence, they find less fiscal room to deal with soft issues like health and education, which are likely to be underfunded as time goes on. But the University has to express the problems in the light of collective and individual needs, and present costs for you to consider and decide whether to accept them, or if not, suggest ways of addressing the issues in an acceptable manner.

"The British Colonial record in the field of PGME had been better than that of most British universities! It wasn't until 1921 that the Athlone Committee recommended that a special hospital be set up, in the UK, for postgraduate medical education, and also an institute of state medicine. The result was the formation of the British Postgraduate Medical School at Hammersmith Hospital in 1930 — of which Dr Ragbeer and a few others are graduates — and the London and Liverpool Schools of Hygiene and Tropical Medicine.

"In 1944, the Goodenough Committee, although inhibited by the official view that no great concentration in hospital facilities should be allowed, proposed that British provincial universities with medical schools should become responsible for PGME and should appoint postgraduate deans. Apart from the support given to London University and appointment of deans — who met regularly, it seemed, but did little — training by British universities has remained haphazard, until more recently. This was foreseeable, as without dedicated financial support, little direction could be given officially by the universities, until

July 24, 1969, when the British Government announced a funding model whereby the university should finance academic training, that is, to provide for its future academics and researchers, and that the National Health Service should see to professional training for its service needs.

"We are not particularly fond of this model, and in fact it may divide the two arms of Government rather than have them work together, as the boundary zones between these two sectors of specialisation may be tenuous or even non-existent, especially in our local environment.[17] But universities have always looked after their needs by selecting their best graduates for academic training. In Britain, it is now clearly stated that the National Health Service must staff its district hospitals sufficiently to allow junior doctors to take time off to pursue postgraduate education, without affecting patient care. Also, the NHS must provide enough senior positions to allow time for junior staff to engage in training, to assist their juniors and to frame graduate education policies, again without affecting patient care. This then is some of our competition.

"From the morass of fragmentation, special interests and differential privileges in England, Scotland and Northern Ireland, specialty Colleges had emerged, one each to take care of certification in the major specialties: General (Internal) Medicine, 1518; Surgery, 1800 (a Guild was formed in 1540); O&G, 1929; General Practice, 1952, and Pathology in 1962. These "Colleges" are examining institutions, whose diplomas and degrees are accepted by licensing bodies in their jurisdiction. In imperial times, this was Empire-wide and extended to some foreign countries in Europe and to some American states. Today, some restrictions apply. These Colleges do not undertake training, but stipulate the training conditions that one must meet to qualify to take their examinations. We have been part of this as we transit from reliance on British degrees to those of our own, with the advantages inherent in being trained in the environment of final practice, provided all other academic needs are met.

"In this context, the single university is particularly burdened by being the main centre with facilities for training (since colonial hospitals, like many in British counties, were rarely equipped for extensive work or even basic investigative work). With imagination and drive, the University would willingly accept the dual role of creating centres of academic excellence and providing continuing professional education throughout its jurisdiction, while remembering its greater duty to

---

[17] Later elaborated by M.S. Ragbeer & C. Burton: *Collaboration between Government and the University on Health Matters (why the "town" and "gown" should woo)*, 1972 CHMC IV, 18 (11pp), Georgetown, Guyana.

learning in general, now that the British Government has explained its position, which former partners tend to accept and follow.

"The UK model is clearly not entirely suited to our situation, where a single university serves fourteen different masters, scattered through the Caribbean, a collection of small states each with a meagre population, and totalling just 4.5 million. The UCWI has been talking and proposing continuing medical education and graduate medical education quite in advance of its independence from London University; indeed, external examiners from Britain have commended our teachers for initiatives, and in some instances have wished they could copy us! Over the years, despite great setbacks and sacrifices, our Faculty has begun to train several doctors for postgraduate diplomas: in anaesthetics, laboratory medicine and obstetrics and gynaecology, and will shortly begin Public Health, with PAHO support, and here I would like to thank them and all those organisations, some represented here, which have helped us in various ways: Millbank, Macy, HOPE and other Foundations, the Wellcome Trust, CIDA, and others. We have supported residents from the start and will continue to do so, including those who prepare for British degrees in General Medicine, Surgery, Pathology, Public Health, Obstetrics and Gynaecology, Tropical Diseases and so on.

"The positive effect of PGME on the quality of clinical service is well-illustrated by the fact that several British *district* hospitals — until now a last resort for any serious scholar or ambitious physician — have begun, since obtaining a subject accreditation for PG degrees, to attract a better quality and larger number of applicants for junior *and* senior posts, and from students doing electives, with great benefit to their health service in both range and quality, which we hope our schemes will achieve, as we accredit national and regional hospitals and other service facilities.

"There is a worldwide shortage of well-trained specialist doctors, especially those who must function alone and without extensive support (material, equipment, personnel, etc.). As I've said, there are hundreds of new residencies in North America, especially in states not previously known or appreciated for a graduate experience, e.g. the southern "Jim Crow" states are becoming likely destinations since the advances made in civil rights. These widening avenues are now embracing our graduates, even the weakest, and they respond in droves: our loss; and they tell us this repeatedly. My office is flooded with requests for transcripts and I spend more hours trying to mollify fresh graduates, who would prefer to stay. I have even suggested that they lobby you, their leaders in the services!

"Many of our smaller members still rely on foreigners, but they are far more difficult and more expensive to recruit than they used to be, when the Colonial Medical Services simply recruited in bulk and offered a global stage on which further training could take place; that alone was a tremendous attraction, and had resulted in distributing some of the best British doctors globally. That situation has ended.

"If we don't train specialists ourselves, no one will; aspirants, i.e. new graduates, wishing to specialise, will go elsewhere, most never to return. We have become, as I've said, a target for recruitment drive for interns and residents by North American hospitals, much like the draft picks for sports teams that they conduct each year, or large Corporations like GM and GE comb graduation conventions for engineers. This process has snared many of our brightest, thus depleting the pool from which you can draw now and in the future. No specialists currently in the Services of our members will tolerate for long a decline in standards, a failure to fill vacancies, or provide for new needs, especially when there is such a growth in hospitals and medical schools in North America, as our colleagues from Project HOPE and other partners, some present in this audience, remind us, and traditional training produces graduates oriented to hospital practices and neglect service to individuals in the community.

"At this stage I would ask Dr Ragbeer to present the main documents. He serves as Coordinator of Postgraduate Education."

"Thank you, Dean Stuart.

"Mr. Chairman, Hon. Ministers, Officials, Ladies and Gentlemen, I thank the Dean and Faculty for this opportunity to present details of our proposals for medical specialty training at UWI, which we introduced last year.[18] I will summarise the principles followed, with background, and current activities at the UWI. You requested further information and more details, including costs. These are presented in the documents listed as "A." *UWI Academic Papers*, and "B." *CHMC Paper 1971*.[19] These

---

[18] Two papers were presented in 1970:

  1. K.L. Stuart, G. Bras & M.S. Ragbeer: *Proposals for Postgraduate Medical Education at the University of the West Indies, 1970, Caribbean Health Ministers Conference (CHMC) II, Paper 6, (36 pp)* Bridgetown, Barbados.
  2. M.S. Ragbeer & G. Bras: *Paramedical Training at the UWI, 1970,* CHMC II Inf. Paper 2b (3 pp), Bridgetown, Barbados.

[19]   **A. UWI Academic Papers (Senate and Council, 1969-71):**

1. M.S. Ragbeer: *Requirements for full postgraduate medical education for the UWI degrees of Doctor of Medicine (D.M.) and Master of Surgery (M.S.)* - Faculty of Medicine paper, 1969.

2. M.S. Ragbeer, G. Bras, K.L. Stuart, H. Annamunthodo, and D. Hoyte: *Establishment of Comprehensive Residency Training in the Faculty of Medicine, UWI, for Specialist Diplomas and Degrees (Doctor of Medicine - D.M. - in Medical Specialties, and Master of Surgery - M.S. - in the Surgical Specialties):* (1) General regulations and (2) Regulations for individual specialties: published in current UWI Calendar); (3) Curriculum for individual specialties and (4). Resource implications.

    B. CHMC Paper, 1971:

were pre-circulated for examination by you and Ministry officers. From "A," you'll see that we've obtained approval for our design of full specialty training, which, by consensus, we've styled DM (Doctorate in Medicine, for the Medical or Internal Medicine specialties) and MS (Master in Surgery, for the surgical ones), with specialty added, e.g. DM (Paed.) = Doctorate in Medicine, Paediatrics; and MS (O&G) = Master of Surgery in Obstetrics and Gynaecology.

"These are easily understood, and the abbreviations do not produce any confusion, ambiguities or horrors. We are aware that some groups, have proposed alternatives, for example, a US-trained neurosurgeon has put to Dr Boyd the idea of creating a College of Neurosurgery to train neurosurgeons, who would earn a Fellowship in Neurosurgery of the WI College of Neurosurgeons (FN,WICN), a cumbersome title; I am not sure how easily most people will decipher that; the surgeon knows of our plans, but has not contacted us as yet.

"The regulations for Diplomas were introduced last year. Just to remind you, these are a level of training between the intern and full specialist, suitable for doctors wishing a limited specialty practice e.g. obstetrics alone, or basic general Anaesthesia, Public Health, or General Pathology etc. and require one or two years full-time. We have persons now on the Diploma track, one each in Obstetrics, Pathology and Anaesthesia, but resources limit us to UHWI residents. The Diploma in Public Health has begun, from special funding by PAHO, and occupies one year, full-time. (Here, you'll permit me to add to the Dean's thanks to Dr Horwitz for prompt responses to our training requests.)

"The definitive documents are A2 and B which give the details requested; B shows an estimate of costs. As the Dean said, the costs are substantial, but these costs will be spread over time, and the full impact will be felt only when all programs are up and running. There are two sets of needs: those required to establish the program, the core or central base, as it were, and include the program leaders, new faculty and new space; and those to be met as programs develop and territories participate at their cost e.g. for residents, or in upgrading facilities to meet accreditation standards. HOPE Foundation is willing to expand its commitment and assist with teaching staff on rotation; this will help enormously to get an early start with the more common specialties needed in the contributing territories. I would ask the Conference to recognise Dr Richard Meltzer, head of land-based programs for the

M.S. Ragbeer, G. Bras & A.Z. Preston: *Postgraduate Medical Education at the UWI: Detailed Plans and Estimates of Costs, with Recommendations of the CHMC Committee for Postgraduate Medical Education,* 1971, CHMC III, 7a, 7b, 7c (37pp), Hamilton, Bermuda.

Foundation (*Ken had invited him to CHMC at the last minute, as an observer, after hearing HOPE's proposal re PGME. Dr Meltzer stood up and was recognised*). PAHO is willing to help further in areas of its mandate. So there is some relief to the financial picture, and who knows, we may get help from other sources, once the programs are approved.

"Regarding needs, we have relied on tables of staff establishment as originally approved by the colonies, and updated since independence. But there is no formal survey of needs for the Commonwealth Caribbean. The Jamaica Ministry of Health confirms that it has enough data on needs to support a start. Most other governments wish to see as much local benefit as possible for spending, and are reminded that they would gain from any training sited locally for resident rotations. These are likely the major islands, but subject to accreditation, and include electives, which can be served in any community that sponsors them.

"This is a mere introduction to what we tried to distil from two years concentrated work. There will be many questions and we look forward to your comments and inputs. I wish to stress in favour of our plan that foreign specialists rely heavily on support services — lab, x-ray etc. — for investigation, diagnosis and on-going care. Our MB,BS graduates are schooled to rely on clinical skills to base management decisions, including investigations, and to begin treatment while awaiting results.

"The adoption of formal postgraduate training *must* be accompanied by Governments' recognition and promotion of our degrees, as they do the British ones, perhaps even give us preference; we hope that this meeting will give us an assurance of this recognition, as it is the first question asked by anyone about to commit four prime years to a choice, when so many alternatives are offered. Recognition comforts applicants and dispels Faculty doubts. This should go far in stemming the costly 'brain drain,' which currently subsidises our rich neighbours and former rulers, so that when their governments and institutions 'give' us aid, they are in reality not donating anything, but paying back and ensuring a steady supply of well-trained people!

"The attraction of an individual to a profession is as much a function of the quality of that profession as it is of the prestige or economic gain it may provide. Members of a profession are the best advertisements for that profession. Their method of advertising is by precept, merit, example and excellence, rather than by advertising, commercial style. Our graduates are our best advertisements, and will amply justify your decision to break new ground. The UWI is already seized with the fact that this would be *the first instance of a multi-national University taking direct charge of full specialty training and granting degrees.*

"In urging your favourable consideration, I wish to emphasise a belief that physicians would be best educated in the environment of future practice, alongside other health care workers, or, if not feasible, at least with knowledge of how they were prepared for their jobs. That way, they can function more easily in teams, especially recognising the leadership role a doctor tends to be given in the West Indies, even when someone else might be more suitable as team leader.[20] This applies even more to academics and teachers.

"In the West Indies, specialists should be clinicians first, able to use what technology was available, but not so reliant as to be useless, or worse, dangerous, without it. The DM and MS are structured to provide the means for a graduate to acquire the knowledge, skills and attitudes to deal competently and independently with problems within his/her specialty, *using the tools available in the health services,* knowing their organisation, but aware of recent advances in the delivery of that care.

"We believe that while we have put together sound schemes in each specialty, *the quality of the entrant* would ensure the quality of the program and of its graduates — a principle applicable to any level of adult learning — and would depend less on the number of teachers and their credentials than on the *soundness of selection,* the environment of training and support given by tutors and peers. A specialty training program is, above all, an exercise in *self-directed learning,* providing opportunity to acquire special skills. So there is every reason to expect that we can produce a product second to none, given basic resources, for we have talented graduates. Bear in mind that the training plans recognise our shortfalls, and provide for up to a year in a more advanced or better equipped centre to receive those elements of training that we miss, whether from lack of staff, as in Radiology or Dermatology, or equipment, or space. Notwithstanding this, we know that certain advances are desirable and we will seek them within the limit of national economies, centralised and optimised for a general benefit and operated more creatively and humanely than in pursuing corporate bottom-lines.

"We are not a litigious society, but increasing exposure to US news and TV, which informs many West Indians, is introducing them to medical malpractice suits. We would ask you to consider appropriate legislation to limit liability to reasonable and 'topical' negligence, in line with local standards, and discourage the frivolous suits that seem to occupy so much legal time and money in the USA.

"We're developing schemes to encourage private individuals and businesses to see the medical services, especially research, as something they should support, at arm's length, and endow, much in the fashion of

---

[20] M.S. Ragbeer, *"Teamwork for health in Developing Countries;"* later presented at the 1974 Joint Meeting of JMA, BMA & CMA, Kingston, and published by ASCOFAME, Bogota, 1974. *Reproduced in Appendix 4, pp. 316-8.*

North American Foundations.[21] Professor Bras used his connections in the US Jewish community to get the Rippel building (p. 95); Mr. Rippel never ceased to wonder why so many rich people in the island were omitting their only university from their wills, yet gave to Americans.

"Thank you very much. We hope we can answer your questions and will note all comments and suggestions."

A full discussion followed; the following were the main points:

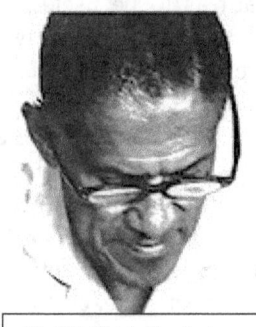

Fig 9-2: Dr. L Comissiong

Dr Leonard Comissiong, Chief Medical Officer, Grenada, noted: "I agree that current MB training does not measure up to the needs. The emphasis that graduates have is on highly sophisticated curative procedures, and here I include our existing specialists who are largely European-trained, and have to adjust to this less advanced environment, to the people, more primary care, and the different diseases. So here is a group of people who can benefit from special programs of orientation and training. The two-stage programs suggested are attractive to small countries; few of us can afford full specialists, except in General Surgery and Medicine. For the rest a Diploma candidate should be enough. I like the idea of pooling rarer specialists among several islands."

Reply: I am sure that once the programs are under way we can tailor short courses to individual need. For many years now, we've had fellows in aspects of medicine, surgery, paediatrics, etc. for one or more months, for refresher or focus courses, supported by some of the organisations here. We've discussed and agree with the idea of pooling for certain specialties.

The Health Minister for Barbados, Ms. O'Rourke, was committed to specialist training and was prepared to meet their share once satisfied that there was an adequate *quid pro quo*, adding that Finance was looking at the matter of capital expenditure in Jamaica. "Specifically though, I have an interest in preventive medicine, which did not seem to play much of a part in the proposals."

Reply: Prevention is an integral aspect in the training of every specialty; it is covered in detail in a separate document, shown in Appendix 1, pages 15-17, and also covered on page 2 of the main document. Primary prevention would be

---

[21] I was delighted to hear of, then see the Tony Thwaites Wing at the UHWI (photo p. 44) since I knew the man and his family, and several of the donors to the project. The unit of 54 private beds is a non-profit facility that offers most tertiary clinical services.

a focus of the new program in Community Medicine, and woven into each specialty plan. Secondary prevention is taught as part of disease management. We don't think it wise to treat it as if it were a separate discipline.

Dr Eldemire, Minister of Health, Jamaica favoured the programs and was willing to commit to a start. "We cannot afford *not* to support this plan, when our students are agitating for it and seem to want it here; for years we have been bleeding from loss of young doctors; once they go away, especially to the US, they stay! We will commit our portion to capital cost. We are exploring sources of external aid.

Mr. Dawson of the British Virgin islands supported the plan but could not make a commitment for 1971, but "we are a small state, and need to have more information for planning purposes." The Ministers of St Kitts/Nevis/Anguilla, Belize, Dominica and St Vincent agreed, the last adding that he "saw no quick benefit to St Vincent, but expected some in the long run; most of the benefit will go to Jamaica, Trinidad and Barbados, but we do support it." All were uncertain of their manpower needs. The Honourable Eustace felt that "most programs would fall short on finances. We have needs for many senior staff, a senior medical officer, specialists in Obstetrics and Gynaecology, District Medical Officers, lab technologists and nurses. We are a small player and likely to be attracted to sharing with other islands; I believe that the document is important to politicians, especially if even small entities can participate in the training of residents through short term postings, electives, etc., as the proposal seems to suggest."

Reply: We hope that even the smallest state could develop 3-6 month electives, which we would be happy to help organise and manage.

Dr Max Awon, Minister of Health for Trinidad and Tobago, thought that the cost of training each graduate was too high, compared with what he had spent to get a specialist certificate from each of the British colleges of Medicine, O&G and Surgery! However "common sense tells me that we must support this, and pay for the infrastructure, but we have to look at costs and make sure that each one gets a fair share; Jamaica will get the lion's share of the funding, leaving less for Trinidad and the Eastern Caribbean." Dr Elizabeth Quamina, his Principal Medical Officer of Health, added, "60% of the shortages in our country's hospitals are at registrar (resident) levels. The University Grants Committee may balk at the proposals which favour the Medical Faculty over others. I've always wondered where our staff go when they leave. We have the feeling, on hearsay, that UWI graduates go back to Jamaica, and we complain that the University Hospital and the Jamaica medical services may be hogging the graduates in its better organised hospital departments, but now we hear that 50% or so leave Jamaica also, and thus they represent a real loss to the region. Do we know where they go? The economic cost must be very high, especially as we try to skimp and save more and more."

Year of graduation	% outside Commonwealth Caribbean in Sept 1970
1965	30
1966	45
1967	59
1968	42
1969	40

Table 9-1: Graduate losses 1965-9

Reply: Most go to North America, particularly since the immigration restrictions were eased in the USA, 1965, and in Canada, 1966, with the opening of new medical schools in both, plus expansion of residencies. We've lost several lecturers to Canada. Jamaica also loses,

but so far, the UHWI is a first choice for the majority of graduates; the Hospital tends to choose from the top, which includes many non-Jamaicans, leaving the Jamaicans also dissatisfied. We have figures for the number of graduates in the last five years who did not return to their country of origin. The 216 doctors lost in the last five years match the total output of two large medical schools, or a loss of over $J2.1 million ($US2.5M), assuming a very low estimate of $J10,000 per graduate, which PVC Preston will correct.

From 1954 to 1970, UWI graduated 568 doctors, 28% of whom are living outside the Caribbean. This excludes those in graduate training, not on migrant visas. Thus you see the extent of lost manpower. With regard to costs, the budget includes the necessary start-up costs, which is not recurrent. We hope that each territory that joins might in some way, in all or in part, benefit, but first we need the resources and facilities. I don't know all the bases of the calculations provided, and will take specific questions to PVC Preston and reply to you.

Guyana Health Minister, Dr Sylvia Talbot: "There appears to be no flexibility, but the short courses as described would interest my Ministry. Four years training appears to be too long and the concentration appears to be on too narrow a specialisation. Community health and health education seem to be missing, although the Dean did point out that these were indeed included in the detailed lists as integral parts of both programs and that the Faculty was considering compulsory courses in community affairs and society for each of its specialty programs and he is willing to extract these and present them as short courses for those already trained, or for any category of staff for the needs of individual ministries. He has also suggested that costs would be less if several of us could coordinate this type of need. Hospitals have to be accredited but there is no detail on how this would be done. Also, what are our priorities? We have few specialists , no pathologist, no anaesthetist."[22]

Reply: Pre-independent Guyana severed relationship with UWI in 1962, when it started a university. But it has had difficulty building and financing it; Guyanese medical aspirants have since then been searching everywhere for an education; a few years ago the Government arranged to finance five medical students at UWI, hardly enough for needs, and the public medical services have lost many doctors and nurses in the last five years. Guyana accepted our suggestion last year to join in our specialty training initiatives, and study of needs. Regarding training time, it would be difficult to find a shorter residency program. One could learn the theoretical side of a specialty by shorter intensive full-time study, but not if you want to acquire a broad range of graded clinical competences, and qualify, on completion, as a consultant, which is our aim. Subspecialty, or narrower fields of training can follow, either here, or by arrangement, in other places. If training were based on competency, it could take less time for the gifted. Accreditation is covered in the Preamble; this would be done in advance, for a set period, say three years, according to criteria, to decide the readiness of institutions for postgraduate training, and periodically thereafter, near expiry of their accredited status and application for renewal.

The USAID agreed that their studies also showed outstanding health problems and while not interfering with ministerial responsibilities would be "responsive to assist with health planning, problem definition, provision of training resources and needs analysis. We are aware of the brain drain which benefits the United States but would doubt whether governments would enact any specific legislation to curtail professional migration." Dr Vanzile Hyde of the AAMC Division of Internal Medicine Education, based in Washington, DC, referred to an American report on *Education and World Affairs*, with a section on the brain drain which was chaired by Dr Charles V. Kidd, but he waffled, perhaps embarrassed, without offering anything substantial, beyond mention of the report. There was no mention of the cost of this subsidy to NA medicine.

---

[22] It was realised that the Minister was new and not properly briefed; she had begun to speak believing that Guyana had equal participatory rights to the UWI. We told her that Guyana did not contribute to the UWI, except for five medical students each year. She was an American, native of St Croix and a well-meaning educator wife of an acquaintance, Rev. Fred Talbot, whom I had met when I worked as a personnel officer in the Medical Department, 1950-1. He had been "afflicted" by the US Civil Rights movement, the Black power expressions in the Caribbean, and the opinions of Walter Rodney and Clive Thomas. The comments rendered above were post-correction, with trenchant criticisms omitted. She had little or no professional experience in, or knowledge of Guyana, and had uncritically accepted President Burnham's word, especially as it was his versus an Indian's, and she didn't know his cunning; her embarrassment was obvious, and later apology accepted.

Reply: We are about to calculate how much has been transferred to the US, Canada and the UK, just the cost of education of the doctors, teachers, engineers and other university educated migrants. This gift may be quite large[23].

Jamaica's Minister of Health, Dr. Herbert Eldemire, acknowledged their need for various specialists but left it up to his CMO, Dr Jeff Wilson to advise on the plan, "by the end of this conference, and what financial support, if any, his Ministry should give;" he urged members not to delay that decision; he had already authorised individual departments to study the plan and meet with the UWI to clarify issues and to present to the CMO and his PS their conclusions on implementation details, including estimates of specialty manpower needs, which his Ministry had studied, in relation to the present establishment of posts, and he would urge fellow members to complete this in their own territories and engage the UWI team to clarify points.

Reply: The UWI is pleased and is preparing answers to Jamaica's questions, some of which could be extracted from the documents. We would be pleased to deal with individual issues, as members wished, alone or in general sessions. If you don't mind sharing them, we would gladly deal with them here.

The Honourable Hunter Francois of St Lucia, said, "My main questions concern accreditation of facilities and the length of training. But you've already answered those. More substantially, I note that the major new money would be for sponsored residents for four years; I take it that capital costs would be met by formula. I follow the general trend and assume these figures are notional and will be refined as we get closer to implementation. Besides, we, like others, must first study our needs for specialists; do we need full specialists? Which? Should we share? Or will diplomates in key areas be enough?"

Dean Stuart: *I want to add the reminder that accreditation of a certain level was needed to satisfy University of London requirements for teaching hospitals. Most colonial hospitals in the West Indies needed upgrading to qualify. We do not find them too stringent, especially re space and services. We recognise that*

---

[23] The loss for just the years 1965-1969 would be US$10,800,000 based on average US medical school education costs of $50,000 per graduate (5 years University). The costs at some private universities are much higher than at State schools. That sum was enough to fund the expansion recommended by the IADB Committee (*Appendix 2, p. 310-3*). My suggestion at a meeting of JCCS that we could raise funds by training foreign students met with a yawn!

professionals in small countries may often have to carry out tasks well beyond their expertise. For this reason most programs demand a thorough basic training with electives that would ease any shift into non-typical services."

Dr. Jeffrey Wilson, representing Jamaica—as well as the Bahamas, his previous post as CMO—focused on the problems of small islands where "medicine for the community would bring greater rewards and satisfaction to a greater number than sophisticated specialty practices, especially in places like the Caribbean with few resources and insufficient power for affordable industry. There is a gap between these two, and the Bahamas, being better off financially than most other islands had adopted many features of American medicine, but with independence, finds that their income has to be spread a little more thinly, and hence would encourage the Community Medicine program."

Dean Stuart: *"The university cannot think in terms of service needs alone, since its primary purpose is education and training. Thus it cannot be committed to a program which does not have a satisfactory academic content. It therefore must ensure the availability of teachers since it is now difficult to get them from overseas due to scarcity and cost, unless willing to import specialists from less expensive sources, like India, as we have done. The university is also concerned about the needs for specialists and has heard them in discussions of Council by various Government representatives. But so far, there has been no concrete determination of needs, nor of priorities, but the university does know the requirements for a minimum performance of particular medical procedures and services. And what governments must be concerned about is the question of whether it is satisfactory for them to have a poorly trained person just to fill a position and to say that this has happened, however politically justified."*

The Director of the Pan American Health Organization (PAHO) or Sanitary Bureau (PASB), Dr. Abraham Horwitz, said that he appreciated the scope and detail of the papers presented and complimented the authors for the diligence and thoroughness that were needed to complete the task in so short a time. "PAHO will support, within their mandate, the priorities of Community Medicine, Paediatrics, Psychiatry, Maternal Health, and to a lesser extent some of the basic sciences. This support however will be more personnel and specific service-oriented than funding, except in terms of specified grants within our mandate. PAHO will therefore review its commitment to the UWI in the light of any decisions made by the Conference. We would like to assist in programs for human resources development, where we have considerable expertise.

"We can help too with assessment of needs for a new specialty particularly with education methodology in basic sciences, and I suggest that a few individuals be added to assist Associate Dean Ragbeer, who authored the papers, and to become involved in particular aspects, as implementation will require many more dedicated hours and specific responsibilities, but from what I see, the presenters have the courage to develop this fully and critically. PAHO would consider assistance to these individuals, as it has given in the past, and will contribute to a Task Force on specialist manpower needs, which several Ministers desire."

Dean Stuart: *Thank you, Dr Horwitz; you have been a true help to us and to our colleagues in Latin America; we appreciate PAHO's support and its work under your direction, and look forward to future collaboration. Dr Ragbeer has indeed given most, if not all of his non-teaching time to this, much appreciated."*

Dr Comissiong asked about psychiatric training and wondered how new methods in psychiatry fitted in with the programs designed for the Caribbean. The Dean responded that there was no specific projection for individual territorial needs at this early stage, but will be considered as the programs develop and specific issues become clearer.

Dr John Bennett (CMA/CESO) suggested that they might consider a grant towards the medical direction of the program, once generally agreed, of $45,000 per annum. He will recommend to the Canadian Government that they study the possibility of making a financial grant with no strings attached and/or specialised equipment. This was a good gesture and suitably thanked. His comments cancelled his 1970 comment of "over-extension" and doubt that the UWI was ready for this. But seeing the documents and the meticulous preparation and confidence of the UWI staff had changed his mind. He had compared us to McMaster and Calgary universities in Canada, with their extensive grants and lavish capital allowances. Yet they had bitten off much less than we had on one-tenth of the materials. He was impressed, and hoped his CMA colleagues would share his view. (*They didn't; see Korcok's article p 190.*)

Finally, with regards to the question of needs, Honourable Hunter Francois reiterated the value of a statistician, thanked Dr Horwitz and formally recommended that a committee be set up to 1) identify needs, 2) set deadlines for implementation and 3) describe a break down for each aspect of the budget. This resulted in the formation of the *Committee for Postgraduate Medical Education* (COPMED) to determine the need of the various territories for specialists; Dr Awon was named Chair, with Dr Alexander Robertson, PAHO, Dr R, Sahoy, Senior Surgical Registrar,

UWI, as core members, and me as Secretary, to conduct a study of the need for specialists in all territories that wished it. The Committee would visit these territories and in each add the local CMO or delegate to its membership. It would be free to involve or consult any or all sources of expertise or data, e.g. USAID, and present a report at the 1972 meeting of CHMC in Guyana.

Other comments were made to clarify detail and the long session was adjourned, as several members wished to "sleep on it."

The same evening, after speaking with a few delegates, Dean Stuart and Professor Bras left, having briefed me and Ken Standard, satisfied they could contribute no more, and more especially that I, as the person left in charge, was unlikely to do any harm, so well received and almost without resistance, except by habit from T&T. The Chair, the Hon Quinton Edness, Executive Member for Health, Bermuda, had reassured our team that the questions were dealt with honestly and he encouraged individual Ministers to obtain further details or explanations in private session with the UWI delegation. I was convinced that were these rich countries, we would get our grant post-haste.

That evening, I met with Dr Wilson; his mien looked troubling. I did not know him well enough to read it; I had met him briefly as a first year clinical student during the Jamaica polio epidemic of 1954, and had admired his unruffled approach in dealing with that crisis. He had already become known for identifying Sickle cell disease, Leptospirosis, Coccidioidomycosis, Myiasis and Visceral Leishmaniasis in Jamaica, in the 1940s. His presence loomed in the medical background after the Polio outbreak, and throughout my 20 years in Jamaica. During this time, he, as SMO, KPH, and Eric Cruickshank, Head of Medicine, UHWI, were the most influential internists in Jamaica, and was missed when he went to the Bahamas as CMO. But our paths did not cross functionally until February 1971, at the CHMC meeting.

Dr Wilson also represented Bahamas that year, which he had recently left for Kingston, on the departure of CMO Dr Samuel Street for a WHO position in Bangladesh. That evening, he affirmed Jamaica's need for specialists, and was sceptical of the UWI's ability to establish and sustain the specialty training as proposed, and worse, that it seemed to rest with me, an unknown "youth," to get it going. He had listened to others in the past months, and had not been convinced that the program was on a sound footing. But he did not allow this initial bias to interfere with the debate. His Minister, Dr Eldemire, had left it up to him to explore his doubts and clarify points of specific concern and come up with a decision, for or against, which he would announce to the meeting. We sat through two long evenings, after hectic daily sessions covering the other issues. We had other interviews with the major delegates, some conducted by Ken Standard, from Social and Preventive Medicine.

Wilson probed every detail of his concerns: aspects of the regulations, specialty specifics, accreditation of hospitals, use of rural hospitals and clinics, country variances, and funding; he probed areas where Jamaica might wish a different option from, say, Barbados, to get to the same goal, and the role of NGOs, like HOPE (though there were some who felt that HOPE was a CIA operation!) Towards the end of the last session on the second day, we finished an intensive session on costing, which Dr. Dick Meltzer of HOPE attended. Dick had been a Professor of Paediatrics at the University of Rochester before coming to HOPE. He had joined the meeting to answer Wilson's questions or concerns about their plans, ability and stamina to participate, proposed duration, and on what basis and to what extent.

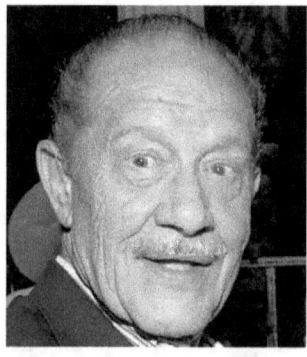

Dr Wilson excused himself, ostensibly to go to the washroom. He had been poker-faced and businesslike through the session and left us guessing. Presently he returned, followed minutes later, by a waiter; he ordered drinks and ten minutes later, Minister Eldemire *(photo, years later)* and Permanent Secretary, Trevor Goldson, came in, looking solemn, and ominously fresh, despite the hour. I was uneasy, although we had covered — satisfactorily, I thought — all the questions then, and dealt with the contentious issues.

Fig 9-3: Dr H. Eldemire (Gleaner)

Two waiters arrived with a loaded trolley, briskly served drinks, then retired, while the Minister chatted amiably, without relieving the tension. Then as the doors closed on the waiters, he raised his glass and said, "Congratulations, Doctors, we're satisfied enough to give this a good go." He shook my hand and those of my colleagues. My elation was understandable: I had lived with this, three years of ups and downs, more intimately than with my spouse! I went over to Dr Wilson and said, "Dr Wilson, you'll make a great poker player, if you're not already one." The mood had lightened considerably. He said, "Call me Jeff."

At the conclusion of the debates next day, and the rest of the agenda, I had contributed by joining the drafting Committee of Drs. Elizabeth Quamina, Leonard Comissiong, and Jeff Wilson, on Dr. Wilson's nomination, to replace Ken Stuart, who had left.

That was the beginning. Jeff and I penned the resolutions 7A, 7B and 7C (*Bibliography*). Minister Herb Eldemire duly announced Jamaica's readiness to start, and Antigua, Dominica, Grenada, Guyana, Montserrat and The British Virgin Islands also agreed to support the programs. The others reserved their positions pending review of the financing, and the readiness of facilities and staff to accommodate residents. No one declined. CHMC support for us would remain constant and university doctors were finally accepted in the group, as colleagues, not as aloof and high-brow itinerants.

In the aftermath, Jeff and I became friends, worked together as a task force of two on implementation details and I served on his Ministry's Advisory Committees on Health, and Government-Faculty of Medicine Liaison; we shared social and professional confidences and experiences.

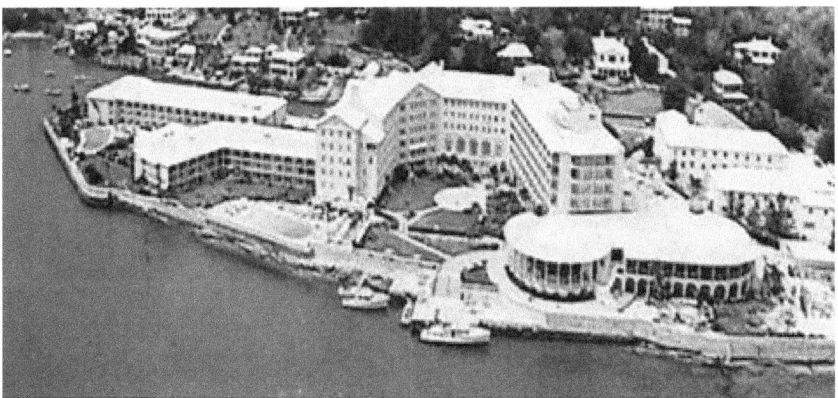

Fig 9-4: The Princess Hotel, Hamilton, Bermuda, site of CHMC III, Feb 1971 (gift by Hotel)

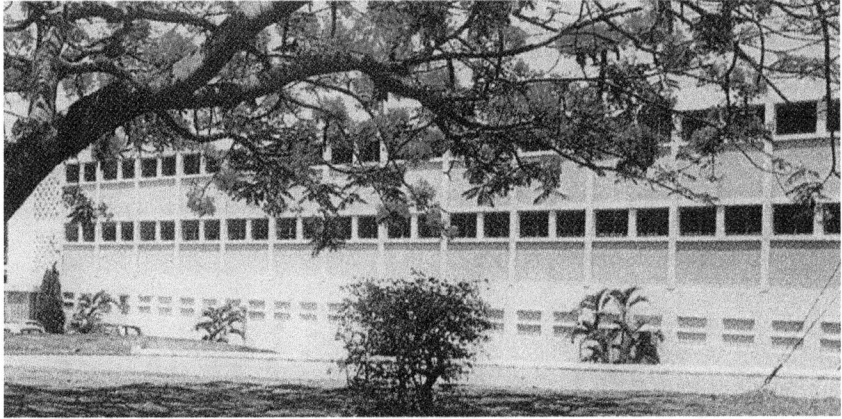

Fig 9-5: The Rippel Building for Medical Research, a gift of the Julius Rippel Fund, USA. The three floors of research laboratories next to the Pathology Department included experimental surgery and electron microscopy; space was rented to researchers, funded by grants or departments. The negotiations for the grant were protracted and deftly conducted by Professor Bras wearing the honourary hat of Faculty Dean of Graduate Studies, from 1967.

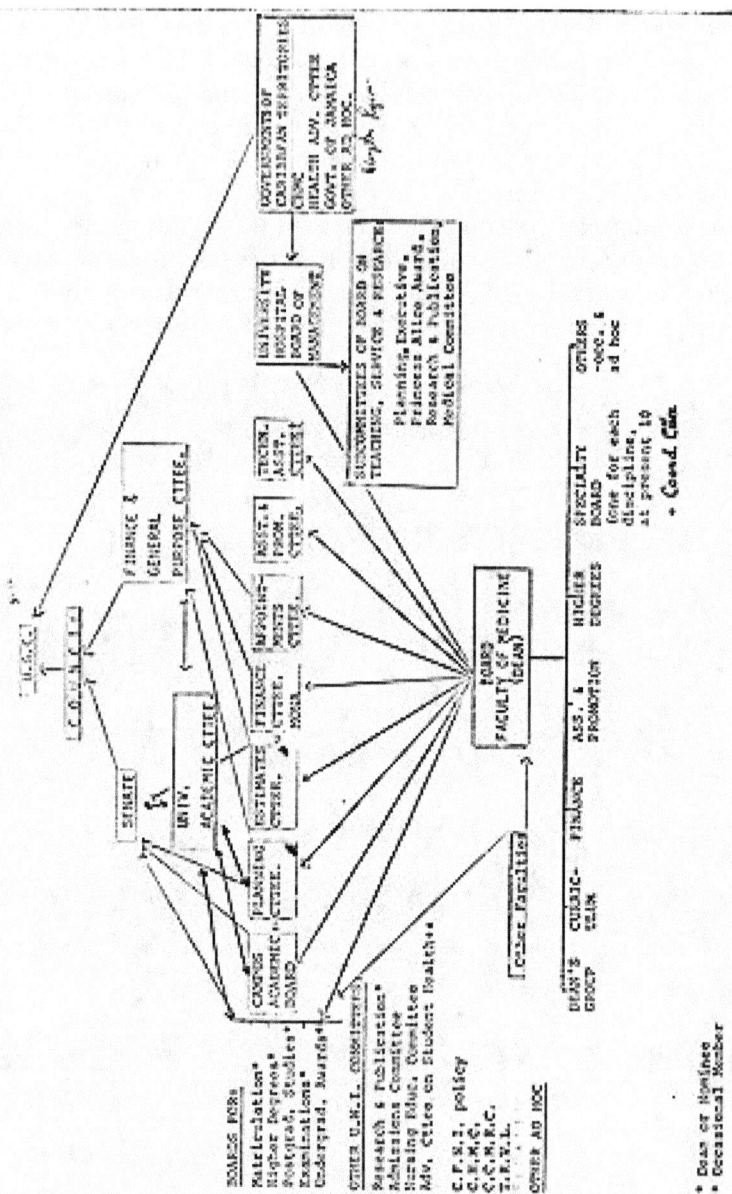

Fig 9-6: UWI and Faculty of Medicine, Organisation, 1971-

CHAPTER 10
Faculty Reforms: Full-time deanship

In the months following the Action Group meeting with the VC, Dean Stuart was pre-occupied with the preparations for the IADB Committee, and I spent much time assembling data for his and the Committee's briefing. There was thus a delay in implementing those recommendations that VC Marshall had deemed administrative. In 1971, the Dean placed the issue of the full-time Deanship before the Faculty Board, which approved it, and informed the VC, who replied, setting out a procedure for selection, which the Registrar, Carl Jackman, duly completed, as the customary Selection Board was deemed unsuited to the purpose. Staff were closer to the issues, the reforms needed, and character of the candidates. The VC had promised a swift response, and to consult them. All members of staff were to indicate, by secret ballot, their choice for Dean among nominees. The choice would be put to the Academic Board, via the Appointments Committee, for a final decision. This was a new step for the University, watched by other Faculties, some considering the change, while others had decided to continue the current arrangement. Careful and wise handling was doubly needed.

I had supported Ken Stuart for three years and had wished to continue as Co-ordinator of Postgraduate Medical Education (PGME), the title under which I worked. I had nursed PGME from the start, and wished to continue as Medical Educator to reform the undergraduate program, and was willing to oversee the launching of Community Medicine. But several department heads and senior faculty, headed by Dr Karl Smith and Professor Standard, persuaded me to stand. I had worked with them for over two years, developing or refining and fitting departmental (or subject) plans into an integrated curriculum, to produce a physician schooled in human behaviour and biology, environment and sociology, aware of the conditions that promoted health, was competent in handling diseases, their prevention and treatment, including the use of tools available and needed for prompt, efficient and adequate treatment, knowing health systems and, above all, how to promote good health.

My work on Final examinations had led to the changes in Part 1, which both Bras and Grant appreciated, also for the time saved in marking papers. Thus, department heads could assess my worth and work, and manner of doing it. They argued that the only way to achieve the objectives we all wanted — at that stage of Faculty affairs, where it was run by a cabal of the most influential and senior department heads (a real Senatus) — was to have someone new and *au fait* with educational principles to take charge of it. I reluctantly agreed, fully expecting to lose:

I was too young and not yet a full professor, and the University could reject an unmerited choice for the first full-time Deanship, a professorial position, for which one had to qualify.

My supporters felt that my work and internal educational publications on examinations reform, critical analyses of objective tests — then incorporated in Part 1 Final examinations and being studied for other parts—the completion of the major groundwork i.e., regulations and final plans for PGME and Community Medicine, plus supervision of two postgraduate students in Pathology, would add to publications and make up an impressive enough body of work for a promotion. But failure would sideline me, and perhaps disqualify me from the positions I really wanted: the Coordinator of PGME or Director of Community Medicine. It was unlikely that Ken Stuart would wish to have me work with him, if I opposed him, human nature being what it was, and he would likely recommend his acolytes for those positions.

If that happened, I would have to leave, as my friend Kassim Bacchus—my critic, tutor and consultant on Education—had urged me to do in 1969, when he had obtained a position at the University of Alberta. But I would not starve, as I had visas for the USA on hold at the Kingston embassy, and could fairly quickly resurrect my US offers, both academically good, the preferred one at Columbia University, NY, where my sponsor, Dr. T. Roberts, still had unfilled positions, and the other in Chicago, with Dr. Pirani's renal ultrastructural pathology research team. But while I would earn five to ten times my UWI pay, I would lose the opportunity I had sought in entering UCWI rather than Oxford or Cambridge (my alternative Arts choices: I had matriculated into both), to help "build and brighten the light rising in the west".

But I was chosen by a hefty margin, 62%:38%. The ballot had been secret, at a special meeting of all Faculty called by the Registrar to obtain their choice, with a mandate to improve, reorganise, and implement changes and new programs. He took the results to the Academic Board via the Appointments Committee, which approved the promotion and appointment. Ken was furious and thought the matter should have proceeded through the Medical Faculty Board, of which he was Chair, a conflict, so Vice-Dean Beaubrun would have had to preside. Ken headed a protest to the VC afterward, seeking to quash the election.

I was then quite willing to quit, rather than having to stitch together a riven Faculty. (In agonising over this, I recalled a timely injunction from one of my high school "landlords," Cecil Tahal, one of two tailoring brothers, when I had torn my only dress pants, required for school functions: *"Mend it the best way you can, so that no one can tell it was mended. That's what we have to do nowadays."* In that closing year of WWII when good cloth was scarce, and the little that could be had on the black market was only affordable by the rich, I had seen many men bring in a jacket or trousers, and once or twice vests for repair. I was 13, and had learned to do this job well enough that only the closest scrutiny could find the lines of repair. Cecil had always been one of my favourite people, a neat and fast tailor, and I had treasured his advice. No, I won't let him down, if it fell to me to tackle that stitching job.)

Ken had good reason to protest, though I suspect he did not know it. The Deanship required tenure. I had no formal tenure, but then I had started a third and indefinite contract in 1971, the equivalent of tenure. Any difference was semantic. Professor Bras, my department head, had overlooked the confirmation of "tenure" with the Registrar. The VC heard Stuart's case, agreed to investigate, confirmed my lack of "tenure," but hearing the rest, had ruled that I had the equivalent and was thus eligible to be Dean; formal tenure was put to the A&P Committee, and approved, Bras getting a little flak, which his carefully cultivated reputation easily fended off. Cruickshank made a joke of it, teasing Bras whenever he could, just to remind him that he too was human.

My appointment was announced in June, 1971. I had a week or so to respond; my wife was both surprised and alarmed by the implications, both for my time commitments and the personalities involved, issued cautions, but was generally pleased that so many in the Faculty had recognised my unstinted burning of the midnight oil. I mulled over the pros and cons, knowing that Ken would accept my choice if I were to withdraw from the appointment. I discussed them with my wife and she approved, saying it would be better for social relations among people who have to work together, and that I could achieve good by doing good! Later, I told Karl Smith and Ken Standard my plan, and decided to pursue it over their enduring objections.

I started by making an appointment to see Professor Stuart in his office that first day, but hardly had we called than he barged in to mine and instantly proceeded to abuse me in a breathtaking tirade lasting several minutes. When he was done, I spoke over my astonishment and told him of my prior intentions, but the attack and unjust accusations of plotting and underhand dealings, and general character assassination had insulted and vexed me. Thereupon, I resolved to keep the role of Dean, and work to implement the plan we had developed. I even added that his action tended to confirm the view some others held of him as self-seeking and unfair, who would deny me a place in the Faculty, in favour of his friends, despite the voluntary help I had given him, the time and labour I had put into educational reform for the past five years, and for preparation of his documents for the IADB Committee.

Also, I had defended him to others before, gratefully recalling his pronouncement to the Faculty Board that my effort had been *"insightful, innovative and meticulous, and sacrificial in that it had taken him away from research work, which was what counted with the Promotions Committee, but the substance and outcomes of his efforts were well worth a PhD in Education!"* That was repeated after the 1971 CHMC III Bermuda meeting, to Carl Jackman. Ken Standard also had praised the " thorough preparation and confident handling of the Health Ministers' issues in Bermuda, and the fine reception we had had." The Hon Quinton Edness of Bermuda, Chairman of the meetings, had given unqualified praise.

But signs of favouritism had begun to appear in the Dean's office, as others had pointed out, and Ken was criticised for misrepresenting or minimising Faculty concerns to the Academic Board, which even his advocate Bras had noted. I had liked the affable professor just as much as the taciturn and exacting Harold Forde, his colleague and countryman, a teacher much admired for his clarity and directness, and his rival even, as top West Indian in the Department of Medicine in 1955.[24]

After hearing of my intention, Ken was dumb-founded, a rare thing for one so articulate and mentally agile. In calmer tones, I told him that I hoped for his cooperation, as the projected Head of Medicine to succeed Cruickshank, then considering a position in Britain. Medicine was a large and critical element in our projections and I wished to proceed without heat or obstruction. It was up to him, what kind of year I would have. He stammered a bit, apologised and hastily left. After a testy period of a few months, fortunately distracted by work on the IADB Committee, our relationship reverted to cordiality, and he was uniformly supportive.

Professor Hoyte had opposed my appointment as Dean, and so wrote to me resigning his function as Vice-Dean, Pre-Clinical Affairs (Basic Sciences), as he felt any Stuart appointee should properly do. He changed his mind and agreed to support me and to resume as Vice-Dean after a frank conversation, in which he found out the real reason for my candidacy, my readiness to decline the position, and the steps taken to do so, when Ken's abuse stiffened my back. My wife agreed to live with it, and secretly liked the idea of being the Dean's wife, and with her love

---

[24]Harold was an excellent clinician and teacher and had left the Mona department in 1955 for Barbados in baffling circumstances, which I would learn when I became Dean and asked him to take on the Associate Deanship in Medicine in Barbados. Remember the racial climate in Barbados then: cricket was the life of the colonies. Barbados had produced three exciting young black cricketers: Everton Weekes, Frank Worrell and Clyde Walcott, who played for the West Indies, and as the 3Ws, were household names by 1955, when the Australians toured the West Indies. A white Barbadian team-mate hosted a cocktail party for the visitors, and failed to invite the three Ws, because white Barbadians did not socialise with Blacks. The snub affected many, confirming the ancient racial divide that persisted in Barbados, though slowly fading elsewhere. Writers who saw cricket as a unifying force in WI colonies had a field day. In the same vein, Dr Forde had been bypassed for promotion for a junior Scotsman, Dr Tulloch; this seemed to have prompted his departure from Mona.

of entertaining, immediately began to plan what gastronomic feats she could accomplish to mend fences. And so we went forward.

Most of my opponents were gracious, if unenthusiastic or dubious, and real hostility came from Bill Brooks, a departmental colleague, Errol (Mickey) Walrond, Surgery, and Paul Feng of Pharmacology, while Picou and Alleyne of the TMRU, and Beaubrun from Psychiatry, were icy, as were a few silent others, presumably most department heads, although later I would learn that several of them had backed me. Brooks' position was expressed at Faculty Board meetings, often opposed to his superior, Professor Bras, and gained traction from the positions of the other detractors, which included the more benign EV Ellington from Biochemistry and James Ling, a classmate, like Alleyne, from Medicine.

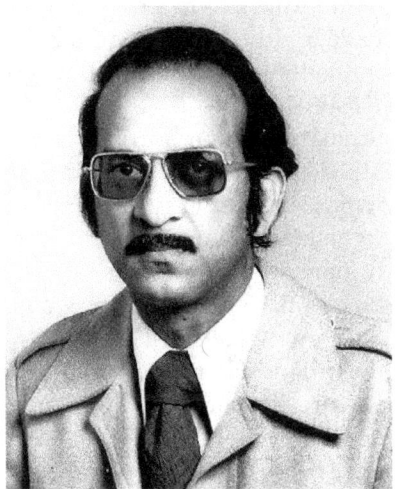

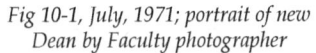
Fig 10-1, July, 1971; portrait of new Dean by Faculty photographer

Walrond was the main surprise, as we had worked together on the Action Group, but he had changed when Ken made him the secretary of the IADB Committee, which had already held preliminary meetings.

I tried to behave towards my detractors as I had done before their estrangement, and felt that their personal grudges were theirs to handle — and I did not consciously alter my interactions with, or regard for them, nor follow their biases; I was cautious, and thus at times some diffidence did surface. Relations with Picou and Alleyne would remain cordial and they restricted professional contact to necessary issues.

Socially there was little obvious change; in any case, wives controlled that side of things, and mine was a good friend of Alleyne's, and quickly exceeded my entertainment allowance to bring relays of Faculty to soothing dinner parties. Beaubrun declined re-appointment as Vice-Dean, Clinical Affairs, and in time transferred his base to Trinidad. (See *The Indelible Red Stain* for a comment on the attitudes of coloured West Indians to Indians, and the colour question in general.) In a sense, the opposition of these men was good, as it made me more meticulous in preparing plans or programs for committees and for the Faculty Board.

Sir Harry Annamunthodo, Professor and Head of Surgery, one of the giants of the UWI Medical Faculty, surprised me with his constant support, as I had thought his friendship with Ken Stuart would make me seem an upstart. But his own struggle for recognition should have told me a different tale. He had trained in the UK at the London Hospital, on a British Guiana Scholarship, and worked in Surgery at King George V Hospital, Essex, with Hermon Taylor, one of the foremost abdominal surgeons in Britain.

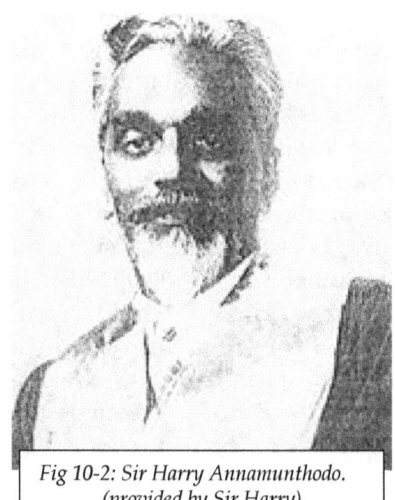

Fig 10-2: *Sir Harry Annamunthodo. (provided by Sir Harry)*

Soon, with his prodigious knowledge of Anatomy and Clinical Surgery, he eclipsed his "boss" in technical skill and the speed of his operations. He rues the fact that he was passed over several times for a Lectureship at London University, and was quite bitter over his appointment at UCHWI as a Senior Registrar in 1953, when so many British types with less than his reputation and experience would get a lectureship at least. Finally, in 1956, he was grudgingly appointed a Temporary Lecturer, and in early 1957 confirmed as a Lecturer.

At that time, there was considerable unrest at the failure of the London-UCWI principals to deal equitably with non-British staff. Ken Stuart and Ron Irvine had also joined the UCWI as Registrars in Medicine; Ken, as Senior Registrar, also felt downgraded. Dr Harold Forde had come on at the same time as a lecturer. The Senior Lecturer in Medicine then was Dr Hugh-Jones, who left about the time Ken came and was replaced by a Briton, John Tulloch, who was soon evaluated by students as far inferior to Harold Forde. So tension developed in the faculty over racial preferment in appointments, and by the end of that decade, would crystallise in the campaign for recognition and reward of these West Indians, and for Louis Grant, who was then agitating for a separate department of Microbiology, and for his personal professorship. These were settled in a few years after the UCWI became the UWI.

It is difficult to appreciate the struggles of these highly qualified and capable academics when one sees the plethora of professors now littering the UWI landscape. They almost equal the number of "Sirs" in Barbados!

Sir Harry was the first to have his status settled when he became Senior Lecturer in late 1957. I worked with him as a student and locum interne a few times, and during one stint at the latter, during my final year, he had Mike Woo Ming as Registrar, making his firm a team of three Queen's College alumni. On my first day of a two-week locum, I was called to an emergency sent in from St Ann's Bay, who, on arrival was hurried through Casualty and sent directly to the operating theatre where Sir Harry was just finishing a case, and could release Woo-Ming to look at the gentleman, since I was in the middle of a procedure in one of the wards. The patient had surgery, was returned to the ward, and given a special nurse, the closest we came then to intensive care.

He turned out to be Capt. Howard Nobbs, our joint QC Principal. When he saw us together on rounds on the day he was well enough to be himself, he broke down in tears to realise he had been "rescued by three of my very own." Capt. Nobbs had retired in 1953 to Britain and was brought by his son to Jamaica's north coast for a winter holiday, when he developed a life-threatening abdominal emergency. The local surgeon, lacking full facilities and an anaesthetist, promptly despatched him by ambulance to UCHWI, serendipitously on our on-call day. Nobbs was in poor condition after surgery but remained stable. Then as he awoke and met his care-givers, the elation of discovery changed his mood and outlook and transformed him; he became chatty and nostalgic, unusual for a reticent man, and recalled incidents in our school life, much to our delight or embarrassment, and it was instructive to see school events and one's own role in them, from the principal's viewpoint. He recovered quickly and well, and enjoyed meeting a stream of old students from various faculties.

We missed him when he left, but was relieved he had mended. Harry used the incident to illustrate the almost optimum performance of a referral service, and the need for an intensive care unit, then being described in the literature, and the health services need for specialists. For Nobbs, everything had happened right, from the moment his ambulance arrived, his son beside him. How often Sir Harry would cite it as service load increased and added delays in response; in just over a decade, he would ruefully remark, as we discussed PGME, "Nobbs might not have made it, had he come in today."

I have nothing but praise for the critical and unstinted support Sir Harry gave me in my deanship, both in regular meetings and offering to take charge when I had to be away and the regular vice-deans were not available, as happened a few times, or threatened when social unrest in the early seventies began to scare away scarce faculty. He commiserated with me re the gun incidents, and would casually drop by on his way from the wards to his office. I spoke to him before my term ended, and bemoaned the misdirection students had received re the start of the Community Medicine (CM) clerkship, while I was away in Trinidad.

He knew how much it had taken, of time and persuasion, to get it and more so, the substantial grant from Kellogg. He was concerned that no successor would be able or prepared to do the jobs I did without additional help or remuneration. My biggest worry, shared with the PAFAMS director, was that the Manchester project would not be carried out as planned. Sir Harry had endorsed the administrative structure, and had a copy of the details for implementation (see chapter on *Community Medicine* and *Appendix*). He had agreed with my choice of Knolly Butler as Vice-Dean, EC scheme, in 1972, and Reg Carpenter, in 1975, to run PGME in my absence, as a stable and reliable hand, but had misgivings re Community Medicine. "The groundwork for the EC scheme is all laid, I see; you're just waiting on Trinidad; I could keep an eye on it. But I leave it to the Community Medicine Committee to oversee that one; I'll remind them to stick to the written plan; yet I fear you will lose it."

I saw him in 1978 at Mona, and showed him a copy of my draft evaluation of the Manchester project. He read the summary and frowned, but gave me only a hint of his deep disquiet. Sam Wray, as Dean, had taken over the management of the project from Owen Minott; subsequently, funds intended for project needs—field-work and clinic supplies, human and material, and UWI specialist staff visits—were diverted to psychological "research;" by-passing the Committee, and depriving students of support. Sir Harry surprised many by resigning in 1980, before reaching retirement age, after 27 years of selfless service.

The Royal College of Surgeons of England recorded the event thus, in their biography of Fellows: "Communal violence marred his latter years in Jamaica, and within the University *he was increasingly frustrated by the deterioration in the high academic and moral standards that he had striven to maintain for so long* (emphasis mine). It was not wholly with regret that he resigned from the Chair in 1980 and spent his last years as a professor at the University of Kebangsaan in Kuala Lumpur."

I can attest to this loss of trust, as reading this, I finally understood his frown on seeing my draft, "Your criticism is deserved; you are wise to stay away, although I had hoped you would come back; the Faculty has fallen into corrupt and incompetent hands." And when I told him that Sam had warned me not to come back, as I had wished to resume as PGME Coordinator or Director of Community Medicine, he said sharply, fury in his voice, "But he told me differently, that you had quit after *declining* the offer of Coordinator!"

CHAPTER 11
Other faculty reforms

The Action Group report had commented on the need for reforms to the Faculty Board and Faculty Structure (Ch. 4). On becoming Dean, my first concern was the IADB Committee's deliberations and its findings, which I would have to present to Council (Ch. 12). At the same time, we began reforming Faculty structure and administration, and its relationship with the University, without which PGME could have stalled in a morass of interdepartmental conflict, and personal biases. By mid-1972, I was discussing with the VC, a divisional structure for the Faculty that the IADB Committee and the Action Group had endorsed. I saw it as aiding function, and one that would conform to the vision of medical education as a continuum from pre-medicine to specialty training and life-long learning, to maintain competence (see fig 4.2, p. 43 and 5.1, p. 56), and to contribute to creation of health teams.

But the Dean's office was a literal mess, a hindrance to efficiency; its filing was haphazard, and key files were in the offices of the various departments heads who had served as Dean annually for 21 years. A requested file—as I found out when collecting material for the IADB Committee—could only be located if I knew the recipient of the communication! Secretaries—there were three—typed and filed. The first, the late Ann Costa[25], assistant to the Dean; the second, Mrs. Dorothy Jung, in charge of all students' activities and files; and the third, Mrs. Johanna Young, would spend up to an hour searching through likely files for the one I wanted, wasting their diligence in these searches. Mercifully, student files were alphabetical, by year of graduation. My inclination was to bury the lot and start anew.

---

[25] Ann Rosemary Costa, my secretary for five years, changed from a sceptic to a staunch advocate of my efforts, and later became the lynch-pin for the PGME program. My kudos to her memorable work does not imply that I think less of the work of the other office staff; they too were diligent, despite having families to distract them, but the Faculty was everything for Ann. She had come to us in 1969 as an experienced person with high school and stenography diplomas, and by 1970 had been immersed in the flurry of events then transforming the Dean's office into an international crossroads. Her initial scepticism soon changed and she tackled the growing problems with dedication and initiative, and also began work, with Mrs. Jung, in their scant spare time, on an Alumnus organisation. By 1974, she had done enough to merit my taking the "unusual step" (as Registry sources had commented) of making a case for her promotion to Administrative Assistant, which normally required a university degree, but we argued equivalence and work performance. Eventually her promotion was approved, the year I finished my term.

We had to reform records management urgently. Here, Carl Jackman, the Registrar, was invaluable; he responded immediately to my SOS, visited, and, stunned by what he saw, sent me Mrs. Irene Walter, an Assistant Registrar, for a fortnight to lay out a plan for organising the office records and filing system, and to train staff. Without this help, we would not have been able to function with any promptness or efficiency. Did previous Deans rely on memory alone, I wondered? I was lucky that I had duplicate files on all the work I had done, on examinations, curriculum and all PGME files, and was allowed access to the relevant files of previous Deans through their secretaries.

We had aimed at having a deciding or major input into all decisions relating to the educational functions of the Faculty, and to have the Dean's office and new committees of the Faculty Board rather than individual departments assume responsibility for academic functions, in the hope that we could pursue a common vision and work towards it cooperatively and professionally. That meant control, or at least a leading opinion on faculty finances; appointments; promotions; leave; organisation and administration; undergraduate and graduate education; curricula; new programs (planning); relations with teaching hospitals and with governments; public relations; publications, research and its funding; and so on. We already controlled examinations, which the central Registry conducted, and continued to urge the Parts 2, 3, and 4 examiners to adopt objective tests (MCQs mainly) for appropriate parts of examinations. But, as before, they hesitated and shifted their reason from concept and style to shortage of staff time and resources, and ultimately, "Why change a system (essays) that works so well?"

In response to criticism, the University had gradually allowed the Dean's Office to have a say in these matters — as it had in educational ones — all of which were handled by individual departments, and a pretence made to interdepartmental cooperation. The first step therefore to reforms was the change in Faculty Board composition to include all members of staff on regular (3-year) contracts, from the rank of assistant lecturer, plus two residents. Later, two student observers were added, to take Faculty news to students, directly and via their paper, *Stethoscope*, after vetting by the Dean's office; that worked well initially, but I was disappointed that succeeding editors in 1974 knew little of curricular and other reforms, including Community Medicine and PGME, even though one of them, as a Board member, had access to all Faculty documents. The changes had been previously discussed by department heads and a few had objected to students being on the reformed Board. But the new Board began functioning immediately and responsibly, not rashly, as some senior objectors had feared. The other reforms agreed were:

1.   The Dean would be appointed for a three-year term, renewable twice, subject to satisfactory confidential internal Faculty and University performance reviews, to be ratified by secret ballot, supervised by the Registry, of a two-thirds majority of Board members voting.

2.   Headships of Departments would be severed from positions of subject Chair, which will also be for three year terms, renewable once after satisfactory performance review and confidential consultation with each Faculty member of the department.

3.   Any tenured member from the ranks of Senior Lecturer and above could qualify for appointment as Dean or Head of Department.

4.   The Heads of Department Committee (the *Dean's Group)* would become a formal Advisory Committee to the Dean and its meetings would be minuted and reported to the Board.

5.   The affairs of the Board would be conducted by several Standing Committees: Admissions; Finance; Curriculum; Appointments, Assessments and Promotions; PGME Coordination; Higher degrees (MSc., PhD.); Planning; Research; Student Health, and others, as needed. For PGME, there would be a subcommittee or Board of Studies for each specialty program, the *Specialty Boards* – each made up of members of that specialty, in numbers to be decided by the Specialty – plus the Co-ordinator of PGME, the Dean or his/her representative, a resident and/or fellow.

Each of the major Committees, other than the PGME Committee, would consist of a core of 5-7 people, nominated by the Dean, as Faculty, not departmental representatives, after consultation with Board members, based on interest and ability, and approved by the Faculty Board and University Administration. The first priority had been the appointment of a Vice-Dean, Clinical, who was trusted by all staff, and unlikely to shift policy without notice or debate. Andrew Masson, head of neurosurgery, agreed to do this. Fourteen years ago, he had been one of my surgical coaches before finals. (He shared a birthday with my last son, while his first daughter was born on mine!)

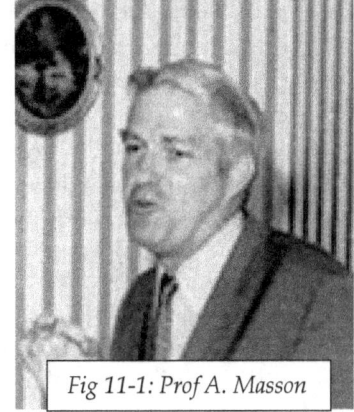

Fig 11-1: Prof A. Masson

"You know I didn't vote for you," he had said.

"Neither did Professors Hoyte or Beaubrun. Hoyte resigned but agreed to stay on as Pre-clinical Vice-dean; Beaubrun declined the offer of Vice-Dean, EC. Everyone likes you, as I do; you know that."

His acceptance brought a fine and respected intellect to my side and he worked, as did everyone on the team, to make the needed changes. His knowledge of the clinical staff and the inputs from Sir Harry, Eric Cruickshank, Rabin Sahoy, Gerrit Bras, Ken Stuart, Colin Miller, Karl Smith and others got the committees appointed in a few months, the time it took to get all interests known. The Dean or delegate would be on all Committees, which would report to the Faculty Board.

I discussed these with Carl Jackman, the Registrar, with whom I had sat for several hours going over the plans; he advised on jurisdiction and strategy. His help was critical. I had also consulted Zach Preston, PVC Finance, and Bursar Hugh Holness, with whom I had worked as a summer student eighteen years earlier, and had gotten to know well, and had maintained relationships over the years. They too took the time to advise on what were possible at Faculty level, what they could delegate, and what was sacred University territory. I had also talked to PVC Leslie Robinson, Planning, and Roy Augier, Chair of the Board for Higher Degrees. I then took my plan to a Heads of Department meeting soon after the newly approved Faculty Board configuration.

Satisfied that I was conscientious in what I was doing, the Registrar tacitly allowed me to review departmental staff vacancies and preview applications, as until then, departments had kept their affairs to themselves, and vacancies were a source of bargaining and trade-offs with others, often just to wait for a particular candidate, a tricky thing then, as doctors were as fickle as any others, and many felt no loyalty to country or alma mater (as I would later find out with Karl Massiah, (p. 206). Thus I came to be forewarned of matters before the University Appointments and Promotions Committee, and after several meetings, I formally requested, and was granted permission for all applications for medical posts be vetted by the Faculty A & P Committee, and also obtained a similar privilege to have all communication, especially on finance and curriculum, channelled through my office.

The reforms had the general support of nearly all faculty below the "Heads" level, and of most Heads, including those who were *assumed* to have been against my appointment: Sir Harry Annamunthodo (Surgery, and the most prestigious Faculty member); Gerrit Bras (Pathology, then Dean of PG studies, a titular appointment, to assist his attempts to raise funds in the USA); Eric Cruickshank (Internal Medicine); Louis Grant (Microbiology); David Hoyte (Anatomy), one of the most influential Faculty members; Mavis Anderson (O&G); David Picou of the MRC (TMRU), who was soon to succeed John Garrow as Director; Paul Feng (Pharmacology); and Eugene Ward (Physiology). Those known to be in support were Ken Standard (Social & Preventive Medicine); Reg Carpenter (Casualty), Eric Back (Paediatrics), and later his successor,

Colin Miller (he was SHO in Paediatrics when I was intern there, and we had become friends; he was a mine of medical information, which I would regularly tap, while he relied on me for administrative and organisational matters). Ken Stuart was in favour (he had supported the changes, including the new Committee structure, when I brought them to a previous Heads meeting); his support remained for the remainder of our relationship, and I would often ask his advice, at first with some diffidence, but that changed with his endorsement for my second term.

The Finance Committee was approved by the two power blocks on campus, the University Academic Board and the Finance and General Purposes Committee, which directed that all departmental submissions had to pass through the Dean's Office, since the Dean could no longer "make the excuse of being an annual, spare-time and toothless" appointee, a situation that several Heads wanted to keep, since they could wangle things directly with the University administration. Administrators, however, had welcomed the idea of being freed from the manipulations of strong-willed medical "heads," as they knew little of the technicalities, intrigues and inter-relationships of the Faculty of Medicine departments, and tended to react to the individual's academic and professional prestige. The Faculty Finance and other committees: Curriculum, Appointments and Promotions, etc., all received the same functional approval; the structural change would follow later.

Interestingly, the most vocal opponent of that administrative structure, was Stanley "Bill" Brooks, a former pathology colleague, as noted, but by 1971, an inveterate, and at times nasty adversary, at all levels of Faculty business, no matter what the issue. He had been lukewarm since my review of essays versus objective tests of knowledge, and cool to the change in examinations and to the diploma level training in clinical pathology, rejecting the concept of "clinical pathology" in favour of individual subject specialties. While that approach was justified for large teaching laboratories, it was not affordable by an island of 100,000 people with 20 physicians at most, which could barely afford one part-time diplomate, while Brooks would insist on three or four full specialists! It was ludicrous, especially as even then, some island CMOs were talking of sharing a diplomate! Even so, he refused to concede that it was the UWI's responsibility to address that need, and backed the gown versus town. He had supported Ken Stuart for the Deanship—unaware than Stuart, like Bras, had shared my view of diplomas—and was livid when I was appointed. Their support did not quell his ire. And so we existed until I had to write him re behaviour.

He had unofficially consulted with his friend Gerald Lalor, and Roy Augier, his neighbour, Dean, General Degree Studies, asking their advice on how my appointment could be annulled. Lalor was a Jamaican creole, a shade lighter than Bill, but in the same stratum, and automatically took his side; this sounds crass, but these subtleties were significant influences among some Jamaicans. Roy was a St Lucian, an urbane and civilised man, dressed in an ample goatee beard; he flippantly answered, "The only sure way, Bill, is to kill him! That's definitive. Otherwise, grin and bear it." Then, seriously said, "You can start a petition, and if you get enough Faculty members signing, you can appeal to the VC. But you have to come good. The VC is impressed with him; first medic, he said, without a vested agenda, and who knew about institutional management and personnel, and stuff about other faculties. He comes prepared to meetings, and the other Deans have fully accepted him. Simple dislike or opposition won't do."

The above is an imaginary sentence, pieced together and based on separate remarks Roy Augier had made to me, unofficially one evening at the Senior Common Room (Staff Club), after his appointment as PVC in 1972, when he casually asked how I would handle opposition among colleagues. He did know of some bad blood, and that Stuart had tried to prevent my initial appointment from taking effect. But he had not heard of any further complaint from him; indeed Stuart seemed quite satisfied and busy with his project in Barbados, and had been pleased that so much had changed so quickly in faculty organisation and administration.

In reply to his question, I said that my response would depend on the type of opposition. "Racists, I ignored or dismissed and tried to treat dispassionately; I had met many in BG (Guyana), and some in Jamaica. With people with different ideas, I prefer a debate, first at home informally after dinner; if that fails or he/she refuses, and the difference stands, I would suggest bringing the issue to a Board meeting and let the Board decide. There were those who couldn't disagree and remain a friend; if his position or talent would help in a project, I would appoint him to the task force; if he refuses, I have no choice but to ask someone else; I would stand by him as a member of the Faculty Board, and I hope he would allow me to be impartial. If he were simply obstructionist for no good reason, I would warn him of his error, and if he continued, I would write him a letter, confidentially, and if that didn't help, I would copy the next one to the VC and to you, and ask for guidance!"

He laughed heartily, slapped my back and said, "Let's have a beer!"

Toward the end of my first year, when the University asked for a faculty review and recommendation for reappointment, the Board discussed the matter in my absence, as was proper, notice of the purpose of the meeting having been given well in advance. Andrew Masson, the Vice-Dean, chaired the full assembly, which was well-attended. Karl Smith and Ken Standard moved for reappointment, recalling that they had made the original nomination a year ago. They reviewed the performance for the year: *"the inauguration of the first full-time dean, the reform of the Faculty Board by expanding its membership to a true Faculty Board; the restructuring of Faculty administration so that all staff could qualify for service on major new Faculty committees, which the University had accepted and encouraged, including Finance, Curriculum, Dean's Advisory (formerly Heads of Department), Appointments, Postgraduate, Research, et al.; the CHMC successes and advances in PGME; successful defence of the IADB recommendations; promotion of Community Medicine; expansion of the EC Scheme; close relations with PAFAMS and Project HOPE; favourable response from PAHO and several other Foundations: Ford, Josiah Macy, Kellogg, Millbank, Commonwealth, Wellcome Trust etc., supporting research, training and scholarship. A most important change is qualitative: we feel the attitude of the administration and the other Faculties to us is changing for the better."*

Ken Stuart had attended the meeting and made complimentary remarks in support, viz., *"He has always acted without obvious bias, and promptly, is inclusive and faithful to the wishes of the Board. The re-organisation of Faculty administration was overdue and the new Committee structure promises fairness and efficiency; his appointments are based on interest and merit, and he's made excellent progress in curriculum matters and in the postgraduate and EC projects. In fairness, we've never credited his hard slogging to get those approvals. Roy Augier had doubts about us, but not now."*

Others who had become Board members since the reforms, remarked on the "democratisation" and welcomed the changes, although some critiqued its slow pace ; the Chair noted that this was beyond any Dean's control, "Things will only move as fast as funds allow." One department head noted, "If we had the finance, things could really fly, both here and in the EC, with plans approved or nearing so." The comments were as Ann recorded, and Professor Masson remembered them. He had thought Stuart's comments marked him as "classy," and put to rest lingering animosities that some of my detractors were too glued to their biases to forego, even after Professor Stuart's endorsement, for which I thanked him sincerely, and for the help he had given over the past year; I held him in the same esteem I had felt when he had become Dean in 1970.

I had expected Brooks to find something to criticise, but after Stuart's comment, he had fallen silent. The vote was by secret ballot, and almost unanimous in favour. Bill admitted that he voted against, and remained quite hostile. Dave Picou, Vasil Persaud and Michael Beaubrun did not attend. There was one abstention, my informant said: my classmate, George Alleyne, who would, with my approval, replace Ken Stuart when Ken resigned as Head of Medicine a year or so later, to spend more time on his research in Barbados. At the same time steps were taken to promote Advanced Nursing Education and Physiotherapy; Professor Louis Grant was Chair of the UHWI Board then, and was charged with opening the Government school of Physiotherapy, which he did with much flair.

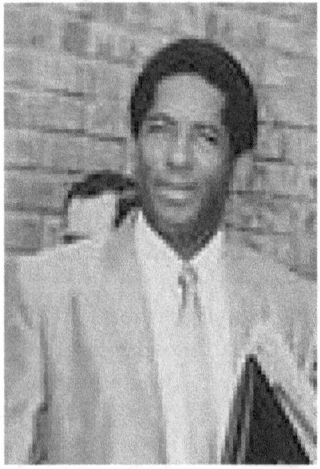

Fig 11-2:

L: Dr Karl Smith, Epidemiologist 1970

R: Prof. Louis Grant, speaking at the opening of the school of Physiotherapy, 1972, Kingston, Jamaica; he backed objective tests (MCQs etc.)

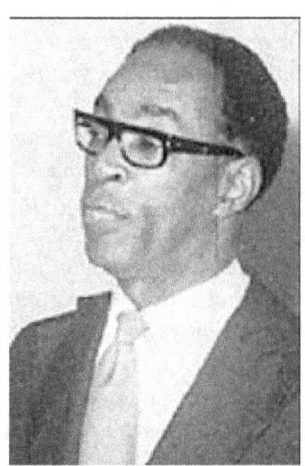

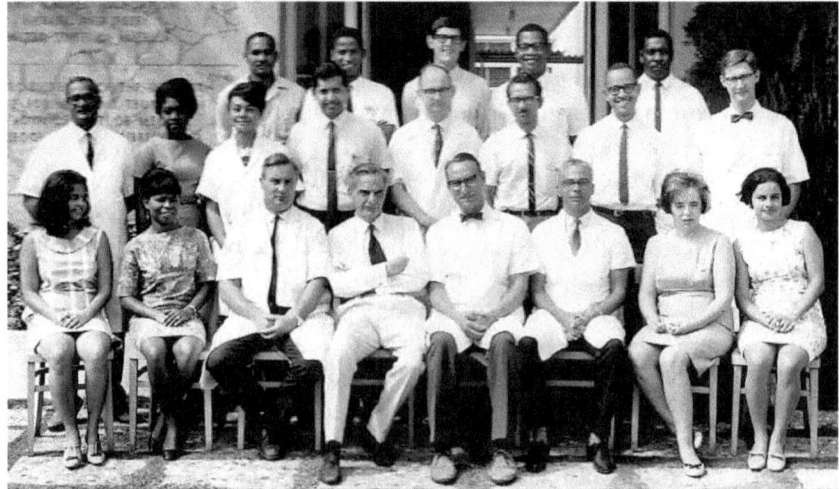

Fig 11-3: Staff of Pathology Department, April 1967, some mentioned in text, who had contributed to the review of examinations and to the MCQ question bank: (Path photo)

Front Row: P. DaCamara, O. Williams (Residents) J. Hayes (Snr Lect.), Prof. Scarff (Ext Examiner), Prof G. Bras (Dept., Head); H. McDonald (Snr Lect., Clin. Chem), M. Thorburn (Lect.), and F. Whitbourne (Resident).
Middle Row: G. Khan (Lab Supt.); B. Lee (Research Asst.); F. Tomlinson (Chief Tech, Haem.); Lecturers V. Persaud (AP), P. Pegg (Clin. Chem), M. Ragbeer (AP); S. Brooks (Snr Lect., AP), P. Milner (Snr Lect., Haem.)
Back Row: C. Benjamin (Chief Tech, AP); R. Jordan, P. Johnson, A. Patrick (Residents); V. Elliott (Chief Tech., Haem.)

CHAPTER 12
COPMED, Task Force on Need for specialists

The Committee for Postgraduate Medical Education (COPMED) was formed by CHMC III in Bermuda, 1970, on funding provided by PAHO, and held its first meeting there. It appointed a Task Force to conduct a survey of specialist manpower needs in each territory that wished it. The Task Force was made up of a core membership of Dr R. Sahoy, with alternates, Drs D. Ashley and P. Arscott, President, Secretary and Treasurer respectively, of the Junior Medical Staff Association, UHWI; Dr A. Robertson of PAHO; and myself as Chair. To these would be added, in each territory visited, the CMO or his/her designate and one or more Ministry officials.

We began the study after a strategy meeting, assisted by a PAHO manpower specialist, who critiqued the plan of investigation and approved for circulation a questionnaire on demographics, health statistics, medical manpower establishment, plans for expansion of facilities and staff, and roles in PGME. This was followed up with visits to Antigua, Barbados, Belize, British Virgin Islands, Dominica, Grenada, Guyana, Montserrat, St Kitts, St. Lucia, St Vincent and Trinidad. Guyana was the first country visited, from March 14 to 20, 1971. The EC islands were visited between October 16 and Nov 5, 1971, Belize Nov 24-25 — at which Professor Masson took my place — and Bermuda, Dec 2-4, 1971.

At each site, the Task Force held interviews, reviewed the data — including the PAHO Quadrennial Projections 1971-74 — met graduates, and obtained the opinions and observations of the Minister and his/her advisors. Meetings with staff, and the local medical associations and professional schools (nursing and paramedical) were held in open forum and dealt with technical and operational issues as well. The team examined facilities, toured sample hospitals and clinics, visited sites of proposed new hospitals in Montserrat, Antigua, Tortola, St. Vincent and Trinidad, and noted plans for expansion or replacement in several others, including Belize. It noted conditions of staffing, facilities and range of services, and discussed needs with specialists, one of the most compelling being Dr Cecil Cyrus, a one man dynamo in St Vincent.

The Task Force presented its Report to a meeting of COPMED held at Mona, on Jan 4-6, 1972. The meeting was chaired by Dr Max Awon, Minister of Health, T&T, and consisted of six other CHMC members: Mr. C. Burton, Barbados; Drs W. Chin, Guyana; L. Comissiong, Grenada; G. Davis, Bahamas; J. Wilson, Jamaica; and Mr. J. Nunez, T&T; four from

UWI: PVC Preston, and Drs Masson, Miller and me; and Dr H. Diggory from PAHO. Dr P. Boyd, Executive Secretary of CHMC, was present, ex-officio. Drs K. Stuart, E. Walrond and R. Meltzer attended as observers.

In reporting, as Task Force Chair, I thanked PAHO for funding, for local help in Guyana, and services of Dr Robertson. Members were impressed with the insights and contributions of the three residents on site visits, and of the young doctors in Government services, graduates of UWI and other schools. There were fewer from UWI in each country than expected from the number of graduates (*see Table, p 120*); those from the UK and elsewhere were on short-term contracts. Among staff, the St Vincent surgeon, Mr. Cyrus, was easily the most impressive, and inventive, with a wide spectrum of skills, a one-man team! (*Bibliography*)

The questionnaires had been completed, as far as reliable data would allow, as a few places had not yet completed an analysis of a recent census. Figures for disease incidence, demographics, and vital statistics were not yet available in two, ostensibly due to lack of staff to review reports, extract figures and prepare them for statistical analysis, which large centres did, increasingly by referral to a government computer service. It is hoped that the CARICOM office would soon help with this problem. The Bahamas completed a questionnaire but declined a visit.

The report noted ways to improve training at all levels of care, and reviewed the aims and development of medical education, practice objectives, manpower realities, the brain drain, and the desire of both young doctors and health services to have a full spectrum of care-givers, from aides to specialists, trained in the local environment of care. A few examples were found of *"well-run health services...in spite of underprivileged economies"* where *"problems were...frankly and squarely being tackled"* in a *"long-term plan with proper priorities."* A few well-equipped units were found and examples of inventiveness and flair.

The main findings were:

1. Hospitals were invariably short of staff, equipment and supplies.
2. *Health officers uniformly supported the plan for PGME, and added Community Medicine as essential in any new curriculum.*
3. The staffing complement in all territories was usually that inherited from the Colonial Office which was constructed for an expatriate professional service. Most were inadequate in all specialties for the health needs of the countries, and some specialties were unmanned, such as Dermatology, ENT surgery, Ophthalmology, Orthopaedics, the surgical and medical subspecialties, and others. The likelihood of the smaller countries attracting any but the retired part-time person in any of these is vanishingly small (see 9 below). The services provided unevenly for urban and rural areas, sometimes neglecting

the latter entirely. We tried to arrive at a personnel structure and training to meet the needs, and to see whether services could accommodate trainees, and if so, how many and in what disciplines.

4. Most services, if not all, were criticised for the retention of the obsolete colonial model of Civil Service staffing (of which health care was part), through local Public Services Commissions (PSC), which had uniform conditions of service, and did not accommodate doctors' irregular hours, on-call, or the possibility of formal post-graduate training, although in-service training was a common obligation. (This matter was brought up again in 1973 in Dominica and resulted in Resolution 18/73 urging the removal of health services appointments from the PSCs.)

5. A recurring problem was the inadequacy of middle grade positions to provide a trainee pool for specialist training, or a structure such as *Consultant-Registrar-House Officer (Resident), Intern,* to provide service and supervision of trainees and allow them to learn optimally from clinical encounters, often different from the patients in the teaching hospital; such an experience might direct their choice of specialty. Also, teaching hospitals had no culture of residents as researchers.

6. In most services new recruits were often shifted without notice among services, the frequency distracting from a line of study.

7. Doctors emphasised the conditions that would attract residents: prompt response to enquiries and applications; improved conditions of service, such as housing; equal pay with foreign peers, who received allowances that natives did not get; better supervision by consultants, who invariably were allowed private practice, and thus had little time for junior staff; less demanding on-call schedules, to allow some study time; reliable drug supplies; designated trainee posts (residencies, see 5); access to libraries, and so on.

8. Some services had few of the "less glamourous" specialties, like Radiology, Anaesthesia, Laboratory Medicine, Family Medicine, Psychiatry, and Public Health, despite the ripple effect they had on the quality and progress of clinical disciplines. While a non-medical virologist or biochemist could fill general needs in a laboratory, one needed a medically-trained pathologist for tissue diagnoses and autopsies; and a radiologist to correlate features on an x-ray film with the clinical condition. Some doctors were referring tissues to the UWI Pathology Department for diagnoses, at no charge. A nurse-anaesthetist might be adequate for a certain level of surgery, but might not be for complex cases such as major organ procedures, thus retarding local development of certain modalities of care. Patients who could afford to, will go to another country or to a private facility, if the country had one appropriately provided.

9. Small countries, such as the Lesser Antilles, welcomed PGME at Diploma level, and would consider joint sponsorship of those specialties where the need did not justify a full time specialist, or if they could not afford to hire one. Doctors have often done short intensive courses in some disciplines e.g. Dermatology, to deal with common conditions, or special ones e.g. Schistosomiasis in St Lucia.

10. Health officers were satisfied with UWI graduates, the quality of their training and their familiarity with the medical and social conditions of the locales, and could communicate easily with patients and the public, which Cubans, Philippinos and Chinese, who were increasingly recruited into some services, could not do, reducing their value and effectiveness.

11. Islands planning new buildings had not engaged UWI engineers or medical experts; nor consulted the University architect; it may not be feasible or economical, as often building loans were tied to technical personnel "approved" by lenders, but the enquiry should be made.

12. In most services management could be strengthened to improve use of resources; ordering of supplies; maintenance of equipment; and eradicate corrupt practices such as extorting money for surgery or hospitalisation, or other procedure, a practice called "bed money" in the Antilles, and in Guyana, and no doubt occurred elsewhere.

13. *Community Medicine integrating clinical and preventive medicine should be introduced to undergraduates and was the wish of all CHMC members.*

14. Health records, medical statistics and libraries were often deficient and epidemiology poorly served. These affect quality of care and are essential for the conduct and success of specialty training.

15. Nursing services were constantly depleted by migration. Ancillary staff such as public health and child welfare aides were needed in most services.

16. There were 203 specialty positions in the region's Government services, including the Bahamas, 33 vacant; 20% of incumbents were aged over 50. In addition, Jamaica had 148 positions, with several vacancies. An additional twenty newer specialists in the islands were senior registrars: 10 in Trinidad, 3 in Jamaica, and 7 in basic sciences.

17. Guyana's inclusion was as a member of CHMC, not the UWI. It was ambivalent on UWI plans, although it had none of its own. The University of Guyana (UG) is severely underfunded, with no likelihood of change under current political direction, which has employed foreign doctors and has promised more Chinese doctors as a likely immediate answer to its specialist needs; it has arranged training of specialists in various places, Cuba foremost, while India has offered help, and several of its nationals are on staff. The current trend to link with Cuban medical schools is favoured by President

Burnham and opposition leader, Dr Jagan, for ideological reasons, as well as Cuba's emphasis on Community Medicine, which we at UWI have proposed to start soon with the curriculum in draft (p. 58).

Comments:

In general the LDCs backed us but could not contribute much financially. Matters for all parties would have been much simpler had they all been roughly equal in population and economy; as it was, finding common ground was a tough task and often interminably frustrating. It was comforting to know that we were not alone, that every organisation I knew faced similar inequalities, but with tiny islands and small populations the difficulties had little hope of future resolution, short of them all becoming future Bahrains or Bruneis!

The Bahamas came on late; their closer affinities with the US, the views of key advisers and Premier Lynden Pindling's own preferences, kept us out, but with the door ajar. We were sure that in time, as a new generation emerged, they would join the UWI; by 1975, they had become independent and more attentive; later agreements would bring them closer to Mona, and a year later they would employ my friend, Guyanese Dr K. Bacchus, Professor of Education, University of Alberta, to head their new premier secondary school, and help plan for tertiary education.

There had been for years an annual meeting of CMO's, but the Faculty was never involved. The CHMC was established in 1967, and members, unaware of the administrative structure of the University and how their governments related to it *(diagram, p. 96)*, began to pressure the Faculty to take a more direct role in the health services, to understand their needs and take steps to meet them, including the training of specialists to meet service needs, and to satisfy those for teaching and research. All of these were affected and got worse as social and political turmoil in Jamaica began in 1971 to threaten the integrity of the structure, and the very fabric of society, as US media were quick to accuse, forgetting their KKK, city gangs, 1968 riots and frequent murders of citizens, presidents, political personalities and civil rights advocates.

By 1971, several residents had enrolled in Diploma programmes. House officers in accredited posts at UHWI and other teaching hospitals were encouraged to register as postgraduate students pending the expected decision to initiate the PGME scheme in the 1972-75 triennium. Jamaica, with a population of 2.5 million, could easily sustain a sophisticated range of specialists but Montserrat with 12,000 could not. Yet, the pattern of health care delivery was the same in both. This dilemma began to be faced, not by the UWI, but by the Health Ministries of the individual countries, which by the end of the '60's were all coming close to internal self-government or independence, with populations in the Antilles of less than 110,000 each. In either political situation, they were totally responsible for health care. (Montserrat, the Virgin Islands, and Cayman Islands sensibly did not opt for independence).

The Less Developed Countries (LDCs) were geographic neighbours and could share scarce and/or expensive resources. In discussions with their Ministers, we proposed at least two notions, neither new, and already raised by Antigua and Grenada at the Bermuda meeting in 1971: pooling specialists (regionalisation of service), and training GP's to certificate or diploma level in the most needed areas of service. Thus, the initiatives that we had begun in the mid-sixties to train diplomates in Anaesthesia and Pathology could be extended to Psychiatry, Obstetrics, Ophthalmology, Public Health, Child Health, Infectious Diseases, Radiology and Dermatology. Pathology, Anaesthesia and Child Health were the most common needs. Pooling would be feasible for consultant level Pathologists, including Forensic Pathology; Dermatology; ENT Surgery; Ophthalmology, and others, as technology developed and became affordable, especially in computers and general communications. Both approaches were feasible and practicable, and steps could be taken to address them immediately; at the same time steps should be taken to develop better travel services than LIAT airline so far delivered.

In 1969, the University Council had decided to continue the regional University for 12 years, with periodic review of funding *(Appendix 3, p. 31)*. But Jamaica wished changes in admissions policy, which the others opposed; this stalled the funding mechanism and the University actually considered reduction of student intake for 1971; a break-up threatened; rumours flew; pessimists fled. We worked in a surreal atmosphere then, preparing long range plans, not knowing whether we would get the funds for them. We knew that the public would not accept the loss of its flagship institution for higher education. So we ploughed on.

We argued in support of regionalisation with dissemination of training to as many territories as could support it, for whatever constructive period, maintaining a high standard, even though that might promote emigration. We resisted pressures to become an 'off-shore' school for rich, but mediocre Americans. But we did support admission of foreign students, at up to 50% of the expanded admissions, in free competition with our own, at the economic cost of medical education. This would help to fund the Faculty, but the idea was almost anathema in the socialist atmosphere of the Manley era, and in other faculties; some University staff accused me of a double standard, and of capitalism, having heard my criticism of the private off-shore schools.

The comparison was "odious," as Shakespeare had said. We were an established medical school with a uniform admissions policy; permanent teaching positions; a stable evaluation system, with intermediate and final written examinations; research institutes and output, an established international reputation and a medical journal, although lame. I stressed the maintenance of standards and that the foreigner had to equal the local candidate in every respect. The matter was shelved on the question of fairness in determining academic equivalence in two somewhat different pre-university systems, and the possible conflict between fee-payers and others. Both were non-issues, as foreigners in most countries did pay a premium for education, and the early UCWI did admit West Indian graduates of US schools. Furthermore, as a fee-payer, like many others, and a student borrower, I was deeper in debt as I progressed, but did not even think of having ill feelings for holders of scholarships or other grants or subsidies, or of my rich peers.

COPMED discussed the findings, comments and conclusions of the Task Force and noted the deficiencies, throughout the region, in the "minor" specialties, including common services like trauma, Paediatrics, Orthopaedics, Ophthalmology and others, even in the four largest territories. It noted the uneven distribution of specialists and the inability of most of the Lesser Antilles and Belize to participate in a structured residency program, though a few could develop in some specialties enough to offer a six-month residency; the likely disciplines would be Surgery and General Medicine and Community Medicine. One that immediately came up was a surgical residency with the inimitable Dr (Mr.) Cecil Cyrus of St Vincent. Most, however, could offer an elective for 3-6 months in selected disciplines in the last two years of residency.

The future of COPMED was briefly discussed and referred to the CHMC. As an *ad hoc* entity, it had done its job and several members felt that some such body should be set up to monitor the progress of PGME. Dr Awon, the Chair, was ending his period in the T&T Ministry of Health. Mr. Nunez and others deferred to the CHMC. The Hon Francis Prevatt was later appointed Minister of Health for Trinidad.

The Committee presented its report, with attached details on each visit by the Task Force,[26] to the CHMC IV meeting held in Georgetown a month later. COPMED recommended that PGME be set up in two centres: Jamaica and the EC, the latter as a coordinated program to be planned as part of the undergraduate expansion now going through the UWI approvals process. Guyana could join with the EC school by agreement, while it waited to establish a medical faculty at UG. Some of

---

[26] M.S. Ragbeer, A. Robertson, R. Sahoy: *Requirements of the Commonwealth Caribbean for Postgraduate-trained Doctors (incl. COPMED Reports)*, 1972, CHMC IV, 18 (88pp), Georgetown, Guyana.

the findings are summarised in Table 12-2, from the Task Force Report, Paper CHMC 17/72. Table 12-1 is from the IADB report.

UWI Medical Students	1970:	10 years later*
Yearly Admissions:	110	220**
Total Student Body:	550:	1100
Jamaica (Mona):	500 (years 1-5)	550
Trinidad & Barbados:	25 each (5th year only)	550*
*proposed expansion:		

** *I had suggested that 50-60 admissions could be foreign students paying the econom cost of education at Mona. Although present political conditions were uninviting, a the presence of a body of white students may be inciting, the country will return normal and the pressure for places will NOT lessen. The time will come when the id will seem less far-fetched. Same with diagnostic and other services (Lab., X-Ray, oth technical and special therapies), which could be centralised, and marketed to the medi community, as Mr. Ashenheim, member of the UHWI Board, had suggested. A feasibil study at least should be done. But the idea of UWI getting into business was anathema.*

Table 12-1: UWI Medical Faculty: Distribution of Undergraduates, 1969-70

Country	Est.	Specialist Registrar	Mid-grade	Non-National	Vacant	10-yr Add.
Antigua	22	7/0	14+ 1 int.	5 Sp.	?	4
Barbados	69	22/18	15+14 int.	9	1	*
Belize	36	17/0+	16 + 3 int.	19	12	Fill vac
BVI	4	0	0	2	0	1
Dominica	16	8/0	8	?2	3	8
Grenada	13	8/0	3+1 int.	4	1	18
Guyana	106	32/10	58+6 int.	34	3	52
Montserrat	2	0	0	-	-	-
St Kitts/N	5	6/0	10-2 in N	3	1	5
St Lucia	23	8/4	11	All Sp.	2	6
St Vincent	21	8/2 snr	11	3/6		?
T&T	?*	62/yes*	*	*		*
Bahamas	86	18+5/0	59+14 in.	?	?	?
Jamaica	?	154	?	?	8	133
TOTAL	**403**	**350/39**	**185 + 41**	**81**	**31+**	**227+**

*Table 12-2: Regional Staff Establishment, and projected needs***

Est. = Establishment; Add. = Addition; int. = intern; N=Nevis; Sp.= Specialty.
*No figures are given, but the need is accepted for at least seven new specialists; final picture awaits decision re development of EC teaching and Faculty expansion.
+ includes 2 dentists. *Numbers exclude UWI staff in each campus territory.*
**All territories were short of space: office, examining and teaching rooms, for current uses and thus future needs; A-V, office, laboratory and X-ray equipment; library materials etc. Similarly there was a general lack of support staff, clerical, technical and administrative.
--Source: COPMED Reports: See Footnote 26, p.119

CHAPTER 13:
Project HOPE, its role and influences on PGME

In 1970, the US floating hospital, the HOPE ship, docked in Kingston harbour, at the foot of King Street. The project, *Health Opportunity for People Everywhere,* was conceived by William B. Walsh, a US navy doctor, who, during WWII, had seen the need for medical care in the Pacific islands, and had gotten President Eisenhower to donate a hospital ship for that work. After planning and refitting the ship, he set about recruiting American doctors for 2-monthly volunteer rotations (expenses paid) to bring US medical advances to developing countries. He would arrange with recipient Governments and a local medical school to provide care as needed and to teach new or improved procedures to local doctors, nurses and technicians, and others as feasible, for a year at each site. HOPE could leave a land-based program, if desired.

The SS HOPE set sail on September 22, 1960, from San Francisco for Indonesia. In 1961, a documentary was made showing HOPE as an example of the benevolent side of American policies, what its kindly citizens could do to spread care and knowledge, to help those in need. The film won an award as best US documentary in 1961, was translated into 23 languages and was a key factor in successful fundraising, which enabled subsequent "missions" to Vietnam, Peru, Ecuador, Guinea, Nicaragua, Colombia, Ceylon (Sri Lanka), Tunisia, Jamaica and Brazil. The ship was retired in 1974.

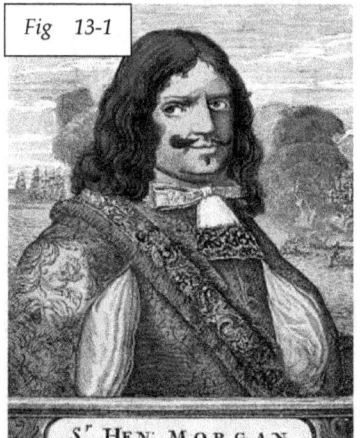

Fig 13-1

Sᵣ HEN: MORGAN

The SS HOPE was in a line of Naval Hospitals, from the U.S.S. *Red Rover*, a converted Confederate paddle steamer, to the largest White Star ocean liner, the *RMS Britannic,* launched in 1914, sister ship to the ill-fated *RMS Titanic. Britannic* served as a hospital from December 1915 to November 1916, when it too sank, after striking a mine. Adding variety to his trove, Bill had a picture of portly Henry Morgan (*Fig.13-1*), the British pirate, who was commissioned to plunder Spanish ships by Sir John Modyford, Governor of Jamaica, 1664-70, and an agent of greedy, cruel and pugnacious British planters, headed by the Earl of Harewood of Barbados and Yorkshire, England, who had established many sugarcane

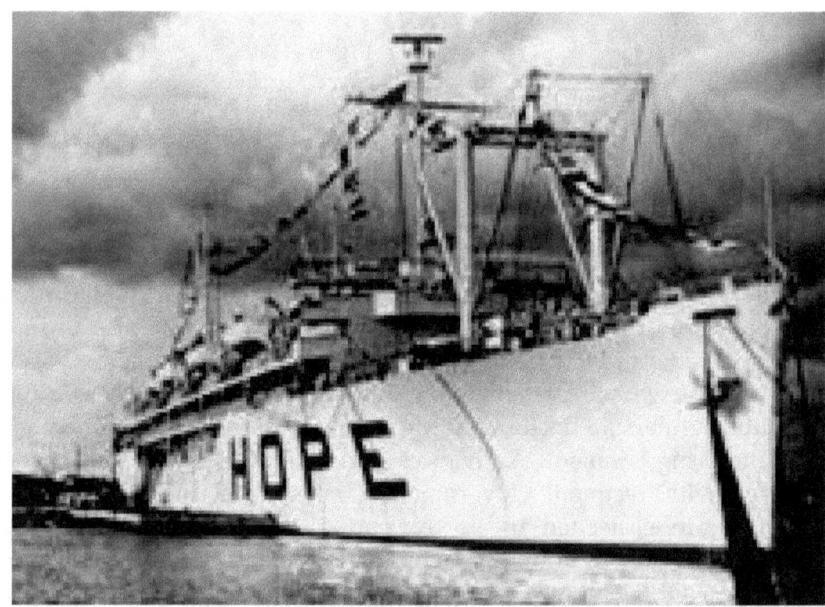

Fig 13-2: The HOPE hospital ship, at anchor

plantations in Barbados, as Mr Cameron Tudor, our QC History master, had related. In Jamaica, with its sparse population then, and no real agriculture, but soil suitable for planting, when the British wrested it from the Spanish in 1655, the Barbadians established several sugar estates and a thriving slave trade. Modyford sanctioned Morgan's raids on Spanish ships and towns, but this angered Charles II, who had become king after the collapse of Cromwell's Commonwealth. Modyford and Morgan were recalled to England and imprisoned in the Tower of London for three years. Morgan was pardoned and made Governor of Port Royal. The Harewoods thrived in Jamaica, sold out and retired to Barbados, where they stayed until 1975.

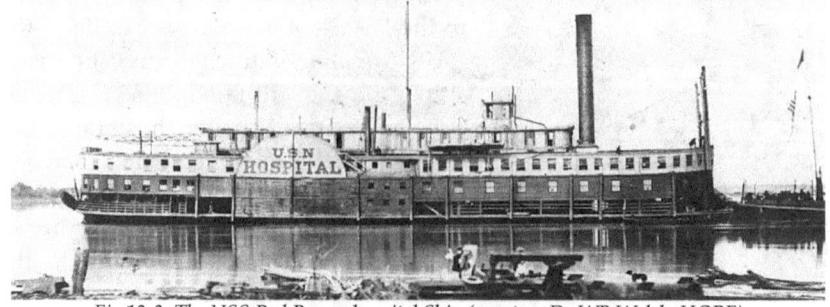

Fig 13-3: The USS Red Rover, hospital Ship (courtesy Dr WB Walsh, HOPE)

Like many on UHWI staff, I had visited the HOPE ship as it lay tied up and secure at the foot of King Street, guarded by local police on shore, and US marines on board. They held daily clinics in adult and paediatric medicine, obstetrics and surgery, and had several operative sessions, each by a particular US surgeon, coordinated with the Kingston Public Hospital. Faculty members were registered as official visitors and given temporary passes. Several of their consultants visited the UHWI and attended teaching conferences, such as the popular weekly CPCs.

Arrangements were concluded in the summer of 1971 for HOPE's land-based program: a contribution to UWI specialty training programs. When the ship left for Brazil, Dr Meltzer and a team of doctors, administrators, and nurses remained in Jamaica to implement their side of an agreement concluded with the Jamaica Government and UWI. As noted above, Dr Meltzer was present when Dr Eldemire agreed to initiate the Jamaican aspect of the program by providing one to two residents in each of the disciplines ready to start. HOPE had undertaken to provide one faculty member and one or two senior residents in each of seven disciplines: Medicine, Surgery, O&G, Pathology, Anaesthesia, Paediatrics and Radiology, while PAHO provided a Senior Lecturer in Public Health. The Jamaica Government would provide living quarters, and other participating governments would support any resident they nominated. Governments would also nominate teaching hospitals and clinics for fixed aspects of the programs or for electives, subject to accreditation; new hospitals would be fitted to accept residents and students. A formal agreement was signed between HOPE and the University, for five years in the first instance.

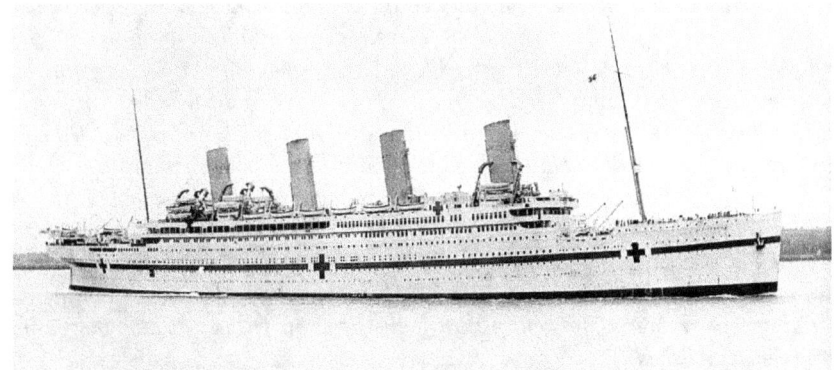

Fig 13-4:The White Star Line's RMS Britannic (courtesy Dr WB Walsh, HOPE

HOPE established its headquarters at a cottage on Monroe Rd., Liguanea, about four miles from the University, and arranged transport for its staff who worked at the hospital. The Director, Dr Meltzer, had an office there but soon found that he needed a desk somewhere at the Hospital. Office space was at a premium, so I established him at the far corner of my office, the position of dominance, according to psychologists. He was an excellent co-worker, stuck to his task when he was there, about two hours every day and gave me noble support, to critique ideas and arguments. An example is this memo he sent me soon after the Guyana meeting of CHMC in 1972, and a series of discussions on training arrangements for paediatrics, and on other issues:

TO: *Dean Mohan Ragbeer*
FROM: *Dr Richard Meltzer*
Project HOPE, P.O. Box 6000, Kingston, Jamaica, March 16, 1972

As an addendum to our recent conversations concerning the appointments and support by Government of a full time member of the University of the West Indies Faculty of Medicine to a post at the Children's Hospital, several considerations should be discussed.

A. The paediatrician appointed to the Children's Hospital post should be of a reasonably senior level, i.e. senior lecturer. One of junior level would be unable to exert the necessary authority to develop an adequate teaching program. This individual would be responsible for the development, management and maintenance of a teaching program for both residents and medical students, for advising and participation in the area of nursing and paramedical education and in the development and participation in the continuing education of paediatricians and other practitioners in and out of Government service. Obviously this person would have to participate in patient care, administration of the hospital and University affairs. It seems apparent that one with these various responsibilities would be unable to carry on any private practice.

B.   It would be well to contemplate the appointment of similar personnel to posts in Surgery and Medicine at the Kingston Public Hospital and the Victoria Jubilee Hospital. It is probable, at this time, that the Government physicians, Surgeons and Obstetricians would be opposed to such appointments but I believe it is necessary if undergraduate and post graduate Medical, Nursing and Para-medical education is to be carried out in the community

C.   A full time member of the Faculty of Medicine should be appointed to the Montego Bay Hospital in a similar capacity. Conferences should be held now between Government and University Authorities concerned with Medical and Para-medical education as to the role of the new faculty in Montego Bay in the overall scheme rather than waiting until the hospital is opened and the paths have been established.

D.   Although the financial arrangements of University and Government services are not and should not be the concern of an "expatriate", based on my experience in similar situations I would suggest that the University pay the above individuals salaries and benefits and provide the same leave and study benefits as other faculty members. The Government should then reimburse the University in full for the cost of the individuals assigned to Government hospitals.

E.   *The method of deciding which direction individual departmental research takes is unknown to me at this time and it may well be that the Faculty of Medicine currently has a workable mechanism to handle this problem. I would suggest, if it is not already in effect, that a committee of research be established to review, advise and approve or disapprove protocols for research projects. This committee should obviously include knowledgeable members from both the preclinical, basic science and clinical disciplines. Such a committee would serve to encourage research, to ensure that individuals or departments do not embark upon projects that do not meet the needs of the University or the area, to set priorities for research within the financial limitations, to coordinate efforts and to, most importantly, advise and investigate sources of funding locally and internationally. I feel sure that unexplored sources of funds are available for many projects in the investigation of such things as the deliverance of health care and other community projects as well as in more esoteric fields.*
    Dick.

We thanked Dr Meltzer verbally and in writing for his ideas, which I put to a Heads of Department Advisory Committee; their reaction varied, but in general was positive; I summarised them as follows:

"To: Dr Richard Meltzer
From Mohan Ragbeer, Dean, Medical Faculty, UWI
Re: Your Memo, "Various thoughts

"Here is a point by point response to your timely and thoughtful memo:

A: Senior Lectureships are the level at which most non-UHWI leaders in subjects will be sought, for the reasons you gave; and to ensure that University goals of education, research and service are preserved in proper balance; they must have the experience and confidence to deal with Government people, notably in T&T, who might see our staff as "trespassing" on their authority, or violating their traditional right to set conditions under which, say, residents work in their units, assignments, time-tables etc. Our approach so far has been for our staff to share academic plans with their Government associates, explain goals and find appropriate ways to work together; we usually fit in with their service arrangements, modified by educational needs and to "protect" residents and their staff. Once trust is established, Government doctors usually defer fully to the UWI staffer. Colonial habits and suspicions linger on. In Barbados and Trinidad, we've seen clashes between UWI and Hospital staff over student assignments, scheduling and the mere hint of competition in private practice.

B: There was some difficulty with the VJH, but we settled with Dr Williams, having earlier done so with the heads of Medicine, Anaesthesia, Pathology, Radiology and Surgery. Indeed, a fine working relationship had existed between us and Government Departments of Pathology, Paediatrics, Medicine, including Chest Medicine, Surgery, and several clinics, all of which have had sessions for students and continue to hold joint teaching exercises and to accept students. We're developing the same in the Eastern Caribbean, including the smaller islands. The credit for this goes to many on both sides; we doubt that any real conflict will develop, not from a structural base, though one cannot predict personality clashes. The joint activities over the years have helped identify areas of need in Government units, for teaching: mainly personnel, seminar room(s), AV and other equipment etc.

C.   We had begun discussions with Jamaica's health officials on a teaching function for the Cornwall Regional Hospital, to which Dr Eldemire had agreed, when he was Minister. Electioneering delayed the planned visit. The new Government had advised us of delays in construction and outfitting. The SMO, Dr Monty Burke is a highly respected internist, and is well-known. He was one of the first medical graduates of the UCWI, favours the education role, and would welcome the added academic staff. We visited recently and saw the obstacles: the building is far from complete and structural changes have to be made to facilitate patient transfer, especially from ORs to the recovery room and wards, as cost-cutting has reduced the width of some corridors and rooms. Splendid German X-ray machines have been installed, but cannot fully rotate on their rails in a narrowed room. Equipment is mismatched: German, American, Swedish, British etc. The electricity supply is not compatible with several items of heavy European equipment, and there are voltage and load problems. We've had similar experiences at UHWI, especially when research granters stipulated buying their national equipment, which was incompatible with ours and we lost grants, though at times a grantor has allowed us our choice. Much remains to be remedied. A revisit is planned and we have submitted recommendations.

D.   The suggested way of sharing responsibility for salaries has already been agreed by the University Grants Committee (UGC). UWI will pay academic salaries for Faculty; the UHWI will pay its middle grade staff; and the Jamaican Government will pay their new residents at UHWI rates; we've recommended the same principle for the EC hospitals, at their rates of pay.

E.   We agree with the idea of a Research Committee as a "clearing-house" for research topics, for ethical assessment of proposals and of procedures, such as whole body radioactive scanning of children, as done for electrolytes at the Tropical Metabolism and Research Unit, (TMRU). Currently, research is problem-based, e.g. veno-occlusive disease, toxic hypoglycemia, neuropathy, cardiomyopathy, infectious diseases, nutrition, etc. The Committee could include fund-raising, local and foreign, as suggested by Mr. Leslie Ashenheim, a businessman on the Hospital Board, although this is a specialised and separate role. Research units exist at the TMRU, Epidemiological Research Unit, and the independent Caribbean Food and Nutrition Research Institute (PAHO). These have no formal nexus with departments but collaborate with them. They – and the Rippel Research Laboratories, now administered by the Pathology Department – could relate to the Faculty Board via the Committee.

Many thanks indeed for these thoughtful ideas. We will no doubt return to them in the coming months, as we continue to tap your expertise.   Mohan

The overall support from Dick Meltzer, John Schaaf, Bill Weaver, Bill Peters, Fred Hubbard (Administrators), and others, was constructive, although they did express frustrations with Government bureaucracy, which muted significantly when I reminded them of the slow grind of the US bureaucracy, which very few of them had experienced; we passed it off as "the nature of the government beast." Dr Meltzer and his wife, Amy, nurse consultant and program advisor, were extremely supportive and maintained their composure throughout their stay on the Project, even during the troubled period starting in 1972, and until re-assigned in 1973 to Headquarters duties in Washington, DC, then to Millwood, Virginia, when HOPE moved into a spacious and peaceful campus there, a gift of 650 acres from the Mellon family, providing it with a stately headquarters, and funds to launch its operations globally. It was also supported by the US government, by what means I was not aware.

HOPE contributed to the Faculty's audio-visual unit and to technical training in the Eastern Caribbean (EC), giving the organisation a wider base and higher profile, as outside Jamaica, it was only a name then. Their work in the EC was based on a survey of needs that I had started, discussed with others, and left the survey questionnaire with Dr Minott in 1975, hoping that the Faculty would get a grant from PAHO to complete it. This did not happen, but a PAHO official did contact me in Canada, late in 1975, *demanding* the data I had obtained, though partial, assuming that they were theirs! I politely corrected him, and informed Dr Acuña, the new Director, who had replaced Abe Horwitz.

Hearing of my status, and knowing me from PAFAMS, he offered a position in Washington, DC. I seriously thought of it; I could read Spanish easily, understood most Latin American accents, and with practice, could bring my conversation skills to an acceptable level. I was encouraged too by academics at Howard, where I had been a speaker in February 1975 at a colloquium on "Black" contributions to medical education. The HOPE "family" encouraged it, but in the end my lack of a government sponsor (Guyana supported mainly Blacks at that time) and family considerations superseded: the children were still "toughing it out." in all-white schools in Ontario; and my wife had declined New York, while family members were leaving DC for Canada.

Interestingly, I had been on the roof of the Howard Johnson Motor Lodge, on Virginia Avenue across from Watergate, taking pictures of the unusual curving lines of its façade, lit by streetlamps whose glow reflected off the white surface. I had noted a few lights flicker on and off in a mid-section of the building, which I would much later learn was the sixth floor site of the break-in that led to the impeachment of Richard Nixon, and that just below me that night, rooms 723 and 419 were occupied by spotters for the burglars.

Dick, as everyone called him, was the most agreeable of men. His wife, Amy, was a Paediatric Nursing specialist and had a supervisory role in the HOPE Foundation. Dick busied himself with helping me set the PGME stage; he sat in on relevant Committee meetings, where he reported directly on HOPE activities. He got along well with all staff and visited each department, especially the recalcitrant or hesitant ones. Dr. William B. Walsh, head of the Foundation—and incidentally a staunch Republican and advisor to President Nixon—had concluded in October 1971 an agreement with us re specialty education, as noted above. We had also planned to introduce a certificate program for Advanced Nursing Education and Administration, and departmental training of nurse practitioners in anaesthesia, public health, and obstetrics.

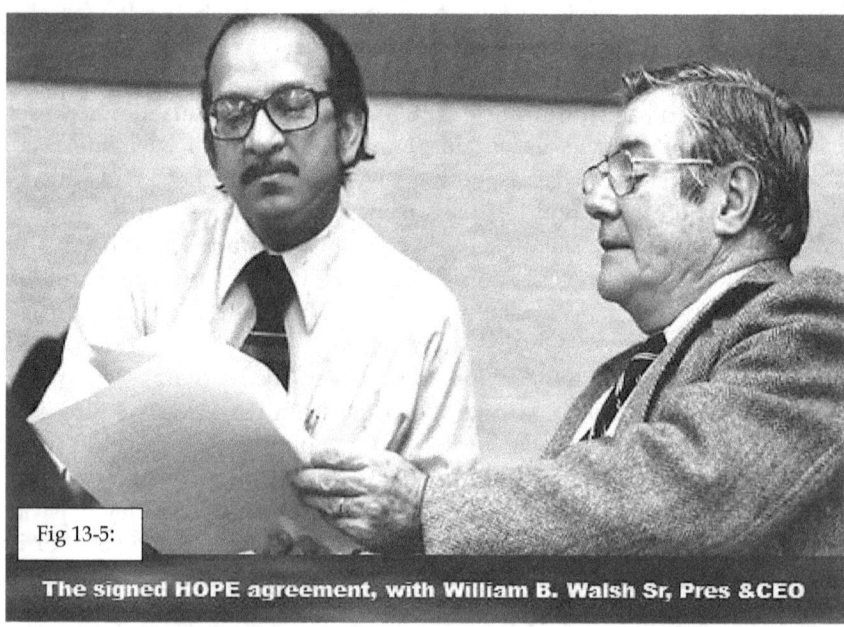

Fig 13-5:
The signed HOPE agreement, with William B. Walsh Sr, Pres &CEO

By this time, we were developing other projects, including Family Medicine and Community Medicine, also of interest to them. HOPE had also agreed to consider expanding on a public health initiative, and had assigned a staff member, Dr Morrow, to S&P Medicine. They had begun a plan with the Jamaican Government, and supported our concept of Community Medicine—a concept new to most US-based specialists, who tended towards narrower and topic-based activities, instead of the broader inclusive ideas our circumstances dictated. US medicine was affordable only in private practice by the rich. Most Americans could hardly relate to the Cali story of prevention of helminthiasis, even those who had seen it during the 1970 ACURI meeting in Cali (pp. 28, 34), and shown in clear detail by the ebullient surgeon Gabriel Velasquez Palau, then Dean of Medicine at Cali. We lacked the resources of the Americans, and were just a collection of unmet needs! We were thus interested in the new Departments of Community Medicine emerging in US schools, starting with the University of Kentucky. With PAHO's help, Kurt Deuschle, Professor of Community Medicine, Mount Sinai School of Medicine, came to advise on the subject. Billeted in the Department of Social and Preventive Medicine, he met department heads, studied our plans and visited our projects, spending much time with Prof Standard and his staff, on the department's work. He wrote a detailed, helpful report and praised S&P and its staff, and endorsed our CM plans.

I had taken Dick and his family on a Caribbean tour earlier that year and introduced him to bureaucrats and politicos at each stop. He had learned much, he told me later, about the small, underdeveloped societies that Americans did not know existed, except vaguely for their resources, or by some better read or travelled, through mechanisms like the Peace Corps and, I remarked, the CIA, citing Burnham as an example. He was apologetic about US strong-arming its interests, often at the expense of the poor and weak. The trip had enlightened him in many ways and he could better understand our attitudes and emphases, and, above all, fears of losing what little we had, of manpower and resources, to the ugly giant from the north. We had worked well together and he had been my sounding board and an astute critic. He understood our aims and my role, and was sure I would "do the right thing".

He had on several occasions been present at his desk when I received phone calls from US citizens in Florida and other eastern states, offering bribes of $5-10 thousand for admission of a son (it was nearly always a son), who was "exceptionally bright and friendly." My usual response was that I was glad he had a bright and friendly son, but we accepted no foreign students. Some, particularly the ones who gave Jewish names, got testy and one lost his temper and started shouting. I had held the phone towards Dick so that he could hear. Another said he was a friend of Mr. Ashenheim, the Jamaican capitalist, hoping that would cow me.

HOPE had heard from USAID about the merger of its grant with that of the Jamaican government to build the Postgraduate Building near my office. They had vouched for me, and I've always been grateful for that, and found out about this action when casually chatting with the USAID officer who had come to see the laying of the foundations of the joint PGME and Family Planning Building in 1975 (p. 214). When the Meltzer's left in 1973, we gave them a Huie painting, a water scene, one they had chosen.

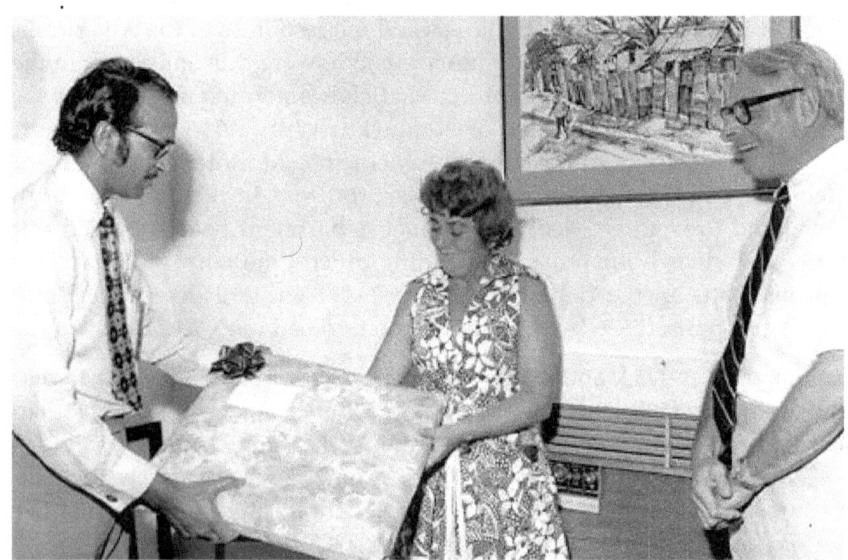

Fig 13-6: Farewell gift to the Meltzers of a painting by Jamaican artist Albert Huie

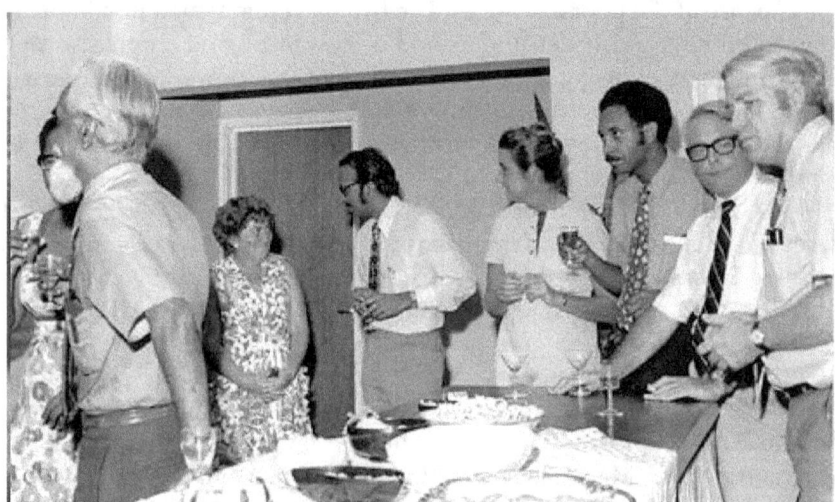

Fig 13-7: Saying Farewell to the Meltzers: D. Ashley (hidden), Sir Harry, Amy Meltzer, M. Ragbeer, HOPE Nursing Director, E. Walrond, R. Meltzer, A. Masson

PS: The HOPE agreement was renewed in April 1977 for three years, expanding into subspecialties e.g. neonatology, cardiology, neurology etc. It included supplying teachers for cytotechnology at the Community College at Papine, and teaching staff in Nursing and Medicine at the Cornwall Regional Hospital. The government signatories were the Minister, Hon Douglas Manley, brother of the PM, Dr Bill Walsh, and Dr Henry Clarke, the newly-appointed HOPE Director for Jamaica.

CHAPTER 14:
Faculty Expansion: IADB Special Committee

After my initial appointment, the first hurdle to be cleared was the work of the IADB Committee on expansion/duplication of the Faculty of medicine. Early In 1971, the University had concluded its assembly of the Committee, which had started meetings in Jamaica on May 24, 1971, and completed its work three months later. Bras had recommended me, in late 1970, for the position of Secretary, as I had already earned my stripes as Associate Dean, and was preparing briefs for the Committee on examinations reform, curriculum revision, and graduate programs. I was familiar with the issues of Faculty growth, and had good relations with departments and with Health Ministers, by inputs and contacts at CHMC meetings. I was involved in technical and other ancillary education (or "allied health" in newspeak) for the health services; and in Nursing education, and had collected data on Nursing Schools. I had written the Ministry to support recognition of Medical Technology and Radiography as professions, to be specifically licensed.

However, Dean Stuart appointed Walrond as secretary, surprising many, but defended as a necessary attempt to develop other talent in the Faculty. This was a good idea, but Bras — who had worked closely with him on the *Crotalaria* toxicity studies in the early days of the Faculty, and on many projects since — was bothered by the failure to consult him for one of the first acts of his Deanship. So were Eric Cruickshank and Stuart's friends, Annamunthodo and Grant.

The IADB Committee had started its work just before the selection of the Faculty's first full-time Dean. Clearly, I had to join the group, and the VC so informed the Chairman, Dr Tenney Spooner. Ken had approved, or perhaps chosen the Committee members, who, as expected, were sophisticated enough to welcome me without obvious reaction, but for Walrond's reserve — an improvement from earlier hostility — which would last the rest of our time as colleagues.

We mustered at the Mona Hotel, where the team stayed and held meetings and interviews, after visiting departments, and touring the campus and hospital. The entire group visited the two EC campuses, and in Barbados went to Codrington College, as it had been recommended to the University as a suitable site for expansion. At Mona Hotel, I formally presented the Faculty position, essentially the same facts that Ken Stuart had given earlier, inviting him, David Hoyte and Mickey Walrond to add comments and personal views. We clarified grey areas and provided specifics, following CHMC thinking, particularly on types of doctor aimed at, curriculum reform, primary care, community medicine, research, service loads and their impact on academics, staffing and space.

That summer was extremely busy for me, starting a deanship full-time, supervising reforms, and drafting many papers for IADB, the Faculty Board and University. I was anxious to ensure that my initial meeting of the Board go smoothly and had prepared a statement which I would pre-circulate, and I would read, *in toto*, if needed, to the Board, at its regular meeting on the fourth Friday of July *(Appendix 1.3 pp. 297-311).*

The team split into pairs, each visiting a group of islands, reviewing survey questionnaires that had been circulated to all member territories, requesting basic health, demographic, educational and economic data, and discussing them and any issue bearing on our mandate, including recruitment of staff, and working conditions. The questionnaire was almost identical to the one that COPMED had sent to CHMC members and that its Task Force had reviewed in Guyana in March; meetings with the other CHMC members would not occur until October, by which time Dr Robertson would join PAHO and be assigned to COPMED.

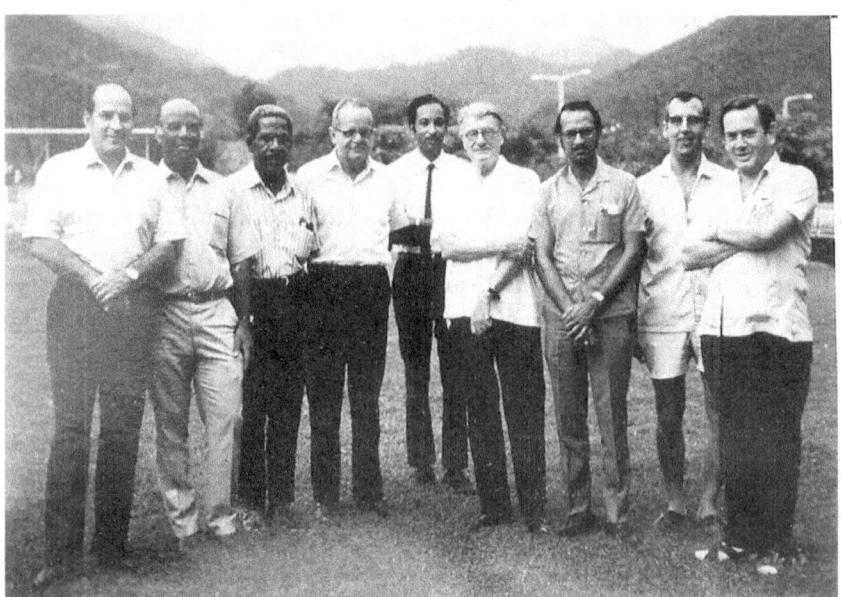

Fig 14-1: L-R: Gabriel Velasquez P., David Hoyte, Ken Stuart, John Bowers, Errol Walrond (Secretary), Tenney Spooner (Chair), Mohan Ragbeer, LG Whitby, Alexander Robertson

I was paired with the Chairman, Dr Spooner, and we drew Antigua, St Kitts/Nevis, British Virgin Islands and Belize, and started from the east, in Antigua, on August 3, 1971, ending in Belize 11 days later. I recalled experiences as a personnel officer twenty years earlier in the Colonial Medical Services, and found them quite helpful; (little had changed in organisation or methods in the island health departments). Dr Spooner was retired, and had been Dean of the London School of Hygiene and Tropical Medicine. He reminisced about his days as Dean, and felt that most young persons were reluctant to serve for fear it would interrupt their academic career, and asked if I had considered that, but didn't doubt that I could survive academically, with the widespread scarcities of leaders and other staff. I told him that it had occurred to me, but I had brushed it aside, wishing for the best, and knowing that we were on a good track, if not the best one for that time, in the Caribbean.

Political leaders were a troubling issue and I had already lived through tragedy in Guyana and its ongoing romance with Communism, now infecting many UWI students in the Social Sciences. I was worried about the possibility of a PNP victory in Jamaica, despite agreeing with some of their social philosophy. My concern had to do with the person of the leader and whether he was too far left and likely to harm Jamaica's sensitive economy, and the likelihood of losing talent, as Jamaicans were fickle under pressure, responding often by fleeing to the UK or USA.

And so we discussed WI politics and the books he had read on it, some before, but most in the months since agreeing to serve on the Committee. He had contacted the Ministry of Overseas Development (MOD, the renamed Colonial Office) and been given a reading list, mostly books or articles on the Caribbean by British authors. Instead, his Caribbean contacts had suggested a different booklist, including Eric Williams' *Capitalism and Slavery* and *History of the People of Trinidad and Tobago*; CLR James' *Minty Alley*; Alfred Mendes' *Pitch Lake*; Clinton Black's *History of Jamaica*; Alec Waugh's *Island in the Sun*; and Kamau Braithwaite's *Rights of Passage*. His earlier reading had included George Lamming's *In the Shadow of my Skin*; Vidia Naipaul's *A House for Mr. Biswas* and *Middle Passage*; and Edgar Mittelholzer's *Sylvia*, all prompted by West Indian students. Parry and Sherlock's *History of the West Indies* was one of the few from the MOD that time allowed him to finish, which he had to, when he found out that the authors were early UCWI faculty. Thus he had covered a fair sample of the literature on colonial conditions in the West Indies. We discussed some of these, particularly the dreadful history of British lords in Barbados and their cruel racism, and the limits of those books as a guide to the modern Caribbean. They were good sources of basic information on economy and social structures, where race, colour and culture remained enduring and divisive themes.

He was pleased with the quality of our inputs, and was impressed with the Faculty and the members he had met, but had misgivings about our economic future. I agreed we were at a tricky stage in development, and needed much dedicated work for progress, but the cooperation we had seen at CHMC, and at the UWI Council so far, was strong evidence for survival, provided that politicians concentrated on policy and stayed away from the details of daily administration, and from inducements.

Our experiences in the islands and in Belize emphasised the magnitude of the task, and how mindful of minutiae the UWI must be. In Antigua, I found that the CMO was Dr C. Bailey, who had served in BG as an Assistant Health officer at the time I was a personnel officer in the Department, and his surprise at seeing me in this unexpected role, matched mine. I had met the Minister, Hon B. Peters, as a student at UCWI in the late fifties; he was trying to invigorate a somnolent service and remove the aged hospital from the risky vicinity of the airport, which was becoming busier as tourism increased.

The island had close to 70,000 people. The hospital had 200 beds, with six specialists and seven medical officers, was recognised for 4 internes, but only two were then funded. There were six places for district medical officers, one unfilled, as was the post of MOH. Two of the junior doctors, the Jarvises, were fresh UWI graduates ('67, and '69). Sadly, they matched the criticism I had heard at CHMC in Bermuda, that the UWI graduate was poorly attuned to the realities of work in the Caribbean, beyond the University Hospital. Both were above average students, but failed to understand and adapt to the scarcities of an island that had, like all the others, suffered from chronic under-provision; they focussed on this, and the likelihood of leaving at the end of the year for North America, even though the CMO would support them for a UWI graduate degree. She became a paediatrician in Canada, and he a radiologist, which, ironically, were specialties that Antigua needed, matching its need for paramedical staff.

St Kitts and Nevis were two mountain tops, the former a perfect cone, the other more irregular. They had shared in the conflicts among Europeans of centuries past, and now stood, abandoned economically, but bristling with the ingrained hostilities of their colonial upbringing and history. Simply put, they hated each other, amply expressed in the annual cricket match, which was taking place at the time of our visit, and for which a half-day holiday had been declared. I don't think that St Kitts has ever forgiven Nevis for supplying a wife for Admiral Nelson, nor has Nevis allowed St Kitts to forget that. The population of St Kitts was 34,227, and Nevis 11,230, having declined by 2000 and 4000 respectively, in the past two years! By 1971, seven nationals had graduated from the UCWI/UWI Medical Faculty. The JN France hospital was only 4 years old, but showed problems of poor construction, with warping wood and leaking roofs, creating an urgent and an unwelcome expense. Another travesty was the Central Supply service, which was capable of serving a hospital many times its size, and sat idle with a porter in charge!

Montserrat is mountainous, in fact harbouring a volcano, the Soufrière Hills. It is a pleasant land with a healthy population of about 12,000, and a hospital of 58 beds in the capital, Plymouth, with ageing structures and inadequate facilities.[27] It will be replaced, plans originally calling for 90 beds, later reduced to 70, but we suggested from the information given that 60 would be generous, and that they should avoid the St Kitts' white elephant. The point was welcomed by the CMO, and later the Minister. There were six doctors, and were assisted in filling posts by incentives. They lacked ancillary staff and usually relied on help for special studies; they, like all of the countries visited, could offer topics for research to elective students, pre-or post-graduate.

BVI were a collection of about 30 islands, with a total population of 10,000 or so, two–thirds in Tortola, the rest in Virgin Gorda and Anegada, with a sprinkling in the others. The capital, Road Town, had a hospital of 35 active care and 10 "infirmary" (chronic care) beds, shortly to be replaced by one of 50 beds. There were four physicians, nine nurses, one midwife and 19 nurse-assistants, trained or in training locally to serve in district clinics. Two added physicians were in private practice. We told them our mission and asked their opinion on PGME. We talked mainly of "refresher" courses (CME) and referrals, and agreed with Dr Thomas, one of the two doctors from the UK, who encouraged us to enjoy the balm that BVI offered. (He had written a book, *Dew Line Doctor*, about his experiences working for years above the Arctic Circle, as a doctor for the USA's *Distant Early Warning* project at a testy time in the early Cold War.) Staff morale was high, despite appalling shortages. Dr Thomas conducted clinics in district bars "because they had furniture" and Mrs. O'Neal, a nurse-midwife, with twenty years' experience, thought nothing of "searching out" articles to outfit her new MCH clinic in Road Town. Their refreshing initiative starkly contrasted with the lack of it in the two disappointing young UWI graduates in Antigua.

Dr Spooner and I shared a hotel room at the old fort which had been bought by a member of the DuPont family *("I'm Elizabeth")* who had just completed a divorce and was recuperating by converting the 8-room bastion on a prominent hillside, into a luxury hotel, and adding 20 rooms beside and behind it. She had a good stock of whisky, cognac, wines and other liquor and was intimate with many, much to Dr Spooner's delight, satisfying his penchant for a scotch before dinner, wine with, and brandy

---

[27]Plymouth and the southern half of the island, including the Bramble Airport on the Atlantic coast, was destroyed by a series of eruptions, starting in July 1995, of the Soufrière Hills volcano, dormant for centuries. The population fled to Britain and the damaged area remains a monitored exclusion zone; current population is about 5,000. Montserrat's Health Minister, Hon. Mary Tuitt, was a loyal supporter of our efforts in the early years of PGME.

after. He taught me much about these drinks, and introduced me to previously unknown brands of single malt whisky, while Elizabeth treated us one evening to a fine dinner and a rare Bordeaux, describing in detail the small chateau that she had visited, which produced it. We were the first professionals to visit, and she had us sign a VIP book.

Belize (British Honduras until June 1, 1973), population 120,000, was at the time in a pathetic state. The capital had been moved from Belize city (pop. 40,000) inland to a new town, Belmopan, built as a stimulus for settlement of the interior, to dissuade Guatemala from its claim to the country. It had 2,000 people, 80% being civil servants. The country's medical staff included 12 specialists, one of whom, the paediatrician, an Iranian, was currently in jail in Iran! The staff included a part-time ophthalmologist; 16 medical officers—2 Indian and 14 Mexican—and 3 internship positions, all of which were then vacant. Nine Belizeans had graduated as doctors from UWI by 1971; one, the anaesthetist, was back home, but he too would be gone by the end of the decade. The disincentives were common to the Caribbean: the North American magnet, unstable local politics, and, as one doctor said, "widespread nepotism, preferment and feather-bedding."

It is doubtful that this group of countries could benefit much from an expansion of medical education unless increased numbers forced graduates into internships and GMO postings, so far overlooked, or deemed inferior to the prime locations. Yet we were convinced that— with improved supervision, prior priming by a more socially oriented curriculum, and frank discussion of politics as a disincentive—as more and more UWI graduates became leaders of society, they would respond to the challenges and fill elective rotations in these countries.

The Committee's final report supported the position of the Faculty members and added substantial details (*Appendix 2, p. 311 for Summary, and UWI CP14 for full Report*). It endorsed the recommendations of the Curriculum and PGME Committees, both of which I had chaired.

Main Recommendations *(bracketed page numbers refer to Report, CP14)*

These were presented under two headings:

1.   Those requiring little additional financing – largely matters for Faculty and Academic Boards and for Senate.
    (a)   Reorganisation of Faculty administration (79-82)
    (b)   Development of a curriculum geared more to the needs of the area (44-53);

(c)   Promotion of closer collaboration between Governments and the University, and thereby between Health Ministries and the Faculty of Medicine (98-101);

(d)   Review of admissions procedures and attempt to identify applicants more motivated to practice medicine in the Caribbean (69-71)

(e)   Improvement of teaching skills in teaching staff by suitable training programs (228-43);

(f)   Establishment of Inter-faculty Committees to study needs for multi-disciplinary programs in health care (p. 40, Ch. 14, 93-97);

(g)   Urge Governments to re-organise health services and improve conditions of service (66).

2.   Those requiring substantial new funding

Remedying deficiencies in current educational and research programs.

(a)*   Establishment of programs in Postgraduate Medical Education, to train specialist professionals in demand throughout the area (72-75).

(b)*   Establishment of a division of Community Medicine based at the Mona campus with responsibility for developing programs for the entire Caribbean, and with a major role in the curriculum (Ch. 4: 54-63).

(c)*   Expansion of undergraduate teaching in Barbados and in Trinidad and Tobago (p. 30), phased (p. 31) in such a way that first, teaching in all three clinical years is developed in both hospitals, then followed by establishment of preclinical teaching in Trinidad and Tobago. This expansion should aim at a final intake of 110 students and could take place within eight years of the time that funds are allocated for this purpose. Simultaneously, postgraduate training should be developed in these centres. The planning mechanism is described in pp. 38-41, siting on pp. 35-37, and phasing spelled out on p. 105.

(d)   The Mona campus preclinical facilities should be expanded sufficiently to accommodate 20 dental students, and facilities sought either in the area or elsewhere for their clinical training.

(e)   Advanced Nursing training should be expanded to accommodate 60 students annually at the Mona Campus.

(f)   Communication between Campuses needs to be facilitated by various methods, including increased staff interchanges for short periods.   (* *Simultaneous activities/developments*)

"Costing was done by the offices of PVC Finance, Aston Preston, and Bursar, Hugh Holness, to indicate the scale of operations (see below). The Committee commented on, but did not critically examine financial arrangements between Governments and University, feeling that this was properly the exercise of another body, even though it was in its remit."

<u>"Conclusion of Report</u>

"*It is emphasised that investments in medical education must be seen not as a contribution to higher education but as investments in overall health services development and in social advancement of the peoples of the Caribbean*" (pp. 103, 104 and 108).

In brief, the estimates were as follows:

1. The EC medical expansion, by 110 students: ($J=$US1.20)
    (i)   Recurrent Expenditures, first 7 years total $J 10,180,524;
    (ii) Capital (Buildings, Furnishings and Equipment $J 7,140,000;
          This included provision for two years at Mona,
          handling an intake of 220 in pre-clinical departments

2. Community Medicine
    (i)   Recurrent Expenditures (approximate annual)   J$ 190,000
    (ii) Capital   J$ 761,680

The Committee had cautioned, echoing the Action Group of 1970:

"*The Medical Faculty of the University of the West Indies (UWI) has reached a crossroads. There are two courses open to it, either to become a modern, progressive institution, or to be stagnant, losing all of the opportunities that have accrued during the twenty-two years of the Faculty's existence.*

"*As we describe and define in this Report, we can only recommend the first course. The judgements may seem harsh, but they are based on our concern for the future of the Faculty and for the health of the West Indian people. To re-establish the momentum of the Faculty, and the kinds of program that are essential to its viability, will require full support from the University and from the contributing territories.*

"* It will also require continued acceptance by the academic staff of the goal of making this Faculty an institution of scholarship and of Commonwealth Caribbean leadership, and complete dedication to these goals.*"

With help from colleagues, Faculty officers and Board members, we presented and defended the recommendations, which agreed with our own. The principles, observations and comments were not seriously challenged, except for the estimates of number of new admissions, which was tentative, and my personal estimates, based on field experience, the island economies and available manpower, was nearer 150, adding 50-60 foreign applicants at an approximate cost of $10,000 p.a. to yield enough to fund up to 50% of the expansion. This last idea (see p. 120) was sceptically received, for idiosyncratic reasons, mainly its "mercenary" nature, obviously entrepreneurial, a concept that was almost anathema in a "socialist" University, despite its grave need of finances; it was unwilling to gain it by enterprise, as if that would defile the purity of academia. Yet it readily sought grants and bequests, which ultimately derived from taxes or profits. Perhaps the climate and basis for thinking of the University as earning its way might arrive one day, and we will begin to patent our finds and market what we know, to protect them from the inevitable American corporate heist of our resources. Already American botanists and pharmacologists have been combing tropical areas for medicinal lore and plants. Why have we not done what any American university might have instantly done with *Crotalaria fulva*, *Momordica charantia* (cerasee, bitter melon), *Blighia sapida* (ackee) and so on? Mentioning these in Chicago and New York, I was invariably asked, "Who owns the patent on these?" Of course, these genera of plants are not unique to Jamaica, but extracts may be patentable, as Dr Walsh of HOPE had casually suggested; the Faculty of Agriculture could advise, suggesting a suitable area of inter-faculty cooperation.

The readiness of the Faculty to take on major new developments was questioned, as by the time the discussions had reached the JCCS (Joint Committee of Council and Senate), and then Senate and Council, the staffing difficulties had gotten worse. But we persisted.

The major question was the projected costs, particularly the proposal to move the Mona preclinical facilities to or near the Hospital, which we defended as probably the most important change and well worth the investment for future development of coordinated or integrated medical education. The existing buildings could be used to accommodate pure science departments, as would be needed for increased admissions.

Learning efficiency was improved by co-ordinating or integrating pre-clinical studies of systems e.g. anatomy and physiology of any organ or viscus, as one could procure models of these, since cadaver organs were not usually suitable. Autopsies offered fresh organs for integrated study of anatomy, physiology and disease processes, and could supply preserved and mounted organs for anatomical study. But purists in these specialties were not enthusiastic then. The UWI was not unique in this reaction, and tended to do what was already accepted. But we should have shed our habit of copying the more prestigious, and try methods that our materials could support to satisfy learning aims.

"We would also prefer to have the Division of Community Medicine nearer to the Hospital for more efficient use of investigative services, sharing of equipment, joint research, easier communications and liaisons between staff, and transfers of patients between the levels of care." The Division would be more interdisciplinary than the University has so far had, in that it would require inputs from other technical Faculties e.g. Agriculture and Engineering, and others like Education, Management, Law and the Social

Sciences.[28] Currently, a simple matter like parking prevented many clinical staff from taking part in pre-clinical teaching! The majority of preclinical staff favoured the relocation of basic science units; a few scientist members preferred being near to the science departments, even though none could point to any collaborative projects, while ample opportunity existed for sharing with clinical colleagues.

The expansion plan called initially for duplication of clinical studies in the two EC campuses, with a gradual development there of basic sciences. Appropriate teaching space should be included in any plan for new hospitals, such as the Mount Hope Maternity complex, which we proposed could be expanded to a full teaching hospital now, to save on site preparation, to meet government needs, and supply current and anticipated beds for the expanded EC scheme. The site had ample room for the preclinical facilities that would be needed later. The argument was supported by academics and the MOH, but Williams kept silent.

We received little in the 1972-75 triennium for structures for the MB,BS program, having hoped for a new clinical lecture theatre of 200 to enable us to discontinue the use of a laboratory designed for 80 at practical classes, which we had been forced to use, over the previous three years, to accommodate the yearly throughput of 110 students. The original request was denied in 1969. Another major issue was the fall in bed:student ratio; we proposed to use facilities outside of Mona, including clinics and health centres, as we developed the program in Community Medicine.

The disappointment was aggravated by the societal deterioration that had changed the prospects for peaceful growth at Mona, negating Government plans for improvements in education and health services, e.g. free education to University level, upgrading of hospitals, and training of 600-1000 auxiliaries for distribution to clinics island-wide. The first major campus disruption and violence came with the senseless strike of the subordinate staff, led by Trevor Munroe, a Mona sociologist, followed by an escalating series of violent break-ins and assaults against householders, as thugs overflowed their Kingston dens and invaded the suburbs, reaching the campus, even in daytime, and assaulting several female staff, including two from HOPE, recently arrived, who had read more tourist literature than the notes of caution from us, and from HOPE, and had left their front doors wide open (see also Ch. 22).

---

[28] I had to give examples of these to the JCCS, where someone queried, "Why Social Sciences?" I instinctively replied that "Medicine is a social science, in lower case!" A hoot of laughter, probably derisive, greeted this. "Does that mean I can become a medical lecturer, and get a better deal?" a sociologist asked. "It means you can teach sociology or demographics, but not medicine, I'm afraid!"

CHAPTER 15
Post CHMC III; Jamaica approves

The next four years were crucial to the survival and success of the DM and MS programs, by securing quite early Jamaica's commitment to them, in word and money (JLP budget, 1971), and to follow-up on an assessment of needs. We had to convert gestures of support from all island Ministries to tangible support such as Jamaica's, and to confirm working relationships and agreements with HOPE and Guyana. I had few expectations from Guyana, as by 1970, the shape of Burnham's dictatorship was quite clear, and he had begun to impose his infallibility by reshuffling his cabinet frequently, thus preventing any one from getting to know "too much." Minister Talbot had been attracted to serve by the wave of *nègritude* crossing the Caribbean, but realising what Burnham's service meant, she felt used, and promptly left to join her husband, who had become his ambassador to Washington, DC.

Dr. Eldemire and Finance Minister Seaga called a meeting soon after our return to Jamaica — which PVC Preston attended. "I remember you; you're the guy with the knife!" Seaga said, enigmatically, while the others questioned with their eyebrows. He grilled us on each line of the budget, from every angle of Jamaica's commitment, before he finally and unsmilingly, but with his famous tic, gave his assent. He enquired into our ability to proceed with Jamaica alone, if the two major Eastern Caribbean partners, Trinidad and Barbados, were to decline. I was frank with him about the former, citing student protests at St Augustine, Black power rallies, army officers revolt, the simultaneous resignation of Chancellor Princess Alice and Pro-Chancellor Eric Williams; but we felt that Barbados would support us as long as Errol Barrow was Prime Minister. I informed him of COPMED, of which Dr Wilson was a member, and the Task Force it had set up to assess needs for specialists in as many member countries of CHMC as wished it, rather like the survey of non-campus territories in 1969-70 re their expectations of UWI, at a time when students were seething re the exclusion of Clive Thomas. Ironically, our survey would start in Guyana in March.

I had known Edward Seaga for 20 years, having met him when we were both second-year medical students at the UCWI. He quit before the second term to conduct social studies in central Kingston, attached to the UCWI's *Institute for Social and Economic Research* (ISER), and later joined the Jamaica Labour Party, under Alexander Bustamante. He became Minister of Finance and Planning in 1968, that terrible year that saw the

US murders of Martin L King and Robert Kennedy, anti-war (Vietnam) protests, and the brutal Police actions against young people of the US Youths International Party (YIP, hence *Yippies*) and Pro-Peace movement that converged on Chicago in August at the Democratic National Convention, when it seemed that Eugene McCarthy, the pro-peace candidate, would lose the Democratic nomination for President. The Jamaican protests had targetted decisions of the JLP (PM Shearer) re social scientists Rodney and Thomas. Seaga's fiscal policies had placed Jamaica on a triple "A" rating with Standard and Poor, and its treasury had about US$170 million in reserve. Seaga was a cautious and strict manager. In the time I've known him, I have rarely seen him smile. But he did, when I mentioned the position of Eric Williams and Errol Barrow in such frank terms, not quite politically correct, but he appreciated that.

In 1970, he had created a revolving loan fund for university students which had added to his social reputation, already solid due to work that was transforming the desperate "back o' wall" slums of the Kingston downtown. These were described as the worst slums in the West Indies, had a precarious water supply, the most primitive sanitary facilities, and stood next door to the largest cemetery in the country. Led by his efforts, "back o' wall" developed into Tivoli Gardens, a relatively neat and peaceful settlement of low-income persons with an ambition to rise in society; children were regular attenders at a new school, and several amenities had been provided, including a playing field. Tivoli Gardens was a good example of urban renewal, in creating a stabilised and serviced low-income neighbourhood in the inner city.[29]

Seaga's marriage in 1965 to Marie (Mitzi) Constantine, Miss Jamaica, was widely acclaimed (3 children followed). So was his knowledge of Jamaican folk music and his promotion of *ska* and *reggae* — the two song and dance art forms, for which Jamaica became known — and of the key artistes, including Bob Marley. Few knew of his promotion and audio recording enterprise, which he later sold to Jamaican band impresario, Byron Lee, nor did many realise how much effort he had put into promoting things Jamaican and the business by that name.

I was careful that I had addressed him formally and not slipped into the familiar, sometimes dismissive way we had done when he was in medical school, largely because his sociological rants were more a

---

[29]But Tivoli didn't quite maintain its stability and peace as the nation had hoped; it fell prey to the late 20th century drug trade, whose local principals used it as a staging base in Kingston for traffic to the USA; it sheltered a drug lord named Coke, who was wanted in the USA, which had asked for his extradition. In 2010, a battle ensued between the Jamaica Defence Force and Police on one side, and Coke's heavily-armed gang on the other, resulting in 74 casualties, mostly civilian, most uninvolved with drugs or weapons, and used as shields by the bandits.

distraction than a help with the volume of new information in Anatomy and Physiology that we had to master. He was, by virtue of his name, in my Anatomy dissection group, along with Otto Sylvester, who kidded him interminably, and David Thwaites. Seaga remembered me as the guy who teased out the tiniest nerve from surrounding fat when most students had difficulty distinguishing the tissues that formalin had made almost homogeneous, at least in colour. At the meeting, he was very supportive and gave me the nod, "I see you haven't lost your dissecting skill. *It's fantastic* that you've brought this project so far in three years; UWI usually takes nine! " He smiled faintly and shook my hand.

Dr. Eldemire was quite delighted, as was Jeff Wilson and PVC Preston, who finally understood the "knife" remark, and his references from time to time to "anatomical precision." PVC Preston explained why he himself had smiled and nodded at the mention of "three years," telling us how at a UWI Council meeting, Seaga had complained that it took the University nine years to get a project from the planning stage to implementation; *"any shorter time would be welcomed as a miracle!"*

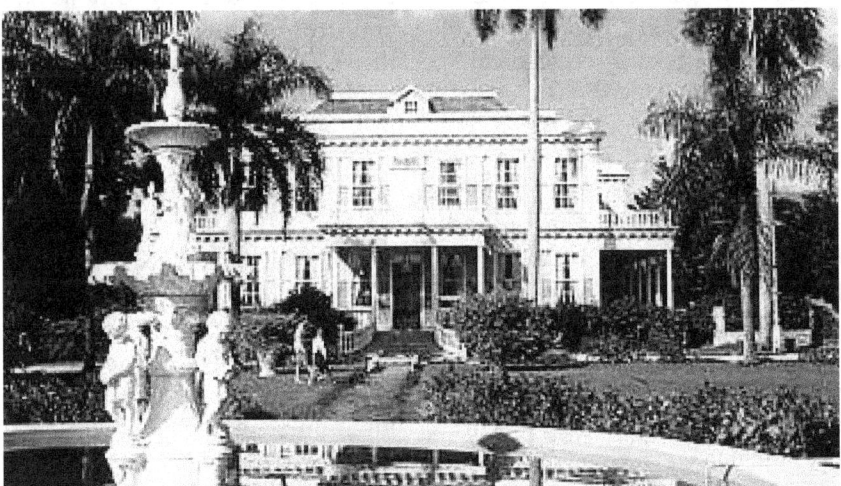

Fig 15-1: *Devon House, built by Jamaica's first mulatto millionaire, was saved by Edward Seaga in 1965, when he was Minister of Finance and Culture, from demolition by developers. It became the HQ of Things Jamaican, and now under a Government Trust, is a favoured local and tourist destination for food, baked goods, ice cream and arts and crafts The other two properties nearby that constituted "millionaires' circle" have yielded to the developer's relentless axe. See text for more on Seaga.*

The JLP lost the elections in February 1972, before the budget was approved. It thus fell to the PNP under PM Michael Manley, Finance Minister David Coore, and Health Minister Ken McNeill to review and endorse, or change it. The survival of our plan rested largely on the solidity of Dr Wilson's standing in the Ministry and the esteem in which he was held there, as much as on confidence in the PS, Mr. T. O. Goldson.

NATIONAL ACCOUNTS DATA 1969 – 73 (J$ million)

	1969	1970	1971	1972	1973
Gross National Product (at market price)	916.0	1014.9	1120.2	1242.8	1487.7
Gross Domestic Product (at factor cost)	868.9	974.8	1093.5	1207.2	1437.7
National Income (at factor cost)	749.3	840.4	932.8	1034.4	1241.8
Per Capita National Income	406.4	449.6	490.7	535.4	631.0

Table 15-1: *The Jamaica economy at the end of Seaga's Ministry, 1969-72. Historically, it was heavily agricultural, like most of the Caribbean, and depended on sugar production and bananas. Bauxite mining began in the early fifties and tourism was vigorously promoted in the sixties, along with a growing construction and light manufacturing industries, which together contributed more than agriculture to the GDP.* Source: *Jamaica Tourist Board*

While we waited during the transition, Ministry officers asked us for a review and a confirmation of the styling of the specialty degrees. I recalled the debates, often heated that this had sparked. Suggestions had ranged from MD (Med., Paed., etc.), and, from one EC source, MSMS ("Member of Society of Medical Specialists)," an entity as yet unknown, and unlikely, as it invited confusion with MS for Surgery, which the surgeons had accepted after wrenching debates. The "Fellowship in General Medicine" (F. Gen. Med., WI,) – for the non-surgical groups – was vigorously defended by the leaders of our Medicine Departments in Jamaica and the Eastern Caribbean, while FGO (WI) for Obstetrics and Gynaecology – as FOG would not do, and F.Obst/Gyn unwieldy – and FGS (WI) for Surgery were discarded.

The titles "Fellow (*F...*) or Specialist (*Spec....*) or Professional Certificate in... (*PC...*)", had their proponents, but were unwieldy; they were linked with the notion of creating specialty societies or colleges to carry out PGME for UWI degrees, but groups in the EC, especially Barbados, liked the idea of royal assent to the designation. (A start to this was actually made by some medical and surgical specialists, but "Associations" – other than the *"Caribbean Association for Public Health,"* and *"Association of Physicians of Jamaica"* by UWI's KL Stuart and KGH's John Hall – would not be formed until 1972).

The final choices of *DM* and *MS* was simple: they created no real acronymic horrors, were preferred to *M. Med.* and *M. Surg.*, and resolved a confusion that *"MD"* would create with the existing MD by thesis. Dr Wilson was cool to the term "MS," a reaction I shared. (He must have been pleased, as I was, when it was dropped years later for the more uniform DM, which had been my initial suggestion to clear the fog of names proposed and debated by the specialty groups.)

CHAPTER 16:
Second Term: the dreamer, an interlude

In early December 1971, I had met Professor Cruickshank at a football field, where his daughter and mine were playing. We sat in the bleachers, almost alone, and he discussed our position, and how pleased he was that I had sailed so easily into the administration and how former detractors had grudgingly changed their attitudes. "But then," he said, "you had come in as an Arts student, and had experience working in the administration of the Colonial Medical Services."

He reminisced a bit. He had come to Mona twenty-two years ago, in 1950, and in 1951 had made a tour of the islands and BG (as Guyana was then), with Chemistry Professor Hassall and Vice-Principal Sherlock, as noted above, to interview applicants for College admission. They had used that opportunity to meet heads of Government, Civil Service chiefs in Education, Health and a few related departments—nearly all Britons, like himself—and the up-and-coming local politicians, likely to lead their islands to independence in the next decade or so, all being well. Suitable details had been added, like the growing attraction of Communism to these politicians. He didn't pay much attention to them, but remembered Norman Manley, Jamaica and Jagan, BG, the latter flagged as an upstart, a communist, "probable trouble; watch carefully." He and Hassall had received letters of introduction to the Governors, and had met them.

He recalled our meeting, astonishingly—even as I did, because of his blue eyes, the first ones I had seen—he, because of the strange admixture of poetry, Spanish, cricket, and geology in Sherlock's questioning, which had made him pay attention. He had forgotten me, until I applied for transfer to pre-med classes, and he thought me eccentric, but later paid attention, on rumours of "Feng's vengeance," and he vividly recalled his questioning me re ciliary reflexes and doubting my account of the location, connections and function of the Edinger-Westfall nucleus, only to confirm that I was right. What an amazing recall, I thought.

I had always felt a bond between us; at each encounter I had been in some kind of need, or awkward position, and he had seemed helpful even when critical, as when I had not signed up for the Allenbury Prize in Clinical Medicine, since I was in a surgical clerkship then, and wanted to do Surgery anyway. He had, with gentle authority, commanded my entry, with less than a week to go; needless to say, I was not prepared, but did quite well until stumped on electrolyte imbalance in a range of diseases; curiously, the questioner on this series was Ken Stuart, then a newly-promoted Senior Lecturer in Medicine.

He was very disappointed that I had chosen Surgery over Medicine, but felt quite pleased to hear from Dr Brahmam of Guyana—whom he had twice welcomed in the department, first in 1960 for a month, then as a visitor in 1970, when he attended a conference at CFNI—of my "saviour role" in the handling of my mother's illness, which would have been fatal, but for my unusual use of bacterial culture, contrary to standard laboratory practice. "That should have been published," he said, "it ranks in the best traditions of medicine! You should still do it."

He wasn't surprised to hear of it, and recalled meeting Capt. Nobbs and the ecstasy he felt on "being rescued" by three past students. What an incredible tale that was, all the coincidences it entailed. Karma, I had told him; pure karma. He knew a little about Hinduism, from his jail mates in Singapore during WWII. He still counted it among the stories that continued to move him, and yet, few appreciated it, in the same way he and I did. He also recalled how pleased his first wife, Anne, had been with the care I had given her when she was Professor Stewart's patient for a few days. I remembered my hesitation on being called to see her, and telling her I'll get the professor. To which she had said, "Never mind him; you're here; do what you must to get me out of this!" Later, I found Professors Stewart and Cruickshank in the former's office, and reported. "When a woman's ill, it doesn't matter that she's a professor's wife!" Stewart advised as Cruickshank nodded, and offered me tea.

He talked of other reactions to the changes. There was, he sensed, a general appreciation of the support, fair dealing and consistency of the Dean's office and the easy access to the now organised materials, a thing he had always wanted, but never could push, as his colleagues, mostly British and "firmly wedded to their personal fiefs, "were perhaps too proud to reveal their lack of experience with organised administration! I told him of my many sessions on "Organisation and Methods" in BG, ten years earlier, at which he raised his eyebrows.

He was pleased that I had developed an easy relationship with HOPE, and had had long talks with Dick Meltzer, who "is very impressed and would have left, were Ken to become full-time! Bill Walsh was sceptical at first, but quickly appreciated the straight talk and had no reservations signing the agreement." Cruickshank knew of the animosity of some people, but had seen the change in Mavis Anderson, Paul Feng and Louis Grant, who had all made positive comments. Ken Stuart had been disappointed, perhaps hurt, and resentful for a few months but "he has praised your dedication, and commented on your lack of ill-feeling for any of the people whose censure had come so quickly, before a fair appraisal." Now, he doubted whether anyone could say that the past months could have been "more productive or more amazing for the positive and speedy reforms." His praise brought a lump to my throat.

He could not understand Brooks' enmity, nor Alleyne's "coolness" except as loyalty to a fellow Barbadian, but he had judged him above that. Feng had surprised him with his turnaround to support me; he had been anxious about how I would handle him, being aware of the "bad blood" that had existed between us, having probed my "failure" in Pharmacology, when my clinical use of that knowledge was "among the best in the class." He had gotten stories informally from several of my colleagues, and had spoken to Feng in one of his turns as Dean. I told him my side of the affair and that it had rankled; but it amused him to hear details of my chat with Feng after taking office. He had been the founding Dean and had had a hand in recruiting most of the staff, including Feng. He had found out early of Feng's "school-masterish" tendencies and had done what he could to curb them, joking that he could easily see Feng wielding a bamboo cane!

"Some older staff don't like residents or students on Faculty Board, as you've heard at Heads meetings; will you change that?" he asked.

"I don't think so; they're observers so far. I trusted students to respond to reason and to address problems constructively. They came in with preconceptions, acquired in our high schools, especially the science students, through didacticism, rote learning and limited exposure to disciplines that broadened our understanding of life around us; I saw this at QC. We put students on the Board so that they could share in debate, contribute to decisions, and explain them to their fellows. If we ignore their opinion, we'll get a fuming Prendergast, not a Hickling."

He laughed, knowing them, but warned that I might have an uphill task with curricular changes; he remained optimistic, yet concerned about the impact of political policies on our work, with Manley hawking social redress for Seaga's tight-fistedness, and the unrest had increased.

He talked about other events and gave advice re "watch your back," and talked briefly about his retirement, "I have to go soon; I'm 57, and don't want to stop working. I didn't want to leave, and delayed looking for a UK job. I have been looking at one in Glasgow and feel much easier leaving, now that I've had the pleasure to see the school produce its first Dean, and a full-time one at that. You know, I was about your age when I started, and quite raw except for my war experiences; those gave me insights into man's behaviour under stress, and deficiency diseases.

"I've always wondered when we would come to this; a full-time Dean was long overdue. I've looked around and wondered who it would be; that the first would be a young man, instead of some hoary-headed wise fellow, quite pleases me. The challenges call for youth and talent; you have both; I'll keep on giving you as much as you ask, or more if I can offer that; but from what I've seen, I'm thankful to have pressed you into service the way I did; I feared it might have affected your academic advancement."

"I was warned about that, but I don't want to leave the Caribbean; I was glad to spend time on exams and curriculum, and to get PGME going, and soon, we'll have Community Medicine and Family Medicine; I knew from my visit to Chicago that much research was required into educational methodology, organisation, management, and the like, and doubted that the university will recognise that work for promotion. Two-thirds of the Faculty agree with me; I have to persuade the others and the University that what I do is worth it.[30] Innovation is threatening to some; I see them at each Board meeting: Ellington, Feng, Picou, Manchester, Alleyne, Persaud, and silent others, even students. In Trinidad, I had to face Bartholomew, and a few others; and Dos Santos, White and Haynes in Barbados. The EC is mostly with me now, or at least willing to listen."

"I'm glad Harold Forde supports you; he's quite outspoken, which others may not appreciate. A word of caution, if I may." I nodded.

"In spite of its youth, this University is quite traditional. To start in new directions, if you want to produce individuals to solve local medical problems, you have to convince it to listen to the Ministries. You know, when they started the first university in Saudi Arabia about ten years ago, mostly with British staff, they declared that the aim of the university *was to train professionals in all fields to solve national problems, within an Islamic context,* and to be aware of advances elsewhere. But UWI did not; it is very British still, and wishes to refrain from close ties with politics, except for funding. Older heads here are wary of academic sociologists, who have connections with groups off-campus, e.g. unions; they say that extramural work prevents contributions to intramural activities, like research and serving on committees. University processes remain highly structured, and often inhibit professional and promotional interests of staff. To train properly for these islands, as you well know, you'll have to include human behaviour, environment, and social determinants of disease; you'll have to work in community clinics, health centres, and other facilities that emphasise primary and secondary care; proceed as you summarised in that document I put to the Board last year. It deserves wide circulation; send it to WIMJ. I've sent it[31] to all Faculty, especially new ones, and to Meltzer. Ken agrees with it."

---

[30] I found out later that having neglected "pure science" for this work, I could not easily get back there, and my educational initiatives were not credited at McMaster, Canada, when I was forced to leave Jamaica, six years later, and ended up there, by chance; they did not understand the realities of poverty, and like Chicago, lived in plenty, so give little credit for achievements in education in underprivileged circumstances, but they happily exploited the experience and guidance I had to offer students, and copied my evaluation methods.

[31] *Aspects of Medical Education in a developing area, the West Indies,* FMP 35a, 1970.

As I thanked him; he added, "One of my biggest worries is that community health centres and district hospitals are so poorly staffed and equipped that most medical students have not seen the like, and may be put off unless introduced to them early by the most experienced or understanding faculty supervisors. We don't have many. And we're not likely to attract any with so many new schools developing everywhere. And it doesn't help that you'll soon lose the steady hand of Gerrit Bras.

"That might have increased the time you need to get the papers that A&P Committee counts for advancement. I had agonised about that, and am glad they recognised your other work. So, here you are, a professor now, and well-deserved. My great fear is that the politics of these lovely islands might turn sour, and destroy all the work you and others are trying to do. Above all, you must be careful. I think you were right to reform the Board, and to give students a voice. But don't expect any thanks from colleagues; and bear in mind always what satirists say of the stages of a project: *rivals, at first, reject your plan; ignore your successes, until established; then seize your work; reject you, and claim all credit! I can see it coming, but don't let it stop you.* Still, I hope I'm wrong, and that your colleagues appreciate what you've done."

He remained a source of good advice and practical help, served on committees, reviewed curricular and Community Medicine drafts, and generally endorsed my proposals for the residencies, and to have the UK MRCP done at Mona. He read my papers on medical education and agreed that *WIMJ* should publish letters, and articles on education. He had raised the matter at a meeting of the editorial board, and blamed himself for not pressing the issue of journal reform; he remained "amazed at how conservative and old world some are, including the new editor, who felt that those things are frills that would lower the scientific standard of the journal!" He agreed with me that "*WIMJ* had a far way to go to become widely recognised." Major journals in English, like the *Lancet, BMJ, New England Journal* and others, all have sections for letters, and even non-medical anecdotes, reports and commentary.

I told him that several years ago, I had corresponded with Eugene Garfield, the founder of the *Institute for Scientific Information (ISI)* and publisher of *Current Contents (CC)*, and had asked him why he had not included WIMJ among CC listings. His reply was that he was building the base for the citations, and additions were constantly made according to criteria. WIMJ was one of several under consideration and would be included when it met their criteria, or if CC expanded enough, to include it in another category. Ron Irvine was editor, and I had told him of this exchange, but as he was leaving, he agreed to pass it on to his successor.

Before he could do more at UWI, he accepted the Postgraduate Studies Deanship at Glasgow University—"a sinecure," he said to me,

"I'll have nothing much to do, not like here." We discussed the dilemma of our tiny states wishing nationhood and craving full services, which most would never have, unless their beauty could attract retiring specialists who were benevolent and wealthy. I asked him whether he had considered that; the mountains of St Lucia or St Vincent were a great attraction, though a bit different in ecology from Scotland, but friendly in climate and people. He had laughed at the idea, not from derision, but from recall of the number of times he had entertained the idea, but given it up for "something more practical and affordable."

I missed him, his friendship, his objectivity and trustworthiness. I have never ceased to wonder how many stories he carried in his head of the many students he has had, if he remembered them all as clearly as the ones he had revealed. His place at meeting tables was never really filled for me. I would hear from him in 1974, when he wrote about my 1973 paper for the Commonwealth Foundation. I reproduce below the start of the Paper, and his letter, as some have said that I made this up!

Years later, I met him in Jamaica at an Alumnus Association meeting when his memory had begun to fade, and his wife (the second) would dutifully supply him with cues. But he had become more convivial, and laughed easily, his eyes twinkling and his smile as impish as it had been before. We had corresponded on the idea of training the entire health care team, under the lead of the proposed Division of Community Medicine, with linkages to clinical and other specialties, which Professor David Stewart would have welcomed. The idea was supported also by Jamaica and the EC countries; my later study of the Ontario Health Insurance Plan would suggest a way Government could fund and operate their health care vision. Events unfortunately aborted that plan.

THE ROLE OF NEW UNIVERSITIES IN THE TRAINING OF MEDICAL ANCILLARIES

PAPER BY PROFESSOR M. S. RAGBEER

Introduction

The Medical Ancillary

The dictionaries which I have consulted for the meaning of 'ancillary' give words such as 'subservient', 'subordinate', 'aiding', 'auxiliary', thus indicating that the medical ancillary should be someone who has a *support* role in the health services, and could include all such personnel whether in health services planning, organization, management, clinical practice, community medicine, public health or in any other health discipline. The ancillary is not then by this definition a 'prime mover' in any particular situation, though he may be the only trained person in a particular role at a particular place at a particular time.

There are at least two approaches to defining who belongs to the group of medical ancillary. The first is to look at the tasks performed by a particular team of health workers, noting the skills required for the leadership position in that team and designating all other roles within it as subservient to that of

Fig 16-1: Title page and first paragraph of Commonwealth Foundation paper, 1974

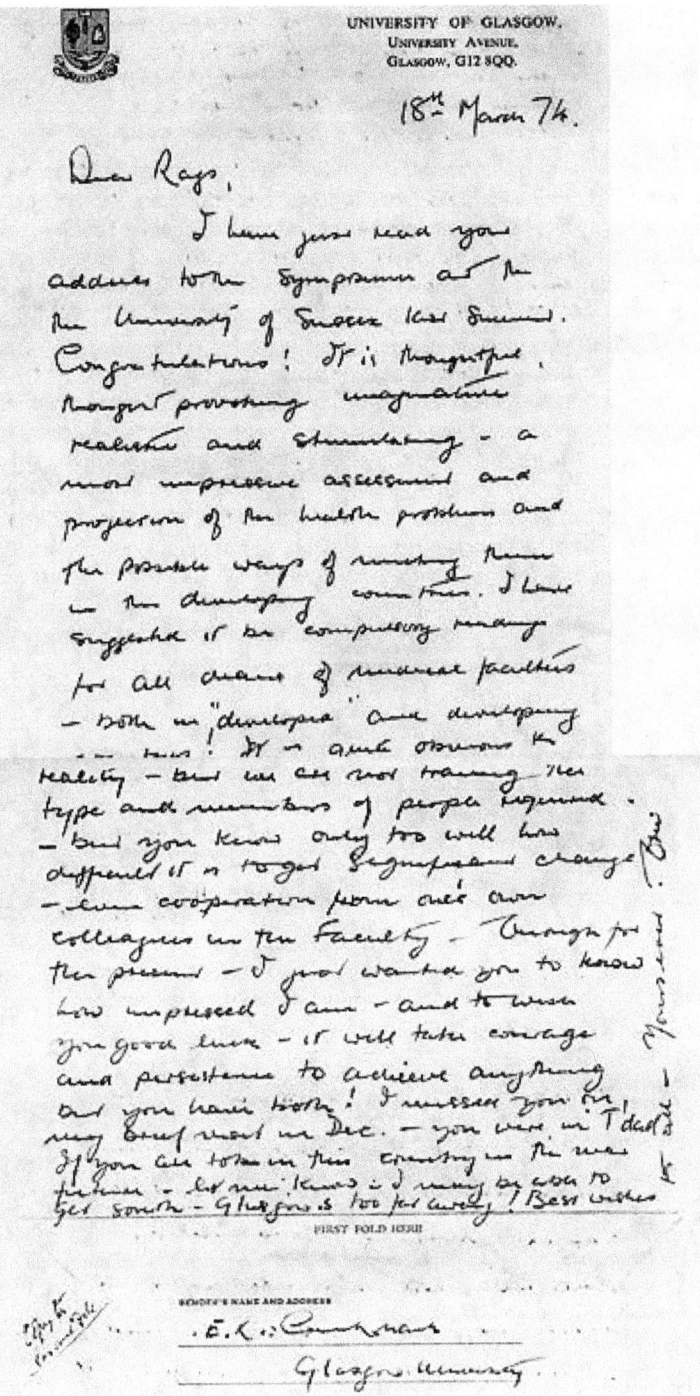

Fig 16-2: Letter from Professor EK Cruickshank on Commonwealth Paper, transcribed below

Fig 16-3: The letter in typescript:

University of Glasgow,
University Avenue,
Glasgow, G12 8QQ
18th March,74

Dear Rags,

"I have just read your address to the symposium at the University of Sussex last summer. Congratulations! It is thoughtful, thought-provoking, imaginative, realistic and stimulating, a most impressive assessment and projection of the health problems and the possible ways of meeting them in the developing countries. I have suggested it be compulsory reading for all deans of medical facilities – both in "developed" and developing countries! It is quite obvious to me after two years back in this country that our medical education is obsolete in meeting the projected needs of the health services of this country in the new generation. We are producing insufficient doctors – and you know reality – but we are not training the type and numbers of people required – but you know only too well how difficult it is to get significant change – even cooperation from one's own colleagues in the Faculty – enough for the present – I just wanted you to know how impressed I am, and to wish you good luck. It will take courage and persistence to achieve anything but you have both! I missed you on my brief visit in December – you were in Trinidad. If you are to be in this country in the near future, let me know – I may be able to get south – Glasgow is too far away! Best wishes (to all.
Yours ever,)

E.K. Cruickshank
Glasgow University

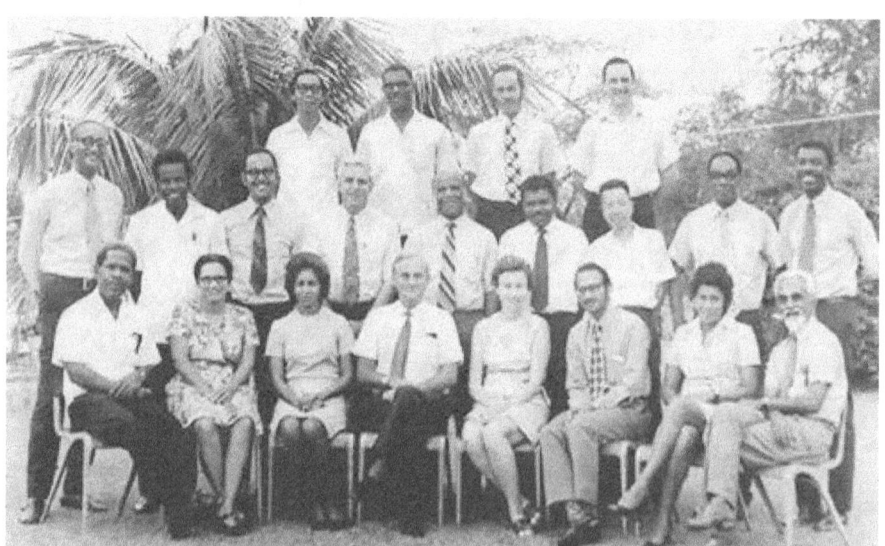

Fig 16-4: On the departure of Eric Cruickshank, 1972, head of Medicine for 23 years, and first Dean: Front: KL Stuart, D. Jung*, Mavis Anderson, Eric Cruickshank,, A. Costa*, M. Ragbeer, P. Morrison,* and H. Annamunthodo.

Middle: M. Beaubrun, G. Alleyne, S. Brooks, A. Masson, D. Hoyte, E. Ward, P. Feng, L. Grant, C. Bartholomew.

Back: D. Picou, K. Standard, C. Miller, K. Manchester   (*indicates Dean's office staff)

CHAPTER 17
CHMC IV, 1972

The 1972 meeting of the Caribbean Health Ministers' Conference was held in Georgetown (CHMC IV). The findings of the Task Force, and recommendations of COPMED were discussed and accepted, and the Task Force thanked. In the discussion, members were surprised at the number of foreigners in Guyana health services, and so many vacancies for doctors, despite 650 UWI graduates so far, including 85 Guyanese (Table 17-2).What was worse, of 579 graduates to 1970, only 54% were in Caribbean. But while 19% of those graduating between 1954 and 1962 had left the region, a huge 51% of graduates from 1963 to 1970 had done so! The majority left for the USA and Canada, and a trickle to the UK. The location of some was not known at the time of our survey; they were likely in North America, or scattered in industry, NGOs and other services globally. Table17-1 shows known location of graduates.

Year of Graduation	No. of Grads	In WI + Guyana	At UWI	In Canada	In USA	In UK	Others
1954	13	8	3	1			1 in Nigeria
1955	16	11	3	1		1	
1956	14	10	2	1		1	
1957	23	19	4				
1958	16	10	5			1	
1959	21	16	2	?2			1 dec.
1960	28	19	4				5N/K
1961	29	17	3	2	3	3?	1 USSR
1962	32	16	2	6	1		7 N/K
1963	32	18	1	8	3	1	1 N/K
1964	35	12	6	8	7	2	
1965	36	20	3	5	4	2	2 Australia
1966	36	17	2	11	4	1	1 Ghana
1967	61	24	4	22	8	2	1 BVI
1968	47	26	4	9	5	2	1 N/K
1969	66	34	10	10	11	1	
1970	74	35	4++	4++	2++		29N/K
Total	579	312	62	90+	50 +	17	50 T269

Table 17-1: Survey of UWI medical graduates (1954 – 1970)

Some Task Force members elaborated on conditions, limitations and expectations, and contributed to the Final Resolution. Ministers accepted a certain loss of graduates, as from any University or country, but a deprived region, like the Caribbean, could ill afford such high losses. They gave helpful criticism and guidance although most from the LDCs were unable to contribute much financially. Among these, strong support came from Dr. Len Comissiong of Grenada, and his various Ministers of Health (the last in my time was Hon. D. Sylvester), whom he carried like protégés; Mrs. Mary Tuitt, Montserrat; St. Lucia's Ministers Hunter Francois and JA Bousquet, and the Permanent Secretary, F. Louisy; Antigua's Lester Bird, and later BA Peters, and the venerable Dr CES Bailey, as mentioned earlier, whom I had known, two decades past, in BG; LB Rogers of Belize and his CMO, Dr Lennox Pike, a 1961 UCWI graduate; FC Bryant of St Kitts; H L Christian, Minister, and D. Shillingford, CMO of Dominica; and Quinton Edness, Bermuda. (Minister B. O. Ebanks, Cayman Islands; Mrs. ME McDonald, Bahamas; and C. Maduro and HP Watson, BVI would get copies and add support in 1974, when CHMC met in Nassau, Bahamas.)

Period.	Tot.	B'd	BG	Ja	TT	Gr	Bah	St V	St L	Dom	B'ze	Ant	St K	US	Others.*
1954-71	650	43	85	310	100	27	10	12	5	14	9	8	5	3	18*+
1954-67	**380**	**27**	**69**	**170**	**49**	**16**	**1**	**7**	**3**	**11**	**4**	**5**	**4**	**2**	**12*+**

Notes:
1. * Other contributing territories (BVI, Montserrat, Cayman Is, Anguilla) plus Bermuda, Canada, Ceylon, Curacao, Ghana, Uganda, UK, and Unknown
2. + Unallocated to country: First row 9; second row 2
3. **Bold** = Graduates with London degrees
4. First row shows totals to date; second shows London University graduates

Table 17-2: UWI Medical Graduates by Country 1954-1971

Others, including PAHO, and its country representative, Dr S. Khanna, were particularly encouraging. Dentists Trevor Mair (Jamaica), and Ivan Ashtine (Trinidad &Tobago) had listened with interest to our suggestions re a school in Trinidad for dentists, and in Jamaica for dental technicians. The USA, UK Ministry of Overseas Development, Surinam, and Venezuela were supportive observers. In later years, others would come from Cuba—which became a major influence in Guyana, and helped to train its physicians. But in Jamaica, as an ally of PM Michael Manley, Cuba was seen as a threat to the integrity of the UWI.[32] The meeting approved the COPMED recommendations, resolution 5/72 stating the major findings of the Task Force, in its preamble. We were hoping to start that year, once the new PNP government in Jamaica had

---

[32] Jamaica had improved its GDP in the eight years of the JLP government, under PMs Alex Bustamante, Donald Sangster and Hugh Shearer, at some sacrifice of social programs, by pushing developments in bauxite, tourism and light industry, and had a healthy foreign exchange reserve, under Finance Minister Edward Seaga. Manley, in a campaign marred by violence, made huge promises of salvation, won the government in 1972, and promoted social programs, including education and health. But mounting violence stalled the economy, exiled professionals, slowed recruitment, curricular reform and UWI plans, e.g. for Family Medicine, which we had hoped Jamaica would fund, and Barbados follow.

given its approval, which the JLP had done in 1971, but delayed implementation due to national elections. Further discussions of the brain drain stressed the lack of PGME as one of the main causes; but COPMED had identified poor conditions of service — notably the long and tiresome recruitment process followed by the islands' Public Service Commissions, a colonial hang-over long due for change — plus the lack of middle grade posts for recent graduates; and others covered in the Report. CHMC resolved (# 6/72) to urge members to adopt measures to reduce negative conditions that fostered a "brain drain."

UWI Medical Graduates by Country 1954-1978

Period.	Tot.	B'd	Gy	Ja	TT	Gr	Bah	St V	St L	Dom	B'ze	Ant	St K	US	Oth *
1954-78	1383	84	122	598	320	43	37	26	23	25	21	20	14	10	31*+
1954-75	1045	70	107	457	222	36	27	22	17	17	15	12	8	7	26*+
1954-71	650	43	85	310	100	27	10	12	5	14	9	8	5	3	18*+
1954-67	**380**	**27**	**69**	**170**	**49**	**16**	**1**	**7**	**3**	**11**	**4**	**5**	**4**	**2**	**12***

Notes:

1.* Other contributing territories (BVI, Montserrat, Cayman Is, Anguilla) plus Bermuda, Canada, Ceylon, Curacao, Ghana, Uganda, UK, and Unknown
2. + Country not stated : First row 9; second row 2; third row 1.
3. Bold = Graduates with London degrees
4. B'd = Barbados; Gy = Guyana; Ja = Jamaica; B'ze = Belize

Table 17-3 UWI Graduates by country, 1954-78

Guyana, represented this time by the Hon Shirley Field-Ridley, a UCWI Arts graduate, my contemporary, now Minister of Education — acting also for Health — was severely critical of the UWI and its "biased admissions policy" against Guyana, and failure to cooperate with UG, or involve it in the PGME plan; Dr Chin, her advisor, who had served constructively on the Task Force in Guyana, surprisingly agreed. The first was easily explained, the second a laughable *faux pas* that Dr Chin's briefing had failed to prevent. The Minister insisted on her version.

Re the first, Guyana had arranged with the UWI to accept each year five medical students, who would be admitted according to standard criteria explained by Dean Eric Cruickshank, and repeated by me in 1969 and Prof Hoyte in 1971, as Chairs of the Admissions Committee. In 1970, Dean Stuart had reminded CHMC delegates in Bermuda that the UWI had dropped its pre-medical year, since the same was available more cheaply in colleges in most territories, producing a surplus of qualified applicants. The exceptions were the smallest Antilles, without advanced level high schools, but the total need was low enough that placements could be made in Barbados or Trinidad colleges by prior agreement.

The Guyanese students did not have that problem. Theirs was a matter of too few funded places, and final choice by academic ranking, which upset Burnham's whims. He appealed by telephone to my *"nationalism and good name (sic) here;"* and when that did not change our decision, he decided to tackle Vice Chancellor Roy Marshall, *"a fellow lawyer who will understand"* (as he said when he called back after seeing our unchanged list). The VC reminded him that the Committee was acting under the authority of the Senate and Academic Board, and that as VC he could not, or would not interfere except for breaches, of which there was no suggestion or evidence. Burnham rebutted vainly about *"special ideological position of medics"* in his plans for Guyana, and key to his desire to build a teaching hospital near to the UG campus. He had instructed his ministers to raise the issue at each meeting of the CHMC, starting in Bermuda, and each time was reminded that CHMC had no authority in the matter. Nevertheless, Sylvia Talbot, when Minister, had persisted in Bermuda, much to the irritation of the Chair, the Hon Quinton Edness, who repeated the lack of jurisdiction. The rebuffed Minister pouted, but later apologised, on learning how uninformed her stance was, and poor her briefing (p. 89).

With Guyana as CHMC host in 1972, the President raised the matter as an agenda item under "matters arising." His disregard for relevance had again embarrassed the senior members of the Conference, but Burnham cared little, if at all, for this kind of sensitivity, and simply bullied on! Perhaps this explained why his team was so antagonistic to the UWI and to me, in particular, because they knew that I would not, nor had not in the past, bowed to aggression. Back in Jamaica, I had reluctantly agreed to the VC's compromise of allowing them to select the final five from a slate of 10, listed in order of merit, which Professor Hoyte, Chair of the Admissions Committee, had presented to Guyana.

I have noted elsewhere Burnham's denial of a place to the top-rated student, an Indian, the younger Drepaul, who, ironically, learned soon after that he had won the Guyana scholarship, and *must* be supported at the University of his choice *anywhere*. He chose Britain, and was lost to Guyana, since he had no obligation to return service, as the chosen five had. Burnham's actions and those of his officials were received coolly by the Conference, barring Trinidad and a few of the Antilles, which followed her. Eric Williams had chosen the matter to criticise the UWI, and as a motive for an independent medical school in Trinidad.

I again had to remind the Minister that UG did not have a Medical Faculty, that we at UHWI, and I personally, had contributed to the start of technical training at UG, which Professor Drayton could affirm. I had up-dated the VC of UG, Dr Dennis Irvine, with our PGME plans, and invited his input. He had regretted lack of funds for "any effort in medical education", and doubted whether Burnham's plans included a Medical Faculty. Burnham grumbled a lot, but seemed deaf on the point of costs. Existing faculties were stagnant, politically pressed, and staff disgruntled; personality clashes were frequent, and it appeared that Drayton, a Jagan acolyte, had left because of that. I ended by hoping that the Minister would consider these things in her comments re the UWI.

My "youth" distracted many of the seasoned men and women at CHMC IV. It had not been an issue before, when I was clearly an aide to Professors Stuart and Bras, two of the heavyweights of the Faculty. In 1971, in Bermuda, they had to leave the meeting early, announcing that I would handle questions, with Prof. Standard; Mary Sievewright would deal with Nursing. Again, my age had come up, but pleasantly. I had grown up being the youngest in class, from high school, where I had to cope with boys and girls 1-4 years older—a huge age spread when you're ten—and I had learned not to think of it as a barrier. It was stated a few times, but needed no defence. Soon, the patronising stance that some members had adopted, changed as I dealt honestly with the issues raised and said "I don't know" when I didn't, and showed respect for minority opinions and the position of smaller states, even the hostile ones.

Dr Comissiong of Grenada, one of the longest-serving CMOs, probed issues consistently, for which some had called him an obstructionist, but we benefitted from his practical knowledge and common sense, which were crucial in finding solutions to the dilemma of small islands in need of special services, but in too small a volume to occupy a specialist in each field. He was one of the first to advocate group sharing of specialists, and closer inter-island cooperation. Hunter Francois of St Lucia, a keen intellect and a valued resource at CHMC meetings, agreed; so did Carlyle Burton and James Williams of Barbados, the latter, Director of the Queen Elizabeth Hospital in Bridgetown, a friend and former cricket team-mate at UCWI. Some of the best discussions at CHMC IV were with these and a few others in the new Pegasus Hotel.

Guyana had lost much, socially and medically, from what it was in 1962 (for details, see *The Indelible Red Stain*, Bibliography). Burnham wished to increase the number of medical students but shied away from discussing funding. He made all decisions, but social services and health care were low priorities. He used the country's resources capriciously for his own needs, e.g. wasting money to fetch dermatologist Dr Norma Shim from Jamaica in a private plane to treat his benign skin rash, and reward her and husband with a 2-week tour of Guyana. The Georgetown Hospital was severely neglected or abandoned and lacked the simplest supplies; most of its capable staff had left or were planning to leave. There were 106 established specialist posts; 85 Guyanese had graduated from

UWI since 1954; most had stayed away, or come and gone. Morale was below the nadir. The needs had increased for all levels of specialisation due to widespread recruitment failure to replace lost staff. They had spread the net wider and most of those obtained were supplied by Cuba — by special arrangement for education and service — and China: 34 in 1972. The laboratory, formerly one of the best in the Caribbean, had faded to mediocrity and unreliability, in just six years post-independence.

Guyana had taken the incredible stance that the UWI was unfriendly and uncooperative with their University. UG had no medical faculty, but a Faculty of Technology, whose School of Medical Technology had opened with a curriculum designed in 1965 at UHWI by Mr. Gool Khan, chief technology educator at UHWI, and myself, then Chair of the Technology Training Committee, gratis, to assist Dr Drayton, a Guianese, head of UG's Technology program. To allow him to study our design in practice, we had to get him a special entry permit into Jamaica, as he had been expelled from the country, thirteen years earlier, as a communist.

The COPMED team that had visited Guyana in early 1971 included Dr Rabin Sahoy, a Guyanese surgeon at UWI, and Dr Deanna Ashley, a Jamaican interne (1970 graduate). At COPMED meetings, and at CHMC, we had become inured to pejorative comments from the Guyana delegates on all UWI proposals. This was comical, especially as their Senior Medical Officer, Dr. Frank Williams, had asked my help in designing a curriculum for training "ancillaries;" this would become their offer to the Texan *Medex Program* a few years later.

Their attitude mystified several delegates, including James Williams — who knew Walter Chin at UCWI — and Hunter Francois, who chose an opportunity during debate on a topic unrelated to the UWI, to comment on "Guyanese hospitality" and the courtesy of the staff servicing the meeting; he reminded delegates to expect varied people and varied positions on issues and proposals, and direct any barbs at those, not on the persons presenting them. *"Lawyers defend criminals, as the Honourable President of this Republic has done numerous times, but he doesn't have to commit a crime to do that. Nor I. It's our profession."* Burnham, who was present at the time, smiled wryly.

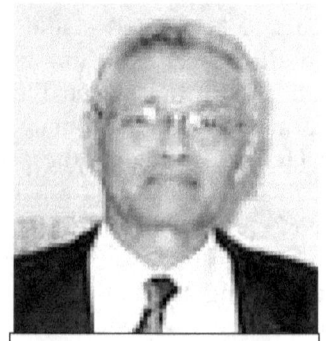

Fig 17-1 Dr Walter Chin, Medical Supt, G H, Guyana

Despite their sour behaviour, we expanded our contribution to other fields, to later Ministers Singh and Harper, the latter a Washington DC dentist and Burnham's brother-in-law, a well-meaning man, with whom I would meet several times during his brief time as Minister of Health in

1974 and at CHMC VI in Nassau; he had realised his unfitness for, and frustrations with the job, and soon left. He was followed by Hamilton Green, Field-Ridley's husband, during whose tenure she died, rather mysteriously. Guyana's descent into despair, medical and social degradation is now legend. (Details are given in my 1993-4 consultancy report for the IADB *Georgetown Ambulatory Care* project. *See Bibliography*). Privately, almost in apology, Walter warned me, "Watch where you go and what you do, especially at night." I was fairly secure, staying in the guarded townhouse of a prominent businessman, about my age and appearance, and driving one of his cars, which was well known about town. I took the precaution of travelling to meetings in the courtesy bus, with other delegates, most of whom were Blacks or Coloureds. I never took any extraordinary precautions, despite the alert. But I should have paid more attention to Dr Khanna of PAHO, if for no other reason than protection from the female attention I had received, which, in my naïveté at that time, I had thought flattering. But, on reflection, and discussion with friends in close touch with Guyana politics, the consensus reached was that it might have been contrived to keep me in sight at all times, and perhaps engineer an accident to get even. This was Burnham's style. The conference lasted five days and I spent the weekend with family.

My chaperone had rarely left my side that week and had played the part of Mata Hari well; I had shared with her little information of any value to her bosses. Besides, my secrets were not the type that harmed governments materially — a little embarrassment perhaps — but Burnham had brushed aside enough of those not to care. I had driven her from Georgetown to a gas station on Vlissingen Road, Kitty, on the eastern edge of town, to get her car, telling her that I would head up the East Coast road to visit family. She drove off in a green Ford compact while I travelled behind her on Duncan Street, going east. At Sheriff St., she turned south, tooted her horn, to which I responded and headed north.

On a whim, I turned off on a side street just before reaching the railway embankment and headed to the nearby home of a family friend whom I had not had the time so far to visit, and would spend an hour there if he were home. I had just made a right turn off the side street heading towards his house, and parked serendipitously just out of direct sight of Sherriff St about fifty yards away, and walking back to the house, saw her car driven north at high speed by a black man, with her sitting behind him, and two other black men in the car. He braked hard to negotiate the embankment which jolted them up and sideways but they settled down and sped on towards the main road. About two hours later, I came on a scene at Turkeyen where a red car was in the trench beside the road, half submerged, its driver side smashed in. A crowd had gathered and some were leaving as Police had arrived, an hour late. All traffic had stopped in response to police signals. Leaning out of the window, I hailed a young man and asked what had happened.

"Is a madman bounce de cyar from behind, push 'e cross de road and dat pick-up hit 'e, spin 'e round and de grey cyar hit 'e dis side and dump 'e in de trench." His hand motions elegantly showed the events.

"Did he get hurt?"

"'e lucky! 'e bang up some and look like he lose 'e senses for a while, but 'e revive by the time people stop and help; he lucky the trench shallah. Dey tek 'im to hospital."

"Anybody you know, somebody from here?"

"No; is an Indian man, like you, same kind cyar; eh, eh, look at dat!"

"What kind o' car hit him?"

"Me din' see 'im; me jus' come; is over an hour now; dat man who dey wid the policeman say is a green cyar, wid three black man and a darkie Indian gyul; they di' movin' fast; 'e say de cyar gat no licence."

I was left wondering to what purpose the elaborate plot. If it were an attempt to settle the score on student choices for the Guyana five — which had excluded two names on his personal list, both unqualified and thus implying favouritism or nepotism — then it was surely overkill. But I learned on returning home that one had become his son-in-law and later got a Cuban MD. Did Burnham feel so miffed that he would over-react in such a deadly way?

By prior arrangement, Ken Standard and I travelled to Suriname, after CHMC IV, to conduct a seminar on training programs for different levels of Health manpower. We spent three fruitful days and made valuable contacts, encouraging the Minister to join CHMC, which PAHO also supported. At that time, the University of Suriname conducted clinical training for students who had completed basic sciences in Holland. It was planning a full program, and was glad to contact and probably link with UWI, a tropical school in their own region, instead of the alternative of Indonesia! They liked our curricular model of team training of all cadres of staff (pp. 54-8), and supported the notion of training specialists in the environment of their final practice. They liked the idea of supplementing standard curricula with additional elements to facilitate a broader professional function, such as overseeing public health needs of a community, always in need by poorer countries. It was cheaper to give specialists the help of ancillaries to allow wider coverage of health and sickness issues. Surinam considered the advantages of closer association, and in time joined CARICOM and CAREC.

From September 25th to 29th, 1972, I attended the 4th World Medical Association Conference in Copenhagen, on the theme, *Educating Tomorrow's Doctors,* an echo of our efforts at the UWI to define the aim and directions of medical education. Among the six aims was *"to develop in the participants a desire to institute changes in medical education based on (health) needs."* Fifty-three background papers from all corners of the globe were circulated beforehand. Each of four plenary themes was introduced by two speakers and then discussed in workshops, followed by a panel to answer questions. I met Prof. (later Lord) Max Rosenheim, my 1957 final MB external examiner in Medicine, and Alex Robertson, who had served on the UWI IADB committee and on COPMED in Guyana. Lord Max gave the first of two addresses on the theme, *"Identifying Determinants of Medical Education,"* the second by Antonio Ordonez-Plaja, whom I had met in Colombia; I was rapporteur for the panel discussion of the topic, which was published in the book *Educating Tomorrow's Doctors,* Joseph F. La Banca Co, NY, USA, 1973.

(I told Lord Max who I was; he naturally didn't remember me, but did recall that one candidate at the oral had asked to sit at a distance and wear a mask, because of a bad cold! He was curious to know how I had become the Dean "so swiftly," and to learn what had become of Prof Cruickshank's *"other* favourite" students. That was a surprise.)

The other topics were *"Instituting change in medical education"* by John Bryant, USA, on *Obstacles to change,* and Diazo Ushiba, Japan, on *Implementing change.* The third was *"Evaluating medical education"* by J T Foster, USA, who critiqued *the current approach to evaluation;* and Socrates Litsios, WHO, discussing *A new strategy for evaluation;* the fourth was *"A look to the future,"* by Moshe Prywes. A summary of reports followed.

A recurrent issue was the need for *Community Medicine* and for poorer countries to avoid having two doctors, one for personal care, and another for communities. It was stressed that medical education must address health care needs of a whole people, while preserving academic aims, quality and quantity of care, and promoting health. It must foster teamwork, including the use of students, sociologists, and the myriad ancillaries that can be trained for the care of communities.

I met Dean Pathik of the Medical Faculty of the University of the South Pacific (USP), based in Suva, Fiji, and described our PGME and Community Medicine plans, and the training of many levels of health workers (p. 56). He liked them; USP resembled us in financing, structure, and the quest for self-sufficiency in health manpower. Specialty Colleges in Australia were pressing him to buy their British style specialisation.

I sent him papers on our training plans; he responded by inviting me and "another Faculty member," to Suva, and was in process of arranging a PGME workshop of "third world educators" when an anti-Indian coup in Fiji deposed most officials, including his administration. (A decade later, USP would join with specialty colleges in Australia, and from what I've heard since, has regretted the move, for reasons of high cost.)

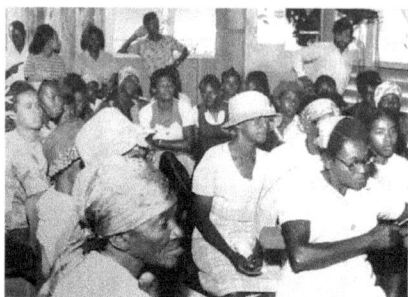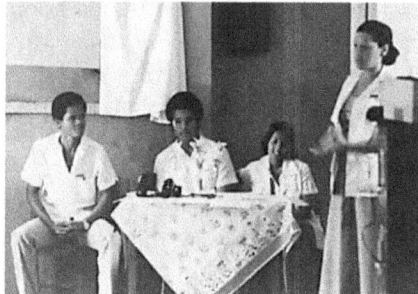

L: Fig 17-2;   R: Fig 17-3

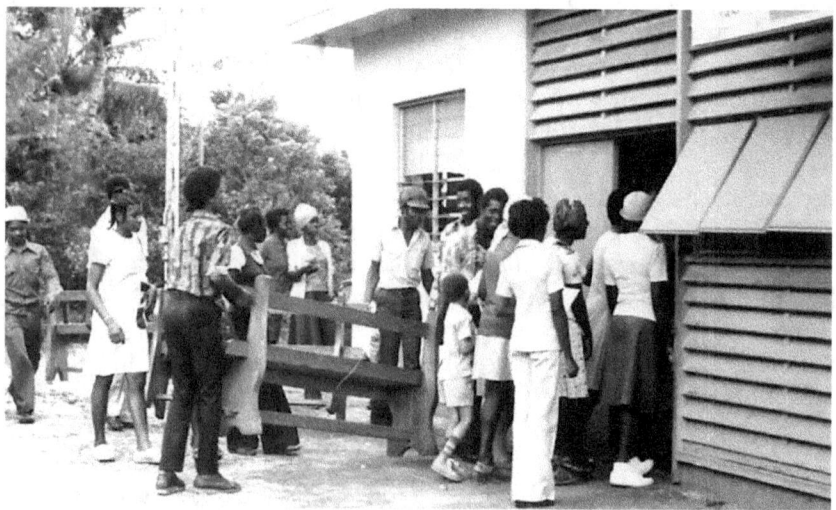

Fig 17-4

In the 3 photos above, students conduct education (prevention) sessions with community members at the Prattville clinic, an example of the way medical students can contribute to primary care medicine and health education; and to expose resident doctors to community problems, and their research. These group sessions are held on specific problems e.g. hypertension, nutrition and diabetes prior to seeing individual patients. In the lower photo, community members attend for information and advice on family planning; large families are a burden to poor households, and crowd health services with preventable problems that medical students rarely see in hospitals except when extreme or complicated. Teenage pregnancy was a major problem, and Vice Dean Smith was engaged in fund-raising for a major assault on the problem. Part of the PGME building (p. 214) was dedicated to Family Planning, on funds provided by Jamaica Government and USAID. (Dean's photo collection)

CHAPTER 18
The Eastern Caribbean Scheme

A decision had been made in 1967 to involve Eastern Caribbean Hospitals in clinical education of medical students and discussions with Trinidad and Barbados led to the first batch of eight final year students starting at the Port of Spain General Hospital in 1968. There were many teething problems, both structural and interpersonal, some of the permanent Government staff clashing in minor or worse ways with the University lecturers, or with associate staff, who were also Government employees, but attached to the "UWI office," which was seen as a place of privilege. The differences affected some students and some rotations, but successes occurred, and at the end of the year, frank evaluations led to improvements and an increased number, plus an inaugural batch to Barbados.

The EC islands had been critical of Jamaica's domination of graduates, who competed for the better experiences at UHWI—from conditions of work and housing to graduate training. Yet UHWI too was criticised for delay in upgrading facilities, and reorganising functions to accommodate more clinical students and internes.

The Faculty had meanwhile planned to have a third of the final year students shared between the General Hospital, Port Of Spain, and the Queen Elizabeth Hospital, Bridgetown, a theme discussed yearly at CHMC, and a move that would please everyone at both points of the Caribbean Sea. Table 18-1 shows the accredited hospitals in the campus territories, their bed complement and number that we proposed in 1971 for the MB,BS and PGME programs.

Country	Hospital	Total Beds	# Teaching
Jamaica	UHWI	500	500
" "	Kingston Regional	600	100- - ->300
" "	Victoria, Kingston	500	100
" "	Cornwall Regional	450	200
Trinidad& Tobago	POS General	920	400- - ->500
" "	San Fernando General	600	100
Barbados	Queen Eliz. General	600	200- - ->300

Table 18-1: Proposed Number of "Teaching" Beds for UWI students

Table 18-2 shows the plan, starting in each location with 25 students in the final (third) clinical year, and adding, by 1973, students in the second clinical year in Trinidad, should we get our finances for staff, space and supplies. Development would then follow as planned.

Hosp./ Year	1970	1971	1972	1973	1974	1975	1976	1977
POS 3	25	25	25	20	20	25	30	40
2	-	-	-	20	20	20	20	20
1	-	-	-	-	10	15	20	20
Beds	100	100	100	160	200	240	280	320

A (above) Trinidad, growth in students and "teaching" beds
B: (below) Barbados .....ditto.....

Hosp.	1970	1971	1972	1973	1974	1975	1976	1977
B'dos 3	25	25	25	25	25	25	30	30
2								10
1								0
Beds	100	100	100	100	100	100	120	160

Table 18-2, A &B: Plan for EC scheme Bed: Student ratio 4:1

Initial success was due to the enthusiasm of students and teachers to blaze a trail. The pioneer students in Trinidad were M. Belfon, C. Caines and J. Juggernauth of Trinidad; V Forsythe and E. Choo Kang of Guyana; J. Glean and L. Bayne of Grenada; and W. Hanna of Jamaica: four women and four men, class of 1968. The actual build-up is shown in Table 18-3.

Country of Student Origin	1968 B T	1969 B T	1970 B T	1971 B T	1972 B T	1973 B T	1974 B T	TOTAL B T EC
Antigua	-	-	-	-	1	-	-	0 1 1
Bahamas	- -	- -	- -	- -	- -	3 -	1 1	4 1 5
Barbados	- -	4 2	2 -	1 3	7 1	5 -	9 -	28 6 34
Belize	- -	- -	- 1	1 1	-	-	-	1 2 3
BVI	- -	1 -	-	- -	-	-	-	1 0 1
Dominica	- -	- -	- 1	1		1	2 -	4 1 5
Grenada	- 1	3 -	1 -	- 1	- -	2	1 1	7 3 9
Guyana	- 2	1 -	- -	2	- 3	3	4 1	10 6 14
Jamaica	4 2	11 10	11 9	18 6	8 1	10 3	2 -	64 31 95
St Kitts	-	-	-	1	-	-	-	1 0 1
St Lucia	- -	- -	1	-	-	2	3 1	6 1 7
St Vincent	- -	1 1	3 -	1	1	1	4	10 1 11
Trinidad	1 3	0 9	1 9	- 15	1 20	1 27	1 23	5 106 111
TOTAL	5 8	21 22	19 20	24 27	17 26	28 30	27 27	297* 141 159 301

Table 18-3: Actual Growth of EC scheme: final year students only: (*diff due to double-counting of 4)
B= Barbados at Q. E. Hospital ; T=Trinidad at the Port Of Spain General Hospital

We had to delay the introduction of 2nd and 1st year clinical students until Trinidad had decided the direction it wished to follow, and not until 1976, did PM Williams decide to support Faculty expansion and build the new hospital at Mount Hope. Meanwhile, on each visit to the

EC, I would meet with students, informally, to get their feed-back and suggestions, as I regularly received from students in Jamaica, both at Faculty Board meetings and individually, from the histrionic to the more sober, contributing in various ways. In Jamaica, Freddie Hickling and in Trinidad, Joanne Juggernauth and W. Hanna, two of the first EC participants, were particularly helpful. I had noted that the ones who were committed and made positive suggestions and criticisms had tended to stay and fight, especially in Trinidad and Barbados, and conversely, but not invariably, that the ones without original ideas or strong desires to stay tended to make a quick exit to points north.

By 1973, student deployment had not reached the levels we had expected in Jamaican regional hospitals, and our plan to start the second clinical year in Port of Spain in 1973 had stalled. Total numbers of beds and students in major hospitals were as shown in *Table 18-4, below:*

FACULTY OF MEDICINE, UWI, TEACHING HOSPITALS		
1973-4	Beds available	Students
University Hospital, Mona, Jamaica	500	280
Kingston Regional Hospital "	600	6
Cornwall Regional Hospital "	200* (400+)	-
Port-of-Spain General Hospital, T&T	980	25
San Fernando Hospital "	600	-
Queen Elizabeth Hospital, Barbados	600	25
*currently open; + under construction		(MMSR,1974)

Table18-4: Actual student participation in EC scheme

It was realised early that the EC scheme could be much improved, for all concerned, by modest investments, particularly in PGME. In 1970, we had argued to the CHMC that "*it is during the four or five years following graduation that medical personnel provide their most vigorous and dedicated service to their local hospital and health programs...(with) career objectives uppermost in (their) minds and the opportunities to reach them most eagerly sought...the local lack of such post-graduate opportunities is the main single determinant of the very high recent emigration rate of our graduates...An annual emigration rate of approximately 40%...means a...contribution of £400,000 from our area to medicine in other countries.*" (CHMC, 1970/6); see also table for Graduate losses, p. 88). Translated into the full cost of medical education in the USA or Canada, the two major destinations, this was equivalent to an annual gift of US $2 million, more or less.

At meetings in Barbados, we dealt with various Ministers, from the reserved to the extrovert: Dr Caddle, Minister in 1973; Mrs. Eastmond the Parliamentary Secretary; Mr. Howell, the Permanent Secretary; Chief Medical Officer, Dr. Wells, who with Drs Boyd, Comissiong, Quamina and Wilson, and Mr. Burton were the major officials on the CHMC; and

Dr. Harold Forde, Associate Dean, (later Dr. Frank Ramsay), plus hospital consultants. We discussed, at length, training philosophy and methods, the planned build-up and the key roles of government health services in the University program, and accommodated their views. Mr. James Williams, Director of the Queen Elizabeth Hospital (QEH), fully supported his hospital's involvement in residency training, and was an exemplary resource for interns and residents.

Other personalities were a neurosurgeon named Bagnall and an internist, Ritchie Haynes, both of whom were associate lecturers. Bagnall advocated formation of a specialist society of neurosurgeons (of whom there were then 5 in the Caribbean) to start a program to train specialists. Dr. Haynes, an ebullient and assertive man, a medical entrepreneur and social adventurer, who used Medicine like a whip, did not quite get on with our Associate Dean, the no-nonsense and scrupulous Dr. Forde, a veteran internist who had begun his service with the UCWI in 1953 as a well-liked lecturer in Medicine, and later proponent of the DM. The Faculty Board had dealt at great length in 1969 with the idea of small "Specialty Societies" and had not supported them as primary vehicles for either education or examinations, and we so informed him. We welcomed, however, their formation, as a good professional and collegial move that could support specialty training, CME, and fund-raising, but we could not see the UWI yielding control of its degree structure to an outside body, nor would the governments fund a parallel and duplicative operation to produce a rare specialist. The comparison with Canada was discussed, but the model discarded at that time, as it was deemed too expensive and too parochial.

At the same time, the General Practitioners (GPs) wanted immediate recognition as individuals and by creation of a family practice degree, into which they could be grand-fathered. We reviewed our plans for Family Medicine; Dr Dyer, head of the University Clinic, had drafted a curriculum covering four years, which the PGME committee judged too long, after six years of medical school and internship. But that plan had included training in some aspects of Public Health to equip graduates to carry on a practice, private or government, and serve as district MOH. Even so, we felt that 2½ to 3 years should be adequate, as I had earlier drafted, incorporating much of the DPH program, and following adjustments to the curriculum to streamline basic training, and prepare students better for smooth entry into any health care function, from primary to tertiary care. Barbadian GPs, led by a 1965 graduate, Dr M. Hoyos, wished recognition prior to approval of a curriculum. This was denied, but they persisted. I had hoped, but failed to involve Dr Edson Inniss (1957), a brilliant man, and friend, who had returned home and set up an independent and successful family practice in Bridgetown.

Curriculum revision, forcefully advocated by the Action Group in 1970, and endorsed by most faculty and students, was a major tool, for Mona and EC programs. The Curriculum Committee had been changed from a ponderous 19-21 members, each fighting its own turf war, to a sleek, purposive team in 1970, which I chaired. In the revision, we took account of advances in sciences, education and learning psychology, and adapted them to Caribbean realities—expectations, experiences, CHMC needs, economies and resources, especially human—and to the need for academic fulfilment for staff. This had been discussed by the IADB Committee and favourably reviewed (see Report).

I pondered that statement, it sounded ambitious. But it was not beyond our abilities: we *were* achievers. This was brought home to me in late 1968, at the Mount Sinai Hospital, NY, while doing electron microscopy; (we had at UWI an old Phillips EM 100C, by then replaced nearly everywhere. At the European Congress on Electron Microscopy in mid-August that year, I had examined instruments on display, to select one, which we would try to get). From Mount Sinai, I visited the nearby Flower and Fifth Hospital, which had pinched Swedish micro-anatomist (non-medical), Johannes Rhodin, and Jamaican EM technician, Shirley Lim Sue, in the fashion of the US to entice and grab the world's best. (Shirley it was who, at this visit, told me of the Walter Rodney riots on the UWI Campus, following his ban from Jamaica by the JLP. He was a Guyanese leftist social scientist at UWI).

Shirley had worked in 1965-66 with Bill Brooks and me. Rhodin's textbook of ultrastructure had become a state of the art reference; he was teaching that to first year students, and allowed them to use one of his microscopes (note, *one of*, while the UWI had just one, a dated model, which students hardly saw!). But Shirley had produced fine images with it, which continued to function, until a new one was triumphantly obtained many years later, followed by a second for the science faculty.

I mention this re advances in science, and their cost. Adoption was a huge challenge, easy to assert but tough to achieve. What we could not do, due to high cost, we chose to substitute. And so we used the products, that is, the electron micrographs, the real learning tool, and followed that lead to seek the essence of progress and to forego the joys of playing with toys we could not afford. And yet there is a limit below which we should not go, not just for intellectual reasons, but for the sake of the care we must dispense. Thus we should have quick access to: an ECG machine and other emergency diagnostic and resuscitative equipment; basic laboratory tests and x-rays; an efficient ambulance service; and trained nurses and assistants, in a system of care based on the principles of health promotion and disease prevention. These we would "preach" to the UWI administration and to the CHMC.

Table 18-5: EC Scheme A: Barbados: Student distribution by country of origin

YEAR	COUNTRY	STUDENTS	TOTAL
1968	Trinidad	1	
	Jamaica	4	**5**
1969	Guyana	1	
	Grenada	3	
	Jamaica	11	
	Barbados	4	
	St Vincent	1	
	Br V .Islands	1	**21**
1970	Trinidad	1	
	Grenada	1	
	Jamaica	11	
	Barbados	2	
	St Vincent	3	
	St Lucia	1	**19**
1971	Guyana	2	
	Jamaica	18	
	Barbados	1	
	Br Honduras	1	
	Dominica	1	
	St Kitts	1	**24**
1972	Trinidad	1	
	Jamaica	8	
	Barbados	7	
	St Vincent	1	**17**
1973	Trinidad	1	
	Guyana	3	
	Grenada	2	
	Jamaica	10	
	Barbados	5	
	St Vincent	1	
	Dominica	1	
	St Lucia	2	
	Bahamas	3	**28**
1974	Trinidad	1	
	Jamaica	2	
	Guyana	4	
	Grenada	1	
	Barbados	9	
	St Vincent	4	
	St Lucia	3	
	Dominica	2	
	Bahamas	1	**27**

Table 18-6: EC Scheme B: Trinidad: Student distribution by country of origin

YEAR	COUNTRY	STUDENTS	TOTAL
1968	Trinidad	3	
	Guyana	2	
	Grenada	2	
	Jamaica	1	8
1969	Trinidad	9	
	Guyana	-	
	Grenada	-	
	Jamaica	10	
	Barbados	2	
	St Vincent	1	22
1970	Trinidad	9	
	Guyana	-	
	Grenada	-	
	Jamaica	9	
	Dominica	1	
	Br. Honduras	1	20
1971	Trinidad	15	
	Guyana	-	
	Grenada	1	
	Jamaica	6	
	Barbados	3	
	Br. Honduras	1	26
1972	Trinidad	20	
	Guyana	3	
	Grenada	-	
	Jamaica	1	
	Barbados	1	
	Antigua	1	26
1973	Trinidad	27	
	Guyana	-	
	Grenada	-	
	Jamaica	3	30
1974	Trinidad	23	
	Guyana	1	
	Grenada	1	
	Jamaica	-	
	Bahamas	1	
	St Lucia	1	27

Tables 18-5 &18-6: EC Scheme showing student choice by country of origin, 1968-74

And so we pushed the EC scheme from 1968, and by 1974 had reached the position summarised for the two sites by number and country of origin of the students *(Tables 18-5 & 6)*. Barbados was praised for its friendly reception, while early students found Trinidad doctors "aloof and arrogant."

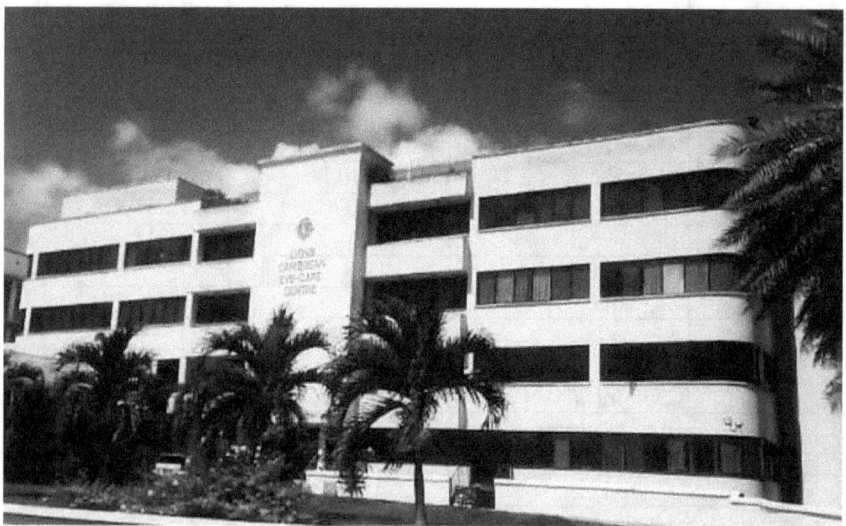

Fig 18-1: QEH, Barbados (CaribDigital)

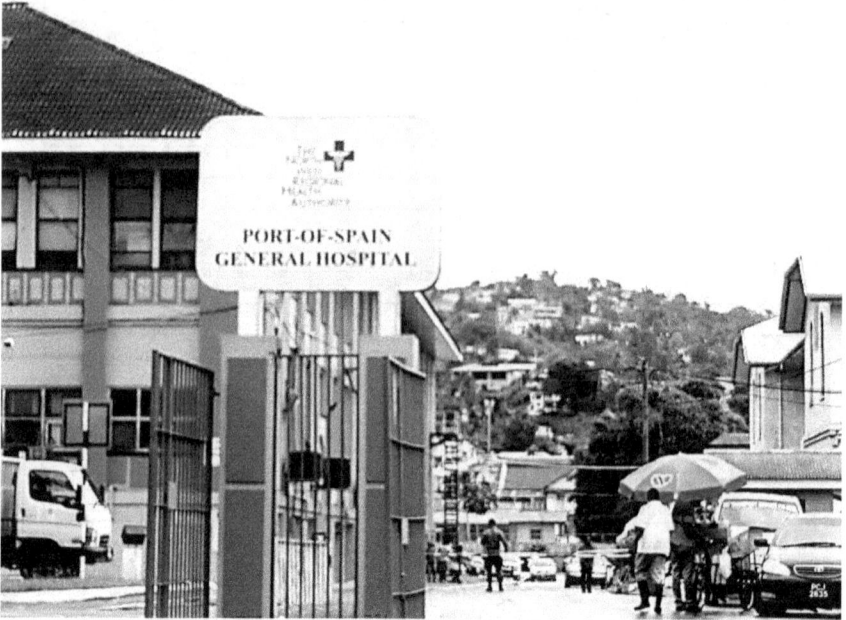

Fig 18-2: Part of Façade and Entrance of POS General Hospital (Photo by author)

CHAPTER 19
Socialism and Specialty Training—
UWI meets with PM Manley

The PNP victory in February, 1972, with 37 seats to the JLP's 16, caused some worry, not because of the PNP *per se*, but because of the perceived financial profligacy that might follow, as judged by the campaign rhetoric of Mr. Michael Manley and his team, especially Manley, with his condemnation of Seaga's "capitalism."[33] The victory delayed us, but it brought in strong personalities as heads of Health: Minister of Health, Dr Ken McNeill, an ENT surgeon, with whom I had worked as an intern, and Parliamentary Secretary, Ms. Mavis Gilmour, a general surgeon and colleague, and wife of Professor John Gilmour, former Head of Surgery, one of my earliest supporters in the Deanship.

With understandable anxiety, we asked the Minister's secretary for a meeting, as soon as practicable, fearing that the PNP would ignore their opponents' decision, especially as Mr. Manley had openly repudiated almost everything the JLP cabinet had approved before the elections. At a brief preliminary private meeting, Dr Wilson assured us that health projects would be spared, as social services were a high priority with the PNP, Minister McNeill and with him; the Permanent Secretary, Mr. Goldson, supported our plan.

But PM Manley and his Minister of Finance, David Coore, had announced a review of the proposed spending moves by the JLP, especially new programs, before preparing a budget. Ours would suffer anxious months of delay, during which we continued to refine the broad measures, and add details to "minor" operating policies.

On my appointment as Dean, Professor Gilmour had paid me a much-appreciated visit and offered support and friendship, a "sounding board" away from the formal faculty, he had said. With the PNP victory, CMO Wilson was almost incommunicado, buried in a series of reviews for the new government. I called Dr Gilmour and explained my fears; he invited me over to his house, "just for a chat," he said, so that he could fully understand the issues. Mavis came in, like someone answering an

---

[33] It was difficult to call Edward Seaga a "capitalist" as he did not conform to the negative associations of that word. He was a socialist, an entrepreneur and money-wise; he had held on to his slum constituency for a decade, and had transformed it from what was described in 1961 as the worst slum in the West Indies, to Tivoli Gardens, (see p. 142 and Fn. 29).

emergency call, for I heard her say as he met her at the door, "Well, here I am; you're not in any trouble, are you?" She sounded quite solicitous.

And so we had a chance to talk; I expressed my fears; she was understandably tentative as government policy had not yet been fully formed. I was a bit hesitant in detailing my concerns as she had previously struck me as being resistant, if not antagonistic to my deanship, being something of a fan of Ken Stuart and not as "familiar with the ways of Indians" as with blacks and coloureds! But the occasion allowed me to prime her with all the elements of the program that she would not have known, save for Surgery, nor easily pick up without going through reams of documents. In the end, she assured me of her personal support, and was sure that the Minister was on our side. She cautioned about the PM. "It won't be long; I heard Ken asking his Secretary to arrange a meeting with you and your team".

At UWI meetings, the Faculty's academic needs caused some stir among members of the Finance and General Purposes Committee (FGP), as the CHMC lobby of their Council representatives had persuaded them that Medicine's requests were urgent and paramount. That view seemed to ignore the needs of other Faculties, as we argued the case for expansion and for changing the educational emphasis to producing a more useful range of professionals than we had done so far, and to revising the MB,BS curriculum to emphasise health promotion and disease prevention, which promised a healthier society and work force.

But the effect was an extraordinary scrutiny of our plans and wants for the 1972-5 triennium, and we had a tough fight to get three new professorships at Mona: Dean, Coordinator of PGME and Director of Community Medicine; a Senior Lecturer for Medical Education; and a Lecturer to fill the vacancy in the department left by the Dean. The Dean's office was allotted a Senior Administrative Assistant, and a Secretary for the PGME program. Capital allowances included four offices for new staff (a renovated area near the main lecture theatre), plus funds for an extension of the small lecture theatre from 60 to 80 seats.

Although fewer than we had requested, these positions proved difficult to fill as social unrest in Jamaica worsened and several senior staff pursued opportunities in the Eastern Caribbean, or extended study leave elsewhere. To avoid an abortion of key programs, I carried on to implement the changes, eking out what help I could get from willing colleagues, or from the HOPE commitment, as long as social unrest did not stall that plan, and to promote the EC scheme with greater vigour.

At the same time, Minister McNeill asked our patience for a few weeks longer while the new government reviewed all spending plans. In the weeks that followed we met with the Minister and his group several times and laboriously went over every detail of the programs. Although he was a member of the Faculty, he had not participated in any of the discussions, nor read any of the documents. These meetings were a repeat of the Bermuda presentations, and of the briefing with Mavis Gilmour; through them, Dr Wilson maintained his stance. At the end, the Minister assured us of his support, which he would put to the PM and Minister of Finance, and in presenting it in parliament, he would take pleasure in emphasising that the opposition was in full support!

Even so, it was not plain sailing. In early June 1972, the University was summoned to meet with the PM and the Minister of Finance for a review of all new University programs to which the JLP had made commitments or promises. The major one was ours. A large UWI delegation attended at his offices, making Manley — dressed elegantly in his tan short sleeve shirt-jack with matching pants — quip mischievously, to nervous laughs, "It looks like you didn't leave anybody up there to teach or mind the shop; but of course, you're administrators!"

Vice-Chancellor Marshall summarised University initiatives and indexed those that Jamaica had supported in Council. PVC Finance Preston then presented the details of each, and after preliminary remarks, he began to speak on Medicine, but Manley cut him short, saying that he wanted to hear from "this young man; I want to hear what he has to say." I was not prepared for this. In our briefing, I was to answer any technical questions and supply any detail requested.

But I gave it all I had, and had done this so often, I could speak on it in my sleep. I told him in a nutshell what we wished to do. Manley began a grilling with "Will this stop the brain drain from Jamaica?" Professor Beaubrun — who was there, had taken ownership of the issue of the brain drain, and had written a paper on it — wished to intervene. But Manley barely allowed him a few sentences dealing with causes and a reference to personal papers, waiving him off, saying, with a smile, "Thanks, Professor, I want to hear what the Dean has to say. He is the man who will be managing my money, if I decide to give it to you."

After a slight pause, I said, "We can't guarantee that, Sir, but every enrolled Jamaican or other resident in the program will be serving Jamaican patients; that means immediate retention of those for up to four years. We expect that people trained in this environment will want to remain here, when they finish. All of those who said they would opt for training here, if it were available in the form we propose, also said that they wanted to work in their home country. In addition, they will be teaching undergraduates and will have an influence on their decisions. Also, individual governments have backed compulsory rotations, after specialisation, through district hospitals and clinics for 2-5 years for anyone funded by them; that would stabilise rural staffing. For Faculty, those who have to teach residents here will have to expand research on Jamaican problems; that should help us to improve the quality and range of services that your government will be able to offer when these residents graduate and join it."

"You sure of that?"

"No more than anyone can be sure of what can happen in a year or four years' time." He laughed.

"That sounds political. You think I'll lose the next one?"

"I'm sorry, Sir, I didn't mean that as political comment. It's the length of the training programs."

"Don't apologise; I'm glad you're straight, man, and not promising magic like some others. Leave the magic to us. I'm the Houdini here."

In the mirth that followed (everybody, especially the University contingent, was nervous as we had no idea where this was going. I could see VC Marshall's face from where I sat. He smiled faintly, and gave a little nod). Manley asked for details on our readiness, state of plans for the building, the position of other partners, and focussed on Trinidad and Tobago, "Now tell me, I see you have a sum for capital, but you're only asking us for a part. How will that play out? You're not going to build our part, let's say I give you money, before you get funds from others; what's their position?"

I explained the aim and rolled out a scroll of the building plan, and told him that T&T and Barbados would contribute, on agreeing to the proposal. The building would be built in stages, and the Jamaica grant would be enough for the first floor, the plan calling for four floors. After that I referred him to PVC Preston, who could more confidently speak on the financial matters. But Manley said, "Before we go there, give me some numbers; how many doctors are we talking about?"

"Since we started, 1954-1971, we've graduated 310 Jamaican doctors or about 48% of the 650 total; T&T, 15.4%; Guyana 13%, Barbados 6.6% and the rest distributed among the other islands and Belize. Half or more of these went on to specialise, at the moment mostly to UK, Canada and USA. This year 46 Jamaicans graduated, and at current admissions, we expect about 45 each year." I passed him two charts showing graduates by year (1954-70), with number of known losses (Fig 17-1, p. 153), and by country (1954-71), including those with London degrees (1954-67, Table 17-2, p. 154), which had been included in the brief sent to his office.

Manley grilled me on various issues including the EC scheme and TRVL. I agreed that a share of TRVL would prove worthwhile once a regional role could be defined for it, such as epidemiologic surveillance, which is poorly developed; T&T would maintain the diagnostic virology laboratory and the facilities and expertise would support education, research and clinical services. PAHO would likely administer it.

He nodded, then focussed on graduate losses (p. 88), tempting me into political comment as people had already begun to blame his socialist agenda for campus unease, but I avoided that and instead pointed out that Jamaica had so far lost about 50% of each batch by migration; most of the class of 1969 had preferred to leave the Caribbean; that was before his time, and Jamaica still attracted graduates from the Lesser Antilles and Guyana. He smiled and wanted to know why we thought our "local enterprise, postgraduate scheme had more merit than an arrangement with the UK or Canada." *(See also p 161, re University of South Pacific.)*

I acknowledged the scepticism of foreign observers shown at CHMC meetings about our emphasis on an independent program, which some had damned with faint praise; but we noted the approval of CMA and HOPE (Ch. 13). Our University basis was unique and gave us service and academic controls throughout the training, whereas the others, like the Colleges and Boards in Canada, UK and USA were only examining bodies, relying on accredited hospitals to supervise, undertake and ensure the quality of training. Although we were not yet officially launched, we did have experience of training graduates for UK examinations, with a very good record so far. Also, as a member of PAFAMS (I had to explain what that was), a group closely attached to US—and some Spanish—methods, we were eagerly watched by educators in Central and South America, monitoring our progress and willing to follow our lead. "They've heard me defend our plan and support our initiatives; officers have visited, and seen what we have, what we lack, our physical layout, and talked to heads of specialty boards and University officers. Many Latin American medical schools have postgraduate training, but few, if any, have anything as structured or inclusive like ours. The simplicity of our Regulations was a surprise."

Apparently, Canadian agencies had dismissed our scheme and wanted to sell him a program, "just like selling potatoes and salt fish," which they would organise and manage, for a fee, since we did not have the "manpower or the finances." He liked the capitalist analogy, and, realising that we had explored joint programs, ended the quiz, commenting encouragingly on our initiatives and the thrust of the program, even though he had called me a dreamer at one stage, and an entrepreneur at another, both good-naturedly, unlike Eric Williams' petulant remark to me two and a half years later (see p. 215).

After finishing his grilling, he said, "Thank you for your information and for your candour." He dealt similarly with the Deans of Education and Social Sciences. The VC and PVC Preston were both pleased with the quality and direction of the presentations, and hopeful. The meeting lasted over two hours. We had to wait weeks for the final word. One day, the VC called me and said, "I have some good news."

In a short time, Minister McNeill's letter arrived, confirming his Government's commitment. That allowed us to start officially in 1972. With the recognition of residencies and Senate approval, since 1970, of all completed Regulations, several persons—who had been induced to remain with us by the promise of retroactive registration—were able to finish in 1974, in Medicine, O&G and Paediatrics, led by Clarence Bankay in Internal Medicine (p. 76). Soon after, two others completed their training and examinations.

But the path here had been rough and troubled. T&T's stance was ambivalent; its Health Ministry executives and Minister Hon. Francis Prevatt, who had succeeded Max Awon in early 1972, were clearly on our side, when we (Butler, Bartholomew and Meltzer) met with them, and after, when the Minister wished to speak to me in camera, since for some reason he did not want witnesses. He probed into personalities, especially the role of T&T staff, and how much say, if any, his Ministry might have in staff selection. I reminded him of the non-territorial policy re UWI appointments, unless such were directly funded by a particular Ministry. It would be useful to discuss this at the next Council meeting, or to talk to the VC informally. He seemed reassured when told that our T&T program did not come under PVC Braithwaite at St Augustine, the Trinidad campus. He said complimentary things about the overall plan, and would let us know after a review of T&T finances, due shortly. Our chances, I concluded, were 50-50 *(See Appendix 8, p. 329)*.

While the T&T Minister supported us, PM Williams and the Finance Minister were cool. They had had enough with internal dissension and infrastructure breakdown, and the PM would not defend investments in "bricks and mortar" outside of Trinidad & Tobago. The political climate that developed in Jamaica had alarmed Eric Williams, who had become increasingly ambivalent about the regional University, despite its campus in T&T, and contribution to the national economy and ego. He had more than once privately wished for his own university, as Jagan had done in 1962-3, and when the OPEC windfall came in 1973, his stance became obvious, despite an honourary UWI doctorate (p. 178)!

But if the position of Governments was erratic, the Faculty had a saga of its own. It had, somewhat tentatively, begun in the early '60s to face the issue of specialist needs in the general medical services. I had joined it when the path was strewn with as much rubble as any hurricane could scatter on Jamaican roads! The first signs came as a difficulty in recruiting certain staff, and the realisation that if a few UC graduates had not pursued an academic path, the University might have been left high and dry when the flight of staff began in the late sixties and picked up speed in the seventies, as social unrest and political violence destabilised Jamaican society. This situation helped us to advance the cause of higher professional degrees in the Medical Faculty, as well as for an extended range of health care workers at pre-university level.

In 1973, I wrote, *"The University, whether old or new, must have a total view of manpower needs for health in the region it serves, and should involve itself in planning and organising training programs for all health personnel. Only in this way will it ensure that all such training takes place in harmony with the education of professionals to create a desirable balance in health teams, to supply essential components of such teams, and to get team members acquainted with one another's roles and responsibilities. It must recognise that the training of physicians alone will not have the desired effect of improving the quality and quantity of care, so long as the team is incomplete, nor will medical students trained in isolation from the rest of the team be competent to lead such teams or work with them for the general good."(Bibliography "The role of the new University...")*

I easily revived a cordial relationship with the Hon. Ken McNeill, which had begun fourteen years earlier, when I worked with him as a surgical intern. I agreed to serve on his Health Advisory committee, and he established a liaison group between his Ministry and the Faculty, of which CMO Jeff Wilson became Chair and I his deputy. We worked on several issues since, and by 1973 made considerable progress in dealing with governments. I had undertaken two studies for the Minister in 1973: estimating Jamaica's need for specialists *(p. 218, Table 24-1)*, and adapting the Cornwall Regional Hospital, Montego Bay, for teaching. Like many Caribbean hospitals, it had major teething problems, but by the end of 1974, the prospects were excellent for its role in medical education, undergraduate and graduate. It was a handsome structure on a beautiful site *(p. 217, Fig 24-4)*. By contrast, we had to wait 17 years, to 1989, before T&T was ready to open the new Faculty Buildings *(pp. 208, 217)*.

The results of the Jamaica manpower survey are shown on the table on page 218, copied from the original document submitted to, and accepted by the Ministry of Health. We noted the limitations, but we had projected needs at the low end of the range in each case, and urged their acceptance as guides. We hoped that the spreading social unrest could be curbed, since most of it was political. We emphasised the heavy competition for teachers, as Saudi Arabia opened new medical schools, the latest in 1969 in Jeddah under an agreement with London University to provide 600 teachers; (one of these was George Stirling, who had been a UCWI Lecturer in Pathology, a decade earlier.) Thus, self-interest alone should convince us to train our own in the Caribbean. We were impressed with the Saudi's "integrated design" in plans for facilities of Medicine and Dentistry, and an Institute for Medical Assistants. They planned to increase native professionals from 21% to 50% in 7 years. We could not compete with their wealth and salary attractions for foreign teachers, underscoring our need to train teachers, and upgrade staff skills in key areas. To this end, we had concluded, in 1971, two fortnightly seminars for staff, funded by PAHO, to enhance teaching skills, one in *Curriculum Development*, the other in the *Teaching of Behavioural Sciences*, both timely, in keeping with our drafts of a new curriculum. The poor or sporadic attendance at these underscored our staff shortages, the need to fill all vacancies, and to increase staffing.

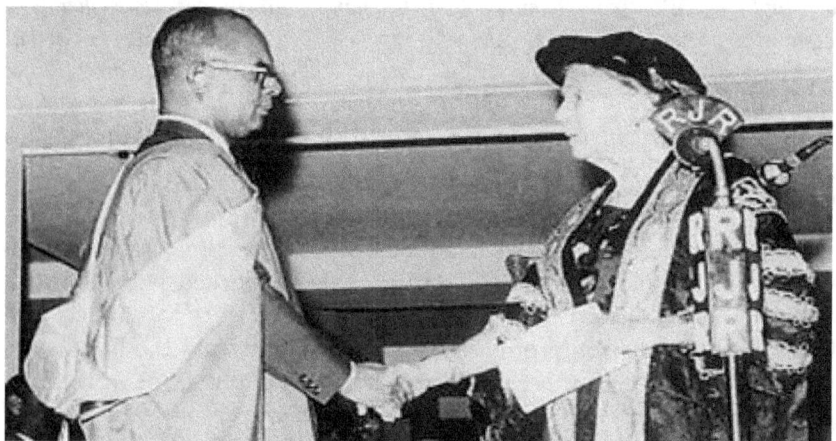

Fig 19-1: *Eric Williams receiving Honourary Degree from Chancellor Princess Alice Athlone. The former served as Pro-Chancellor for a decade. Following militant protests by students between 1968-70, both resigned in Feb 1971, Williams immediately, Princess Alice when Hugh Wooding took over.*

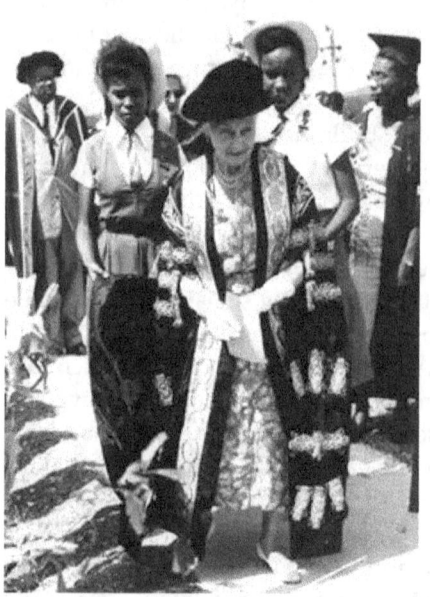

L: Fig 19-2

UWI Chancellor Princess Alice is attended by high school students carrying her train; this was the service refused in 1970 by UWI students on the St Augustine campus. They also refused to do the wine service at a formal dinner on the campus, and in the same vein snubbed the Canadian Governor General Roland Michener at St Augustine in 1969. PM Manley had cited the events illustrated here and the subsequent resignation of both from the UWI Chancellery. He had always had a good feeling for Eric Williams and respected the dignity of Princess Alice. Their resignations left 'a bad taste in the mouth.' (FM Dean's photo collection, figs 9-1 and 9-2)

178

CHAPTER 20
CHMC V, VI, and 1st meeting of CARICOM MRHs

In Government services, UWI medical graduates were praised for their clinical skills, but criticised for having poor "people skills" and "little or no orientation to communities, or understanding of the administrative, managerial and financial problems of the territories." This was hardly fair, as none of these elements was the stuff of a standard London curriculum, which they had failed to critique when the British ran the UCWI. Governments generally expected our graduates to be fully competent to handle all problems, including forensic and community issues—something they did NOT expect of those trained elsewhere—and even thought that all UWI graduates should be equipped to perform certain specialist functions, like some of the early graduates. Several Council members found it difficult to accept that further prolonged training was needed for a specialist qualification. In fact one member of Council, as late as 1970, opined that "Sir Harry (Annamunthodo) was crazy to suggest that it would take six years to train a surgeon after graduation." His Minister of Health repeated that thought at each of three later CHMC meetings!

Politicians were in general uninformed as to requirements for different degrees, and had they enquired, they would have found that it often took up to ten years or more to specialise by the traditional in-service method in their own services. That was acceptable, because the aspirant was providing service locally, but a residency scheme would take them away from the smaller islands that lacked accredited facilities. Some opined that the UK could produce a 'specialist in two years after internship, implying that the 1-2 year courses for some diplomas applied to all specialties, ignoring the prerequisites, which often covered several years. These would criticise the UWI and North America at each CHMC meeting for taking four to five years to get the same result.

But we were at pains to point out—and here we were joined by some Ministry doctors like Jeff Wilson, Jamaica, Elizabeth Quamina, Trinidad and Len Comissiong of Grenada, among others—that even the major UK specialty degrees only qualified the person for a Registrarship, which would in time gain him/her the experience needed to obtain a consultancy, while our specialist, and the North American, would be trained to *start* as a consultant. We had to deal with this and other misconceptions on the way to convincing governments of the number of years of funding needed for each specialty; we emphasised the service

179

given by the resident in that time, outlining ways in which they could be assigned to serve in the Lesser Antilles. We had planned for this by including electives in the final two years and helping the Antilles to develop sites and facilities for them. Similar electives would be designed for residents on a UWI-Government basis.

CHMC V was held in Dominica on February 5-9, 1973, at the Goodwill Parish Hall, and chaired by deputy Premier R. Armour. Because of ill-chosen references by early speakers, we briefly reviewed the evolution of western medicine from the early Salerno medical school in Italy — derived from earlier Arabic schools in North Africa, themselves derived from Indian and Greek medical practice — and evolving from humours, magic, witchcraft, blood-letting and so on, to modern practices dominated by science and technology, which we try to adapt to our resources, creating wants, in skills and equipment, affordable or not. We had to choose wisely, and, in medicine, advance in clinical knowledge and in humane practice, both affordable, and learn to innovate, to get the best of the 15% of national budgets spent on health care.

We showed our detractors that the fledgling PGME in Jamaica had, by 1973, already enrolled 36 graduates in 9 specialties, who might otherwise have migrated. In my review, I asserted that we could, with patience and determination, be among the world's best medical schools. We were not vying with Johns Hopkins, Case, Columbia or Harvard; we could consult them for advanced and costly technology, but we could teach them much in clinical and community skills, which we could cultivate to the highest level, at low cost, and emulate the Cuban gains in preventive medicine, and so share, and even market our strengths.

In 1972, the UWI Council had approved the expansion plan, to begin in the 1975-78 triennium, for a full EC school based at Mount Hope, Trinidad, with integrated basic sciences and clinical training, including veterinary science, a dental school for twenty students, and a branch clinical Faculty in Barbados. The facilities would be designed to promote integration, along curricular lines shown on pp. 54-58, so that the Faculty could influence or control all aspects of medical manpower development, even though it might not directly train non-matriculants, except as may be done by departments. But it could assist with such training at schools for medical ancillaries, or in local technical colleges, now functional in Jamaica, Trinidad, Barbados and at the University of Guyana.

The St Kitts Minister, Hon. F. Bryant, supported by the Hon K Mohamed of T&T, and Hon D. Singh, the new Guyana Minister of Health, rebuked us — a Kittitian ritual set from the beginning of UCWI by the St Kitts PM, Hon R. Bradshaw, and repeated by his Ministers since — asserting that UWI "*must cooperate with the Ministry of Health, not the other way round*," that it should "*train all levels of workers*" and that "*research*

<u>must</u> be subject to our (MOH) direction." All reasonable! But last year he had queried the time needed to train a specialist, and ridiculed the idea that "it would take ten years from *graduation* to produce a surgeon." (What we had said was "at least ten years from medical school entry!") He complained that we were trying to run the Ministries, rather than cater to their needs. While I consulted my colleagues (by note) re a reply, the Barbados Minister, Hon Dr R. Caddle, rebuked them, saying, *"Politicians should clean their slate first before demanding subservience from the UWI!"* He reminded them of the "moat and beam" in the New Testament, Matthew, Ch. 7, 1-5!

With our team's support, I responded to the Ministers, stressing first that migration of skilled peoples was occurring globally, from smaller or poorer countries to the expanding economies of North America, Europe and elsewhere, and that it also affected the UWI and the Medical Faculty. *"Yet we must continue to produce a range of doctors to a high standard of education, for the territories' needs and hopefully our own; no one would want any less; our graduates will often be left on their own here, and must feel secure in the theories and skills they had learned. The UWI has been doing that, and so far no one has complained. I agree with the Hon Bryant's view of the need for joint study of health problems and training needs of all territories, but we have inherited a curriculum which needs adjustment to Ministries' needs, not a change in quality. In fact, North America and the UK are so delighted with the quality of our product, that I believe we could earn income by training some of theirs! If our contributing territories wished, they could change or expand our mandate by resolution of the UWI Council."*

We reminded them that we have a clinical elective plan for final year students, which could cover some local service and research by their own students. *"Few Ministries have taken advantage of this; several students had enquired, but had cancelled, as replies from the Antilles had been too late. Ministries should note that students are on a strict time-table, and need prompt answers to queries, to conclude their learning plans, if Ministries wished to participate in them. They must understand the pace of student learning and know something of their syllabus, and how precious their time is. The Faculty is right to ensure that facilities are suitable for training, to attract students to spend a rotation in them; in return, Ministries will get competent assistance, although still in short supply throughout the Antilles. A good bonding experience with gifted seniors, some we know, like Dr Cyrus, might induce students to return after graduation.*

"It is also proper for the University to indicate what would promote and what hinder positive development. How better to illustrate that than to look at the spread of Faculty expertise at this table; these professors are known to you, for their research into the health problems of our communities; they are here not only to represent the UWI, but to share with you what they have learned of the pressing medical problems in the region and to discuss solutions. This is a

proper role for the University, to discover new truths, inform those in power and assist in applying that knowledge; and it has done so for twenty years. Prof Stuart was foremost in the team that identified 'bush tea' poisoning in Jamaica and will deal today with hypertension, a major cause of morbidity; Professor Beaubrun has dealt with the 'brain drain,' and today will focus on mental health issues; Professor Standard is well-known as an advocate for preventive medicine and supports its role in our planned Community Medicine program; Professor Hoyte is one of our ablest educators and a rare species, a medical anatomist at the forefront of integrating basic sciences and clinical medicine, which is a foundation for education of the future doctor we all need, i.e. the family doctor and the community physician. Dr Sievewright is a world figure in Nursing and will update you on her efforts to obtain funding for Nursing facilities. Dr (or Mr.) Butler is a respected surgeon and our newly created Vice-Dean for the EC Scheme whose role will expand as the program grows. Mrs. McGhie is here to share her expertise on health education. In the past, Professors Sir Harry Annamunthodo, Gerrit Bras and a number of others had been before you, and are active in health and manpower issues. Our local staff in T&T and Barbados engage with Government counterparts daily to tackle local problems. We hope to expand that, even though we're facing grave social ills at Mona.

"These, ladies and gentlemen, are large talents, not to be restrained in their academic or clinical thinking or corresponding actions, if you wish the best from them; so when you wish a research input, whether it's St Kitts or anyone else, ask them; they will respond, knowing the people and the places, and gladly discuss the issues. We're in the same boat at Mona. The University must fill its needs for teaching and research staff, or founder. It too suffers a brain drain."

On recruitment and retention of staff, I recalled my service as a personnel officer in the Colonial Medical Services in BG, where I had suggested that the recruiting and management of medical staff should be placed in the Ministry of Health, not the Public Service Commission, noting the many differences from, and clashes with the conditions of service in the colonial office. In the interim, local personnel officers should be allowed to apply prompt and appropriate solutions to administrative problems, instead of the ponderous regulations designed for uniformity in a world-wide imperial service, intolerant of local deviation, however sensible, except in emergencies. *"Those regulations are still in place in most countries, as we saw last year. I would urge Ministers to discard outworn practices and develop a unique set of rules for recruiting and managing health workers (and I daresay, others), more in line with local needs, and vest those in an upgraded personnel division in the Ministry of Health. Ministries could consider using a common recruiting agency through CHMC, since each island is unlikely to need or afford one of its own."* (Later, Barbados severed Hospitals from Civil Service control and assigned the QEH to a Management Board, like the UHWI and Kingston Regional Hospital, but the ponderous and frustrating recruitment procedures remained.)

We informed the new Guyanese Minister, Hon D. Singh, that at UWI we viewed Guyana as a regional ally, and had done for it as much as we could, without funds. *"We had urged last year's Minister to persuade your President to allow the VC of UG to work with us on graduate education. We knew of the President's interest in CARIFTA and the Non-Aligned Movement. Perhaps he might develop health manpower training into an agreed conjoint activity, so that together we can cover the full spectrum of needs. But whatever the route chosen, some funds had to be found for it. We have already assisted in planning training programs for technical and auxiliary cadres, at no cost to Guyana, knowing your struggle to meet personnel needs. Your government has two choices, either to develop your own programs or to contract with another educational authority to supply the training."*

A silence followed that made me wonder whether I had gone too far, although I had been as gentle as I could; but then Professor Hoyte squeezed my arm and Beaubrun smiled briefly, as Dr Wilson spoke. He thanked me for the remarks and told the meeting that UWI cooperation with the Jamaica Ministry was at a high level, and had not always been so, but he welcomed the co-operative approaches, the changes planned for the curriculum, and suggested that UWI and its research must be "unfettered," and that it *did* address problems of the region, neglected earlier. Any reluctance to probe problems was due to lack of funds or appropriate facilities. This was one reason why he hoped to reach a formula to establish a headquarters for PGME at Mona and expand it in the Eastern Caribbean. He agreed with the need to shed some colonial practices, and to modernise rules and regulations "to make them more suited to the conditions of newly-self-governing states."

Professor Hoyte endorsed my comments, *"The Dean is himself a considerable talent. He is, like Professor Standard and Dr Minott, a UCWI graduate, and many from other faculties now staff your services, and soon will run governments. He is unique in being a chance transfer to Medicine from second year Arts, an experiment, in fact. You've heard him briefly on medical history, and is very well-informed on medical education and curricular matters; he'll speak later, on the need for a regional forensic service. You may not know it, but it was out of a review of forensic autopsies that he noted the high incidence of fatal heart disease in East Indians of Guyana. That was ten years ago, a new finding, and it complemented a similar observation by Dr Wattley in Trinidad. That subject remains to be researched. Perhaps the Hon Minister from Guyana is aware of this. It is a fertile field for cooperation between Trinidad and Guyana, and a proper subject for the new EC Faculty. Indeed, an epidemiologist from UWI, Dr Ashcroft, is just about now working on that very problem, and a British researcher, Dr Miller, is probably also in Guyana collecting data."*

The Hon. Singh, caught flat-footed, and not knowing of it, chose not to comment. The lunch break gave an opportunity to soothe any bruised egos and the Chair resumed the afternoon session by thanking us and praising the work of UWI staff.

Discussion of our proposals re Community Medicine stressed the needs for primary care and noted the changes in curriculum to facilitate training. It had helped us that Dr Matthew Beaubrun of the Caribbean Medical Education Council (CMEC) had spoken to several EC ministers in favour of our plans, and assisted further in arranging interviews with them. The Beaubrun family was a major social and business force in St Lucia and known in the Antilles. (Dr Karl Smith had once told me that all the doctors in Dominica were members of the six or seven large land-owners in the island. This pattern held in most of the others.)

In a post-conference session with the Hon J. Compton, Premier of St. Lucia, at his office in Castries, we discussed Community Medicine; he would support an elective, and try to develop a local learning centre for primary and community care, if he could meet the conditions, perhaps at the *Schistosomiasis Research Centre*, which would be closing soon. It was housed at the hilltop Morne complex, which we had visited with Dr Peter Jordan, the Director. The Premier endorsed our primary care proposals, and I later sent him literature and plans, including curricula. We agreed that he would keep in touch, directly and through the Vice-Dean, EC, or Dr Matthew Beaubrun, who had arranged the meeting.

The establishment of the new EC "school" might be more convenient for the Antilles, since administration from Mona might prove unwieldy as student intake expanded. It was likely that if current political thinking prevailed, the Faculty would be triplicated as finances permitted, with a Dean at each campus, and at Mona, a University Dean—*or PVC, Health Sciences (HS) Education*—since Faculty training schemes would inevitably grow to include all health workers.[34] CHMC supported these initiatives with resolutions: PGME, Res. 12/73; Community Medicine, Res. 13/73, 20/73; Advanced Nursing Education, Res. 14/73; Brain Drain, Res. 15/73; management, Res. 17/83; removing medical staff hiring from Public Services Commission, Res. 18/73; Forensic Medicine, Res. 22/73.

But the resolutions were not acted on with any consistency or dedication, prompting reminders from the Secretariat. The Forensic Medicine paper resulted in contact with Mr. Kenneth Jones, a British forensic scientist, who, in January, had started a survey for the British Ministry of Overseas Development (MOD), of needs for forensic services in the EC and BVI. His visit to Dominica overlapped the days of our meeting. I met with him, and later found that Health Ministries had no

---

[34] I discussed this informally with VC Marshall in late 1973, and again with VC Preston in 1975. Both saw merit in the re-structuring but suggested a deferral of any proposal to Council until the EC scheme was established, and Trinidad committed.

knowledge of the purpose and nature of his investigations, and that the western territories and T&T would welcome his survey. I suggested that they contact the MOD, UK, directly and urgently, since Mr. Jones would be in the Caribbean until March 19th. His report would be sent to Ministries of Home Affairs. (Mr. Jones sent me a copy of his very comprehensive report on March 5, 1975, which covered in detail how a regional forensic service could develop, with two centres for the EC, one in St Kitts, the other in Barbados, near the QEH, and later, at Mount Hope, in Trinidad, and one near to the campus at Mona). A later seminar on Forensics held in 1974 at Montego Bay, facilitated by Dr Lentz, an academic from the University of Pennsylvania, supported this plan.

An important presentation (Doc 23/73) by Dr J. Sejda, PAHO Zone adviser on epidemiology, dealt with the high incidence of microbial diseases in the region, and the need for surveillance and preventive measures, including immunisation; a cholera epidemic had reached West Africa, and required actions in America to avert the threat. He suggested that the Trinidad Regional Virus Laboratory (TRVL) — then limping along awaiting a decision on its future — become an epidemiology centre for regional education, service and continued research. TRVL had been founded in 1953, jointly by the Rockefeller Foundation and the Trinidad Government, under American virologist Dr Wilbur Downs. In 1964, it became affiliated with the Microbiology Department of UWI, with Dr Leslie Spence, a West Indian, as Senior Lecturer and head, later Professor, replacing Dr Downs, who had retired, having gained a global reputation for TRVL and himself. The unit maintained its status under Professor Spence, finding and characterising several new viruses.

In 1968, Rockefeller had decided to end funding of virus research in Trinidad, which had to take over the laboratory, until arrangements could be made for its continuation. Williams was peeved that Jamaica was not interested in partnering, despite his reminder that T&T had invested heavily in Jamaica. But Jamaica felt it was too far to get any benefits from viral research or routine epidemiology, 1000 miles away. As funds declined, Professor Spence left for Toronto.

Dr A. Jonkers, a Rockefeller virologist — who had come to TRVL in 1961, with Dr E. Tikasingh, a T&T microbiologist and entomologist, and Dr Aitkens, a virologist — became acting head and continued the field work, though curtailed, and kept the laboratory going. CHMC passed Res 19/73 urging each Caribbean country with over 200,000 population to set up an epidemiology unit within its Health Ministry, and update immunisations and reporting of communicable diseases. In 1975, TRVL became the Caribbean Epidemiology Centre (CAREC) run by PAHO (p. 215). In 1977, it welcomed Suriname as a contributing member.

The aftermath of CHMC V saw strenuous efforts to get our new programs going, particularly Family and Community Medicine, and a revised curriculum implementing the ideas on pp. 53-8, and to advance the EC scheme, PGME having taken promising root in Jamaica. The value and status of allied health workers were acknowledged by Jamaica's MOH, which granted professional status to several: Laboratory Technologists, Physiotherapists, and Radiographers initially, later others, and thus made them registrable. Other aides and assistants were also recognised as needed contributors to health care. My office had supported the submission by the Society of Medical Technologists, WI, (SMT,WI), and up to 1972, I had served as Chair of its Education Committee and Examinations Board, *ad personam*. It was well-organised and capably administered by Vic Elliott, its Chairman, and Mr. Gool Khan, Chief Education officer *(see group photo, p 112)*, both of whom had advised technical groups in the EC. Jamaica had taken this step, while its CHMC partners were still considering the issue. We had supported physiotherapists, radiographers and other technical grades, as listed in the IADB report, and their training at the recently-founded Community College at Papine, near the UHWI.

Our work became known to Commonwealth groups. In spring 1973, I received an invitation from the Commonwealth Foundation to speak at a Seminar at Sussex University, Aug 31 to September 2, 1973 on *"The Role of the New University in the Training of Medical Ancillaries."* The paper was published by the Commonwealth Foundation *(Bibliography)* and a copy sent to Philip Boyd, Executive Secretary of CHMC. Hon. Ken McNeill quoted it at CHMC VI in Bahamas, 10-14 June, 1974, as a blueprint for joint action by Governments and Universities in broadening the scope of manpower training to cover all health care needs. He later sent us a letter of congratulations *(Appendix 15.4, p. 359)*. His Ministry had agreed to fund the training of nurse-practitioners in Paediatrics, General Practice and probably Psychiatry, to add to the program for nurse-anaesthetists already started. It wished also to train 600 community health aides in the first phase of a project to provide basic, essential and simple services in community health centres.

With its interest in manpower development, and pursuing objectives of the World Health Assembly, PAHO convened a *Pan-American Conference on Health Manpower Planning,* in Ottawa Canada, from 10-14 September, 1973. The host, Health Minister Hon. Marc Lalonde, boasted of Canada's self-sufficiency in health manpower, but the plenary address did not permit questioning. The meeting allowed me to get first hand data on Cuban methods, and from others outside CHMC with comparable problems. I led the Working Group discussing *New Health*

Occupations, (Appendix 1.2, p. 295), which fitted neatly with views expressed in my Commonwealth Foundation lecture.

Colleagues from Latin America and Surinam were there, and shared our views on Community Medicine. Dr Ramón Casanova gave details of the Cuban build-up of manpower and its high achievement of national health coverage and primary care goals. Dr Wim van Kanten of Surinam updated me on advances made in the Paramaribo medical school since Standard and I had visited in 1972, and Matron Rita Somaroo of the Academic Hospital, Paramaribo, gave full details of their plans for Advanced Nursing Education, in the face of nursing losses by migration to Holland, due largely to partisan political pressures, unrest, and violence, as in Guyana and Jamaica. We had much in common. The emigrants included their chief pathologist, and several physicians.

I told them of the visit to Martinique with Alan Butler and Matthew Beaubrun, after the Dominica meeting, at the invitation of Dr St Cyr, the Chief Surgeon and Head of the City (Fort de France) Hospital, where we discussed an affiliation with UWI Medical Faculty, the concept of *nègritude* that Aimé Césaire had popularised there, before WWII. Spurred by independence and US civil Rights, it was now spreading in the Caribbean and the mainland, and had caused unrest in the EC, especially Trinidad and Guyana, after the visit of racist Stokely Carmichael (p. 18).

We also discussed Francophone interest in independence. I liked the idea of affiliation, as with Surinam, but I spoke against independence, after hearing details of current economic status, social mobility and educational opportunities inherent in internal self-rule status. The only gains would be poverty and social struggles as the islands began to face the high costs of independence, as each Anglophone island was discovering, with distress. The French islands remained with France.

Speaking for Surinam, van Kanten regretted the time that they *had* to spend to persuade politicians to settle differences, rule for all, and build a country. But for the instability, he would have had us back. They felt isolated politically, and so we discussed CARIFTA, which they wished to join; I knew that Burnham wanted to extend the Caribbean Common Market to include Cuba, Haiti and Santo Domingo (the Dominican Republic). Why not Surinam? It might help with the border dispute.

Carlyle Burton, head of the Barbados civil service, delivered the concluding address in Ottawa, in which he hoped that we could *"look forward to the solution of perennial domestic rivalries and suspicions, and to the time when it can be seen that without loss of face, the autonomy of the university can be preserved through service to the community."* He had echoed my thoughts. This was a role that I supported in my Commonwealth Foundation paper (p. 177). I saw it as enhancing, not threatening the status of the University, but so many at UWI thought it almost belittling.

It was also a corollary to Marc Lalonde's revealing what he called the *"Health Field concept"* of causation of disease and mortality, which we had begun years ago to emphasise, not in those words, in our lectures in Pathology, as pathobiology, environment, life-style choices and health service facilities. To me, it was fulsome self-praise with new words for an old concept. In fact, in the fifties our clinical histories on each patient had to include notes on diet, family, social and economic concerns, work, recreation, etc. ("life style"). In those days, student files were reviewed and probably marked. The trend towards probing personal and group issues gave way to the mass of data flowing from pathobiological advances, and the flood of new antibiotics and other drugs, which displaced prevention, and made it almost obsolete!

Our views on Community Medicine were welcomed by certain Canadians, notably Bill Cochrane from University of Calgary, and we visited them and the Family Medicine unit at the University of British Columbia. No one we met was interested in paramedical training, since, in Canada, that was done in Community Colleges, which did not want to lose turf by risking formal curricular union with the higher body.[35] Travelling allowed me to start work on a book on Medical Education, with Dr Alberto Cristoffanini of Universidad Austral, Chile, for PAFAMS, to be published in Spanish and English *(Appendix 12, p. 341)*.

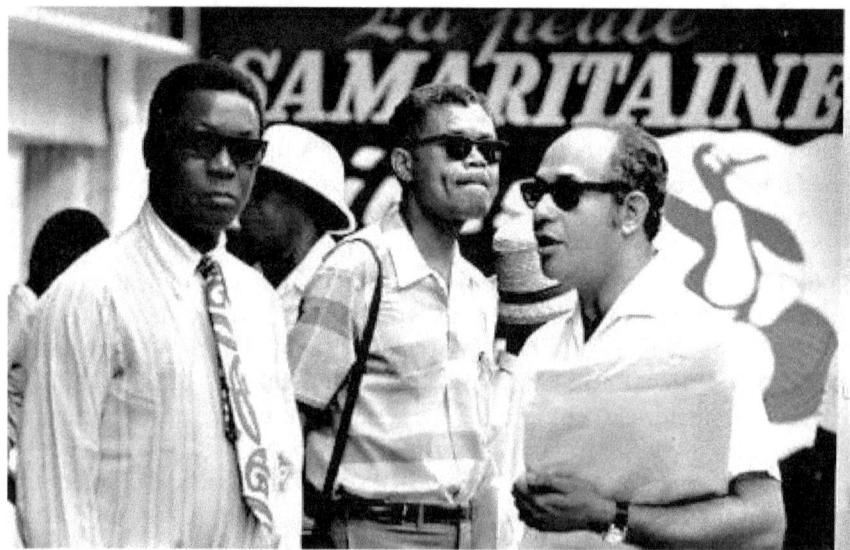

Fig 20-1: *Vice Dean(EC), Butler, and Dean's advisers. Prof George Ling, Head of Pharmacology, University of Ottawa, Canada, and Dr Matt Beaubrun,Caribbean Medical Education Council, leaving Martinique after the post-CHMC V seminar on Caribbean Medical education.*

---

[35] Decades later Mohawk College and McMaster University in Hamilton ON, would develop closer liaison and conjoint programs in certain fields, e.g. engineering.

CHAPTER 21
Assessing the programs — as others saw us: the dreamer

Apart from the continuous review and feedback that we received from our colleagues in the University, Governments, PAHO, HOPE and from time to time, British external examiners and members of PAFAMS, we were visited by several persons and agencies, most of which were North American, and sceptical of our ability to undertake PGME and other innovations. In 1971, however, John Bennett of CMA (p. 92) had been so impressed with our plan that he suggested that CMA might approve a grant towards Faculty administration. We heard no more from CMA; after hearing me at the *Fourth PAFAMS Conference on Medical Education* in Toronto, 28-30 August, 1972, styled *Education for Decision Making*, the CMA maintained its positive opinion, but the Association of Canadian Medical Colleges (ACMC), which co-hosted the meeting, was so sceptical they commissioned Milan Korcok, a free-lance medical journalist, to investigate.

His interview was in 1973; the report, p. 190, entitled *"Medical brain drain from Caribbean subsidizes Canada,"* appeared in CMAJ, 1974: 110, 1089-1092. It presented a choppy account of the Faculty and of my views. He had, as if to preserve existing biases, left out most of the more important and fundamental points, caveats, expectations and program details, including positive developments that would have made our plan coherent, thoughtful and plausible, as John Bennett had concluded in Bermuda. Instead, his article was superficial and projected the prevailing Canadian scepticism that any serious new discovery or advance could be made in a poor country. A few excerpts from his article illustrate:

"... Dr Ragbeer feels the Caribbean area can become self-sufficient in terms of specialist physicians...within a decade... Some Canadian observers who have been involved in development of Caribbean Health Services have a jaundiced view of this degree of optimism. They doubt the possibility of self-sufficiency for a good long time regardless of the postgraduate programs, regardless of the "social consciousness" of the emergent student population. ...Canada in the course of one year provides between 200 and 2000 physicians to provide health care and teaching assistance in one form or another....IDRC, CIDA, CMA and CUSO are among active contributors of personnel, equipment and/or money." Another exaggeration was *"students are... run off their feet providing service to the point they don't have time to take structured instruction;"* I had ascribed this to student leaders at Mona, but they denied that.

He had wildly exaggerated Canadian support, which was usually scattered throughout the islands, mostly near resorts, consisting *mainly* of tax dodgers. Many came to the Social sciences and Humanities Faculties; few under the aegis of the Faculty of Medicine, which was giving the USA and Canada about 50 residents yearly, costing some $10 million, much more than Canadian aid to us, as the title of his article conceded. In 1972, I had asked CIDA for support, and renewed the request in 1973, when we reported on progress to CHMC. They made an offer, which we had refused, as the terms diluted our agenda, and gave Canada more say and more benefits than we got: all help and materials must be Canadian, even if cheaper locally or elsewhere, and we would have to train, house and pay travel and other local costs for the technical help offered. The HOPE aid cost Jamaica just housing. I had said this to Don Ferguson, a Canadian aid agent (IDRC), who privately agreed that the terms were onerous; so did VC Preston when I reported it; *"short term gain for long term loss,"* was his comment. Korcok had obviously stuck to stereotypes, and could not believe that we were serious about self-sufficiency.

Another flagrant piece of condescension was the doubt that we could achieve our aim: *"...foreign observers maintain a high skepticism about UWI's attempts at self-sufficiency in the foreseeable future. Specialization is impractical in countries where primary care is so obviously the major deficiency. They say the search is counterproductive in that a person trained to such heights will be an unlikely candidate to ever stay home;... the forging of a new health system in which young people would want to work will remain just a dream."*

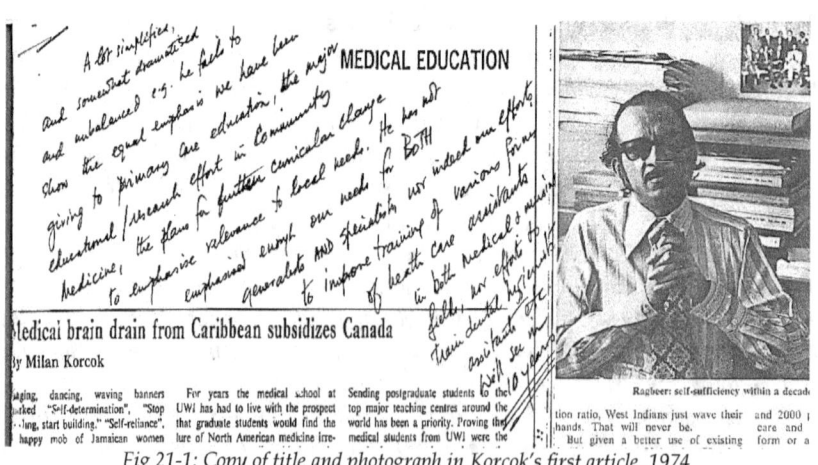

Fig 21-1: Copy of title and photograph in Korcok's first article, 1974

Korcok grudgingly conceded, *"Though Ragbeer's projections may be optimistic, the thrust of his argument is hard to contest – that changes and development has (sic) to be stimulated from within."* Despite repeated correction, he maintained that the UWI Faculty ran the islands' health services, and blamed the services for "poor accounting" to understate their external aid! In 1974, I wrote, re Korcok's article, *"A lot simplified, and somewhat dramatised and unbalanced; for example, he fails to show the emphasis we have been giving to primary care education, the major educational/research thrust in Community Medicine, the plans for a new curriculum that would prepare students for any line of practice, teaching or research, from primary to tertiary care, and emphasise relevance to local needs. He did not emphasise... our needs for both generalists and specialists, nor indeed our efforts to improve training of various forms of health care assistants in both medical and nursing fields, nor efforts to train dental hygienists, assistants, etc. We'll see in ten years!" (See fig 21-1).*

A decade later, he returned for the kill, to review the doubts that he had previously publicised; he wrote instead, tail tucked between legs, *"Jamaica's medical school, high quality on a low budget"* (Fig 21-2).

Jamaica's medical school: high quality on a low budget

MILAN KORCOK

Like the nations that are its bene-

sewage services taxes the financial resources earmarked for health care and social services. But then the English-speaking Caribbean nations have learned that despite the help

sion. So when North American medical leaders casually lump the UWI medical faculty in with the offshore schools, men like Dr. Samuel Wray, dean of the UWI faculty of medi-

Fig 21-2: Title of Korcok's second CMAJ article. CMAJ, 1984: 131: 66

It contained a catalogue of the measures developed and implemented in my Deanship, and how well they had turned out. But, even then, he got the school's name wrong, and failed to mention his earlier patronising criticisms, or that the various successes were the very ones I had shown him ten years earlier, crediting only the "Faculty" (or perhaps his sources chose to do that). Yet I recognised each verbatim piece of my writing and other quoted work, all without credit. An embarrassed Sam Wray, whom I met at a PAFAMS meeting in Bogota, and agreed to cover for him there, as he had come down with "a cold," chalked it up to "Korcok's error." In fact, the Faculty had forgotten the days when every new development was left to me as Dean; was it, I asked in pique, in the hope that I would fail? Instead, in the face of PM Manley's social adventures that scared more Jamaicans away, I stuck to it for three years heading three offices: the Dean's, Coordinator of PGME, and Director of Community Medicine!

At a meeting of the Administrative Committee of PAFAMS in Rio de Janeiro in 1976, I had been asked to comment on progress of the UWI program in PGME. One of my colleagues referred to a 1972 article in the *West Indian Medical Journal* on PGME (*Figure 21-3*), and to another published in 1976; he expressed surprise that I had succeeded in implementing the specialty training program at a time when many Latin

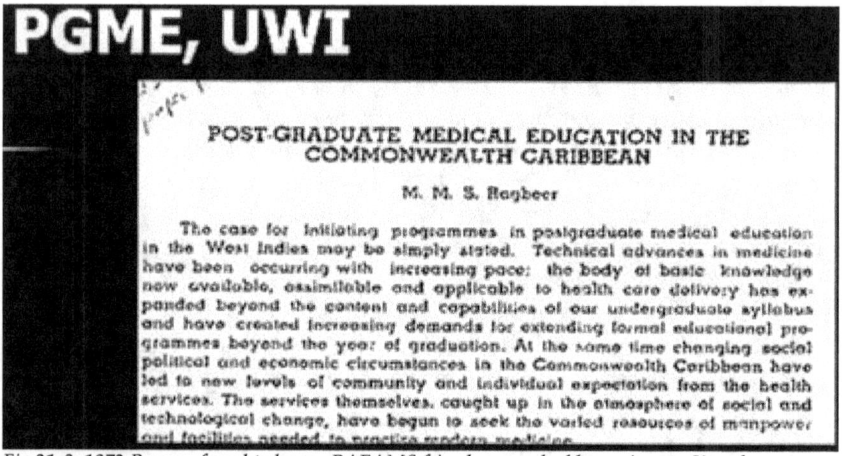

PGME, UWI

POST-GRADUATE MEDICAL EDUCATION IN THE
COMMONWEALTH CARIBBEAN

M. M. S. Ragbeer

The case for initiating programmes in postgraduate medical education in the West Indies may be simply stated. Technical advances in medicine have been occurring with increasing pace; the body of basic knowledge now available, assimilable and applicable to health care delivery has expanded beyond the content and capabilities of our undergraduate syllabus and have created increasing demands for extending formal educational programmes beyond the year of graduation. At the same time changing social political and economic circumstances in the Commonwealth Caribbean have led to new levels of community and individual expectation from the health services. The services themselves, caught up in the atmosphere of social and technological change, have begun to seek the varied resources of manpower and facilities needed to practice modern medicine.

Fig 21-3: 1972 Paper referred to by my PAFAMS friend; a copy had been given to Korcok.

American medical schools were grappling with the problem of primary care medicine, and the difficulty in finding enough teaching beds for undergraduates. I told him that we had the same problems with change, and had to go about solutions gingerly, to avoid the many ruts along the way. "More than that," he said, half smiling, "you couldn't succeed in what we think is one of the most daring medical education programs in Latin America and the Caribbean, by being, as Americans say, "chicken!" He had assured me of ongoing PAFAMS support, "even though we cannot help with funds." Figures in Table E-1 *(Epilogue p. 261)*, show the output of specialists, with an 88% retention rate to 2008, virtually ending the "brain drain." Korcok and other nay-sayers should have noted that by 1984 there were over 50 specialists with an MS or DM degree, and 130 or more with diplomas. Twelve PhDs and 25 MScs had been completed in the basic sciences, and 4 were on the way to an M.Phil. When I reported this in 1984 at the PAFAMS meeting in Bogota, to an audience knowing of our struggle, the applause was brisk.

In Rio, I spoke in defence of Community Medicine to Dr Carlyle Macedo, then head of manpower training for PAHO in Brasilia; he accepted my argument that the personnel solution for a Caribbean island was more in line with that of Cuba than Brazil or the USA, achieving the USA's indices for life expectancy and infant mortality at one-tenth the cost. (Later, he would succeed Hector Acuña as Director of PAHO.)

Dr J.Z. Bowers of Josiah Macy Jr Foundation, and a member of the IADB Committee, was, like CIDA and IDRC, cool on PGME, doubting that we could do it alone. He supported training of ancillaries, "loved" my paper (p. 150) and, like Professor Cruickshank, felt that the "left hand side" of our curriculum and skills plan (p. 56), a non-university area, should be actively promoted. We agreed on the need for ancillaries, and I told him of Jamaica's intention to train them *and* specialists, and had contributed towards a building, eight residents, nurse practitioners, and health care aides. But aides could not supply specialist services, and we had an obligation to complete the upper rungs of the skills ladder (pp. 56-57) where fewer, costlier, but essential personnel were needed to run the health care machine. In April 1974, noting the progress we had made in PGME, and nearing our first examinations in Internal Medicine and Paediatrics, he relented, offered commendations, and invited me to speak at a seminar in Paediatrics he had arranged with the Barbados Paediatric Association, to coincide with a UWI Council meeting, thus allowing Faculty members from Mona to attend. He supported our plan to start Family Medicine training and would consider contributing to a brainstorming meeting on the matter. I couldn't give him a date as Dr Dyer was yet to give me his recommendations (p. 279).

As customary on visits to the EC, I met with students and interns, who wished to discuss concerns:

A. *They were disgruntled, mainly in Trinidad, due to:*
1. lack of supervision leading to the belief that they could go directly into a private practice after internship, since they had grown accustomed to working unsupervised, with no knowledge of outcomes;
2. difficulty in getting some members of senior staff to assist;
3. night duty exceeding one night in three;
4. virtual absence of liaison between staff and Ministry (MOH);
5. the policy of MOH not to make appointments to the Port of Spain hospital until peripheral posts were filled.

B. *Their Interests:*
1. They were interested in PGME; we discussed the pros and cons. I reminded them that the program had already started and had just graduated its first physician. Some doubted whether T&T was ready to participate, in view of A1 above.
2. Proper training of GPs was essential as local GPs referred everything, since they seemed unable to perform even simple procedures. This applied less to UWI graduates with Mona training. We discussed, and they welcomed the plan re Family Medicine (FM) and Community Medicine (CM), but didn't think that any would spend four years to train in FM, when they could complete it in Canada in two. I agreed that it was too long.
3. They and their colleagues in Barbados had noted that few Barbadian students had taken part in the Barbados program between 1968 and 1974 (27/143, nine of those in 1974, much to the relief of the Barbados MOH); this was a baffling observation,

which had more to do with social barriers in that island than medical conditions. Jamaican students had taken up 63 of 143 Barbados slots, the others 48. By contrast, the 158 places in Trinidad were taken up by 105 T&T students, 30 Jamaicans, 6 Barbadians and 17 from other territories. Random interviews of students opting for the EC did not show a clear correlation with the political unrest in Jamaica.

Vice Dean Butler and Associate Dean Bartholomew were fully aware of the issues, and had brought them to the attention of department heads and the PMO, but had to face the sloth embedded in the civil service, where, incredibly, all might agree to change but seemed paralysed by the persistence of colonial hindrances that should have been expunged a decade earlier from their operating manuals. This was the same issue we had urged members of CHMC to revise urgently, and amend or discard much of the Colonial Regulations.

In 1972, however, the doubters were many, supporters staunch, even though we lost a few professors. But at least, I could savour the appreciation from Chancellor Hall, my undergraduate residence after Gibraltar Hall, when the Warden and Hall Committee decided to honour "high-achieving alumni" and named me one of the five *Super Lions* awarded that first year, 1972, along with Drs Ken Standard and a KPH urologist, Lawson Douglas. The other honorees were PJ Patterson, later PM of Jamaica, and Eric Abrahams, Jamaica Tourist Board. (Fig 21-4).

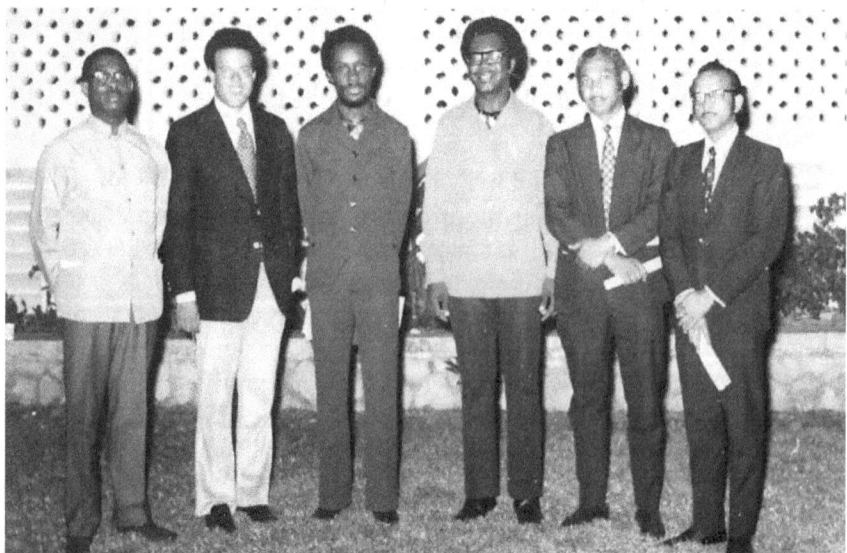

Fig 21-4: The first "Super Lions" of Chancellor Hall, UWI, 1972, with Hall Warden Winston Wright, third from right. From left, Prof. K L Standard, Mr. Eric Abrahams, Mr. P J Patterson, Dr Lawson Douglas and Dean M. Ragbeer. The selection committee was chaired by PVC Leslie Robinson, a meticulous mathematician.   (Photo by Anthony Ham Phong, medical student.)

CHAPTER 22
"Quenching Fires"

There were many fires to quench, as the campus became restive with the surge in gun battles between rival political street gangs in West Kingston and the increasing tempo and temerity of the violence from gunslingers like *Feathermop, Burry Boy* (PNP) and JLP's Massop. It crept into the campus, and threatened housing areas. Security had increased and we were deeply concerned with the safety of temporary staff from HOPE. But before these, the most serious for me and the Faculty was the "impeachment" in 1972 of Keith Manchester, a bright young scientist (a year younger than I was). He had been appointed head of Biochemistry in Prof. Cruickshank's deanship, despite lack of administrative or leadership experience, a choice forced by scarcity of applicants. He soon proved incompetent as head, with no latent skill in administration, suspicious and adamantly unwilling to learn or delegate. But he was stoutly defended by TMRU's Picou and Alleyne.

He had a record of good experimental work, done solo, with more than a hint of unwillingness to share, which blossomed in the first year of his contract. Complaints of biases and arbitrary and exclusive use of departmental resources for his own work, of failure to consult, of frank denial of requests from some staff, of overloading of some staff with teaching, of preventing use of refrigerated centrifuges—admittedly obtained with his research grant—but not all was black and white, a terrible phrase, as he was white and his main complainant, a suave black man, Dr Chris Kean, with impeccable good manners. The complaints had reached two earlier Deans: Eric Cruickshank and Ken Stuart, having been filtered through Vice-Dean Hoyte, who had signed off, saying that he was too close to the issue, and in any case tended to side with Manchester, as his critics had become too subjective or insistent.

The matter had dragged on, and hardly had I become accustomed to my chair, met a delegation of biochemists and organic chemists: Chris Kean, E V Ellington, Alan Fincham, Gerry Quashe, and Murchison Wilson. I promised action, but maybe not satisfaction. I called Manchester for a meeting, suggesting his office, but he declined, and complained to the VC re jurisdiction: was he responsible to my office, or direct to the VC, as the formal structure stated? I had agreed, but noted that I was trying to help with an issue within my responsibility for staff and student welfare, curriculum, examinations, etc. I was glad that he contacted the Vice-Chancellor, whom I had briefed on the issue, as I understood it, and on what I had done. A day or two later, the VC phoned to say he had told Manchester to see me, and that he had directed me to investigate and report. I could enlist any faculty input. Reluctantly, Manchester agreed.

We had met before on several occasions when I was Associate Dean for Education, and had had friendly and useful discourses. I generally considered him a sociable, though high-strung and secretive person. In our short phone conversation, he had said something damaging about his staff referring to the "aberrations" of two of them, who were known homosexuals, but neither flaunted his choice, or abused anyone; in fact their interpersonal relationships were as good as anyone else's. He accused one or more of the others of surreptitious and improper use of his centrifuges, so he had taken to detaching the heads whenever he left his laboratory, or otherwise disabling them.

When we met, he became very hostile and inflexible, so I told him that I would have my secretary come in, or I would tape-record the interview. He agreed to the latter. But I warned that we should address the complaints dispassionately, that I was neutral, and my performance would also be on record; my wish was to promote the integrity of the Faculty, its staff and property, without prejudice. He began to answer the question of resource use, including the specific one of centrifuges and equipment needs. I indicated that I would be willing to fill an urgent need, but he declined to give me a list, and maintained that he was the *only* scientist in the department, had become its head, and thus had first call on *all* its resources — people and equipment — and that the others should be willing to do as he chose, and not pry into his work!

He complained that he was disliked by all except Hope Calogero, the youngest staff member, and that the others were incompetent, did little work, and had not published much since he had come. He denied the allegation that his restrictions and sequestering of equipment had contributed to that. He had answered the complaints to Professor Hoyte's satisfaction, and had thought the matter settled. He went off on a tangent from that, in fact several sequential tangents, so that after a while, he was lost and couldn't trace his way back. The interview lasted over an hour, exhausted my tape, so the last ten minutes were not on record; however, I made full notes and verified them with him. I told him that in view of his accusations, I would meet with his staff, together or separately. I met them individually, as they had chosen.

Accusations were repeated and consistent among staff; even Hope Calogero, who took his side, agreed that he "tended to be high-handed." I asked Prof. Hoyte whether he had any opinions about Manchester's state of mind, as many of his actions and behaviour suggested a personality or behavioural disorder, and I would seek an opinion from Professor Beaubrun, of Psychiatry, after clearing with Manchester.

Hoyte had not thought his behaviour too strange for "a dedicated researcher", nor was his secretiveness unusual for someone who felt he was on the edge of a key discovery, a new enzyme or metabolic pathway, something like the Cori cycle. Manchester on the telephone rejected the idea of Beaubrun (I had told him the conversation was being recorded, which he accepted resentfully), ranted about conditions generally, the scarce resources, the likelihood of colleagues stealing his work, stressing his "ownership" of departmental resources, and lastly, my incompetence in that matter and in everything else, or words to that effect.

The VC, with a career in legal academics, responded by suggesting to me that my report raised questions of administrative competence, and behavioural pathology, that he would consult others and that he would make sure that Manchester and I were party to the findings. Professional opinion, including Professor Beaubrun's, with my tapes on record, and Manchester confirming his part, led to the conclusion that I could seek his dismissal from the headship on medical grounds, under University regulations, by "impeaching" him before the Academic Board.

I took this, a most serious step, after consultation with Department Heads. Manchester had underestimated me, and had widely claimed that he and his clinical friends would ruin me, after our exchanges. He chose Prof. Hoyte as his advocate, which Hoyte, gentleman that he was, accepted after warning me of his conflict, since he was also a Vice-Dean. I told him I was glad that Manchester had chosen him, since he was generally regarded as one of the most knowledgeable, methodical, fair and eloquent members of the Faculty. He stood for principle and agreed that department heads "must manage the resources of the department," which, however, included proper training of users of equipment.

But Manchester had neglected to ensure the general academic progress of the department, and to promote the welfare of his staff. His choice of method had produced discord and unhappiness in the staff and stagnation in his department, except for his work and that of Gerry Quashe, who had an independent grant, and generally avoided the "confusion," as he had told me in testimony, though he was aware of the general unrest and almost toxicity in the department.

In the hearings before the Academic Board, I used the ploy, towards the end of my testimony, of needling him, after I had presented my case and been cross-examined by Hoyte. I admitted the tendency of some department heads to regard departmental resources as proprietary, but he was unique among Faculty heads in being so inflexible. I criticised the concept as invalid, and was not surprised that it had contributed to retard the academic progress of his staff, and thereby reducing the discipline to a "one-man show." In this, he had failed in a prime role as "head": to lead a team of scholars and teachers.

At this, he exploded and called his staff lazy and incompetent, praised himself, and accused me of bias and weakness, and "too lazy to find out what was really happening." Hoyte tried to silence him on that score, but Manchester was on a roll and continued ranting, blaming, insulting, and accusing his staff, person by person, and me for listening to them and "encouraging" them, when Hoyte knew, from the beginning of the affair, that I had done all I could to placate the staff, without having a fund to finance a separate laboratory. Manchester's rant of incompetence had included most faculty members!

The assembly was stunned; silence blanketed the room, except for his voice. Then, that too was overcome by the silence, and he sat down. Hoyte gently put his left arm around his shoulder, and comforted him like a child. Manchester's face was red, his eyes wide and staring, his breathing rapid and shallow, panting like a pup after a run. I felt sorry at that time that he had so revealed himself. The child, frantically protecting his toys from bullies, who would rob him of them, and do them harm.

VC Marshall dismissed the "litigants," to allow the assembly to consider a decision. Manchester was relieved of the headship, and terminated, with a year's leave, on the grounds of illness, and a recommendation for psychiatric review and care. I went to see him, with Prof. Hoyte; he received me with a stare, almost unknowing, and was quiet and polite. He seemed depressed. I urged his colleagues to see him and otherwise give whatever support they could. I had to take over as head of Biochemistry until a replacement was found, as none of the others wished to assume the headship, even temporarily. Thus, I had to serve and did so for the entire year 1973, in addition to my job and two enforced "headships" of PGME and Community Medicine. Finally, Chris Kean agreed to act as Head, enabling me to revert to my three professorships for the remaining two years as Dean!

In recommending the acting headship, I remarked in jest that I had saved the Bursar a minimum of US $200,000 over a 3-year period. Zach Preston, then VC, smilingly acknowledged this in 1975, when he chaired the meeting that denied me paid leave, which he had backed, based on eligibility for sabbatical. Three were granted that year, when PVC Lalor, my nemesis, in charge of the rankings, blithely announced my exclusion, having placed me sixth on his list of six! I have no doubt that those three and some unnamed slush fund benefitted from my toil.

In the late sixties, students were caught up in the Black power movement; Afros and long sideburns began to sprout everywhere, even on white heads. Caribbean 'nationalism' was flaunted by many, and overwhelmed some Jamaicans, especially with the intensifying socialism of Michael Manley, whose victory over Edward Seaga happened just when I had hoped to get the latter to sign the PGME approvals. But the trend had odd effects on some people, one of whom was George Locke, a somewhat eccentric friend, of the 1961 class, whom I had gotten to know through a shared interest in photography and audio; he was a member of the University Photographic Club, of which I was Secretary when he joined. His mother was a nurse in the US (?NY), who pampered him, filling his wants, trivial or not, for audiovisual and other toys.

He had disappeared from Jamaica after graduating in 1961, and had returned in 1971-2, having completed training in Neurosurgery, in Britain and Canada (Alberta). He was seeking a position at the UHWI in Neurosurgery, but there wasn't a vacancy then. He had also applied directly to the University for a lectureship, the usual route for applicants, since up to then all applications were handled centrally, and decisions on filling posts were made by the cumbersome and tardy method of Registry screening, referral to department concerned, striking a selection board, notifying the Faculty Dean—more from courtesy than for any decisive input, yet every position had a teaching function of importance to the Dean's duty as chief education officer; as expected, departments guarded their roles quite jealously.

Although lectureships were available by direct application to the University Registry, I was tacitly allowed to "divert" the medical ones to my office for screening by the Faculty Appointments and Promotions Committee, one of the new ones approved by the Faculty Board. I had also obtained a similar privilege to have related communications sent to me; thus I came to be forewarned of matters before the Committees. George Locke's application was one. It had originally been referred directly to the Department of Surgery. He was informed that there was no vacancy and that his application would be kept on file. Jim Cross of Trinidad had been appointed earlier as a second neurosurgeon. Locke had established contact with the Kingston Public Hospital and it seemed that some arrangement had been made to accommodate him pending a check of his references.

His criticisms had revived an older rant against the Head of Surgery, Professor Harry Annamunthodo, the cause and sequel of which I have so far been unable to ascertain. I reproduce it here just to show the kind of chauvinism that was displayed by over-enthusiastic nationals, and which I had to deal with several times. I could not find the letters alluded to by the writer, who had sheltered under the sobriquet, *Sinnombre,* (Nameless); his letter had appeared on November 16, 1966 in the *Daily Gleaner,* Jamaica's major daily, and a well-reputed paper.

"*The Editor, Sir:-*

The alien enclave at Mona is once again being vocal and verbose than constructive (sic). The Professor of Surgery has for the second time in a year accused the Jamaican doctors of being more interested in "the few" and their Trade Union activities than in the health problems of the community.

The Professor of Surgery should have refrained from his holier than thou outbursts as:-

He is a foreigner who has never practised medicine in Jamaica and can know little or nothing of the problems of the Jamaican doctors.

His emoluments (taking into consideration leave pension, house, entertainment allowance etc.) come to no less than £6,000 per annum, which is more than most local doctors earn. This job security frees him from the worries of his less fortunate professional brethren.

It is unseemly (and in some cases unethical) for medical men to write this type of attack of one of their colleagues in the lay press.

Of course the Medical Association functions as a Trade Union (the dirty word). So do Medical Associations in all parts of the world. Surely The Professor of Surgery must have taken part in "negotiations" more than once in his time in Jamaica. Or is he above soiling his hands with filthy lucre?

The background of the Professor's effusion is the smug mentality of the foreigners at Mona. By and large they suffer from Mona inertia and a feeling of superiority very common in many egg-head types. Far from helping to improve our country they are continually shooting off with disturbing and divisive diatribes.

I am, etc.,

Sinnombre

What is important here is not so much the identity of the writer as the tone of his criticism, the personal attack and the focus on "foreigner," which rankled, as the surgeon was a Jamaican citizen. How happy we would have been if a few foreigners had responded then to our need for other staff! The qualified Jamaicans had long fled or were thinking of fleeing. The writer had made many errors and presumed a level of idleness among UHWI surgical staff that was, to say the least, fanciful. So when George Locke wrote accusing the Faculty and University of bias in appointments, of appointing "unqualified" people, and of overlooking his training in neurosurgery, it reminded older heads of this earlier letter, not likely from George. He declined my request for a meeting.

A columnist for the *Daily Gleaner*, Morris Cargill, a lawyer, who wrote as *Thomas Wright*, commented on Locke's complaint, and wrote us, asking for a response. I discussed this with Sir Harry Annamunthodo, head of Surgery, founding member of the *Association of Surgeons in Jamaica*, and knighted in 1967, who gave me the above background, but had heard nothing from Locke. After consulting the Vice-Chancellor, I wrote to Mr. Cargill.

University of the West Indies

Dean's Office
Faculty of Medicine
Mona, Kingston 7

Morris Cargill, Esq.
Charlottenburg,
Highgate, St Mary

12 October, 1973

Dear Mr. Cargill,

Many thanks for your considerate letter of September 4th, 1973 regarding the Locke affair. I was out of the country on Faculty business when your letter came, and illness on my return, followed by pressing problems on campus, of which you are aware, have prevented me from giving the sustained attention, which your letter and Dr Locke's require for a reasoned reply. I hope you do forgive me then for the long delay in replying.

I am saddened to read Dr Locke's letter, not so much by the tone of it, but by the pathetic obstinacy with which he has chosen to pursue the matter, even though he must know that his arguments are based on assertions and semantic niceties, rather than upon an objective evaluation of facts.

I will not answer Dr Locke's letter point by point, but will present you instead with the facts as they are currently available, and in so doing hope to cover the areas of difficulty or disagreement.

Neurosurgeons, like most other professionals, are trained by different countries in different ways. All training programs however have one basic general aim, that is, to ensure that the professional who, on completion of training and establishes practice as a neurosurgeon, is knowledgeable and skilled in neurosurgery and possesses certain desirable attitudes to his patients, to the community, to the profession and to learning in general.

In any system, the ascent up the ladder of professional responsibility requires that the trainees show certain definable aptitudes and capabilities at successively higher and more complex levels of training. All systems therefore set minimum standards of professional competence before recognition is accorded. Training programs aim to satisfy or exceed these minima, and are in general conducted under the auspices of a nationally accredited examining body. It is recognised that trainees will become – or at least some of them will– future leaders in the field, and should therefore be able to think for themselves, to continue their education, once on their own, to contribute to the education of others and to the further development of the profession. Various stratagems and devices are used in different places, according to local experiences, laws, styles and resources, to achieve these ends. Therefore it is not necessarily profitable to pursue the argument on differences between the techniques of one system and those of another. What is important is that all are concerned with pursuing excellence in training and in professional activity, and that the person who is accepted as a neurosurgeon within a system is therefore a recognised and qualified neurosurgeon within that system.

In Canada, all postgraduate training is regulated by the Royal College of Physicians and Surgeons of Canada. Neurosurgeons require five years of residency training after internship (see attached regulations) of which thirty months are in neurosurgery, after a basic year in surgery. The remaining 18 months can be spent in a variety of options related to the practice of neurosurgery. These are minimum requirements. A candidate satisfactorily completing the program may apply for and be granted permission to take the examinations. If he passes, he obtains a "certificate" and can describe himself as "certified". He may thereupon apply for admission to the R.C.P.S.(C) as a Fellow; certified applicants are automatically admitted upon paying the appropriate fee, and thereafter can use the letters FRCS(C) after their names.

U.S. training is similar in concept. The examining body is the Board of Neurological Surgery, which stipulates a minimum 4 years of training after completion of preliminaries. Those who wish to take the examination must do a further two years of practice. Foreigners are not required to do this compulsory additional training (but see regulations attached). Passing the examination leads to receipt of a "certificate". No special letters are used after the doctor's name.

In the U.K., the custom has been for the prospective neurosurgeon to undergo training first in general surgery for about four years, qualify for the Fellowship of one of the Royal Colleges of Surgeons (England, Scotland or Ireland) then join a recognised neurosurgical unit (usually in a teaching hospital) for advanced training in Neurosurgery. In such a unit, under the tutelage of consultant neurosurgeons, he will be guided in the acquisition of the necessary knowledge, skills and attitudes required of the future consultant neurosurgeon. The period of neurosurgical training occupies in most instances three to four years, unless the individual has had prior accredited experience in neurosurgery or is especially apt or unusually gifted. In such instances the special training period may be shortened. The trainee is assessed continuously and the teaching unit will issue to any employing body the appropriate letters attesting to satisfactory completion. As no special diploma or certificate in Neurosurgery is issued, the individual is not "certified". He may seek accreditation by registering his qualifications with the General Medical Council, which will not register him as a neurosurgeon unless satisfied that he is one.

It is worth noting that the recommendations of the 1971 "Joint Committee on Higher Surgical Training" in the U.K., (excerpted by Dr Locke) include "certification" of specialists by the Royal Colleges, and are not significantly different from existing practices in that country.

Considerable nonsense is peddled, even by professionals, about the international value of medical qualifications, both basic and advanced. Professional (as distinct from academic) degrees, certificates, diplomas of one country are not automatically recognised by the licensing bodies of another (with the notable exception of certain British degrees in ex-colonial countries, *and vice versa). Normally a North American qualified neurosurgeon would not be eligible for a consultancy in the British National Health Service, purely on the basis of his North American experience. The reverse holds equally true for the British-trained person who wishes to work in North America.*

Our own system in the Commonwealth Caribbean is derived from the British. Most of our doctors were trained in it, whether here or in the U.K. Indeed, the UWI was nothing more than a transplant of London University. Others of our doctors were trained in the U.S.A., Canada, and in various countries of Europe, each country contributing its own peculiar variation on the basic theme. I would hesitate to issue judgements on the comparative value of each product to us in the Caribbean. We are now developing our own graduate training programs, with the same general aims stated earlier. We began some of them in January, 1972 and are developing others.

The final demonstration of one's specialist competence in any field of medicine must be the acceptance of peers, and of the community of medical professionals, both local and international. Such an acceptance will only come from confidence in the quality, reliability and validity of the specialist service offered. Quality will derive from painstaking effort and from a constant striving for improvement through actual problem-solving, not from empty proclamations or self-advertisement. In medicine as in everything else, the Caribbean has its fill of those who are content to talk and who believe that mere talking means achievement.

Neurosurgery has developed in the Caribbean through the quiet dedication of a few men who persisted, despite great odds, to build sound units of international acceptance. For example, neurosurgeons from Project HOPE who were among the most prestigious of American neurosurgeons during the visit of the ship here in 1970-71, were full of praise for the University Hospital's Neurosurgery Unit, its achievements and the collaborative efforts of UHWI-KPH teams. The UHWI unit has, over the past several years, been visited and given a good name by senior Canadian and British neurosurgeons. These are matters of record; indeed, in the HOPE personnel assistance program neurosurgeons are now on a low priority!

I would repeat therefore the information I gave you earlier, which you were good enough to publish. The persons I named are all bona fide neurosurgeons, accepted as such by their colleagues, both in neurosurgery and in other fields of medicine, locally and internationally.

I sense that Dr Locke is seeing "training by internationally recognised standards" as an end in itself rather than as a means to an end, and is emphasising it as the sole criterion of the real specialist, rather than seeing it in proper perspective. Perhaps he has forgotten that medical specialisation is still young and growing, and that specialist disciplines were developed by medical pioneers who had the wit to recognise areas of need, and the character to set about the arduous task of defining such needs and devising means to meet them. Such men trained themselves and set the standards! I hope that Dr Locke is not

203

suggesting that this type of innovation must stop, nor that we here must sit content to follow slavishly the patterns, styles and dictates of someone else. Surely we can show initiative, inventiveness and set high standards for the rest of the world. There are great challenges here in medicine for those with real intelligence and understanding.

For your confidential records, Drs. Ghouralal and Bagnall are, like Dr Locke, "certified" neurosurgeons, the former trained in the U.S.A. and the latter in Canada. Drs. Cross, Masson, McHardy, McKenzie and Supersad were trained in the British pattern. Dr Cross, for example, has worked in the U.K. as a locum consultant for the same gentleman, Dr Norman Guthkelch, under whom Dr Locke had previously served as a registrar.

In the past two years the University Hospital of the West Indies unit has performed some 580 surgical procedures, a commendable achievement. The Head of the Unit, Professor A.F.Masson, was almost singlehandedly responsible for the development, over the last twelve years, of the unit, which, in spite of difficulties, has been described as "an excellent neurosurgical service" by a well-known British neurosurgeon. Professor Masson himself has been highly praised for his pioneer efforts, for his personal knowledge, ability and character by high-ranking American, British and Canadian neurosurgeons.

The U.W.I. Medical Faculty is not yet a third-rate institution; mere assertions will not make it so. Indeed, a defence of our reputation is not necessary. The statistics on graduate losses to foreign countries speak for the quality of our products, and show the paradoxical position that while we are desperate to reduce this loss, we have to quote its occurrence as evidence of our standards!

I hope this long letter will help you get the matter right. If you need further information on, or clarification of anything I have written, please let me know.

With best wishes and personal regards,

Yours sincerely,

Mohan S. Ragbeer
Dean, Medical Faculty

cc VC Roy Marshall

In 1972 and 1973, interpersonal problems were common, at all levels of organisation, especially where older "colonials" clashed, through imposition of their norms on the younger independents and across racial lines. In Trinidad, at TRVL, a key part of our EC scheme, the domineering attitude of a senior administrator, Mrs. Lumsden, almost cost us two rare young lecturers: a microbiologist, Merle Balbirsingh, and a biochemist, Barbara Hull, both Trinidadians. The Director, Pierre Ardoin, had given up trying to understand or correct it. Dr. Balbirsingh had written me, and to her department head at Mona, Dr. Dorothy King, who had asked my help to intervene and settle the problem.

In her office, I advised Mrs. Lumsden about responsibilities and boundaries. But she remained obstinate, insisted on having her way, (*"we've always done it so!"*) and continued to conduct affairs as she had been allowed by past Caucasian bosses, despite the changed professional needs of the two scientists, a local Indian, and a dark coloured lady, her social "inferiors" in Trinidad society. I had to remind her of her role as their supporter and team-mate, not employer. She was naturally peeved at this, but after complaining to Dr. Ardoin, and learning more of the fate of TRVL, agreed to try my way. I took the two complainants to lunch, which Mrs. Lumsden declined, and explained to them what I had done and expected. On a later visit, I noted the improved relationships, but Mrs. Lumsden told me that she had decided to retire shortly.

In developing teaching activities in the Port Of Spain General Hospital (POSG), we had to overcome uncertain hospital policies, and the proprietary attitude of some consultants. The Ministry of Health (MOH) complained that the appointment of University staff created schisms. For example, the pathologist, Dr Jack Arneaud, who had started his career at Mona, and was then POSG's head of the Pathology Department, was displeased with the appointment of a University lecturer in Anatomic Pathology, Dr Prabhakar, complaining that Dr Prabhakar was nibbling at his referral practice, and giving service to a private hospital. We settled with Prabhakar, who showed us the very low numbers involved; he agreed to forego the referral income, and the private hospital visits, until a policy was agreed between the University department and the Government, while Arneaud conceded that he was entitled to any income from cases referred to him directly. At UWI, we did not charge for referrals from Government health services. I referred the matter of private fees to Professor Brooks for a ruling on policy.

In the Queen Elizabeth Hospital Laboratory, Bridgetown, Barbados —a critical need, like Radiology, to support the entire array of specialties—the head of the department, Dr. Errol Dos Santos and his associate, Dr. Harold White, both of whom I knew well professionally, were, like Dr Arneaud, concerned that they would lose income, if a UWI pathologist were appointed. We were able to dispel those fears, but found it much tougher to recruit a pathologist, when we eventually had the position approved. Barbados at that time also needed a radiologist, whom our friend in Bristol University, Prof. H. Middlemiss, head of its Department of Radiology, undertook to provide, as he had done for UHWI in seconding Drs Bateson and Moule. I visited Bristol in 1972 and met staff in other disciplines, interested in joint teaching and research projects, and quite fascinated with our program to train specialists. They agreed to help recruit for Barbados an anaesthetist; psychiatrist; ophthalmologist; orthopaedic surgeon and an ENT surgeon.

I was assured by Karl Massiah, a Barbadian, who had completed Orthopaedics residency training in Toronto, that he would accept the new Government position, provided we could get a University position in Pathology for his wife, Pamela da Camara, a Guyanese, who had also completed training in Toronto. Both were 1965 UWI graduates, who had begun specialty training at Mona – I was one of da Camara's supervisors in Pathology *(photo p. 112)*. They had been very vocal in support of the DM and MS programs, vowing to return to serve their *"alma mater."*

We secured the Pathology position, with Bras's support, after intense personal lobbying; I faced heavy criticism from Faculty specialists, who claimed that I was biased in pushing for the lectureship to be specified as "Pathologist" and not transferable. Massiah – who had been kept abreast of my efforts to secure the position, and to settle conditions with Dos Santos and White re consulting income – replied to my triumphant note, however, by *declining* on *their* behalf! Dr AJ Dutt was eventually secured for the post in Pathology.

In Jamaica, much had been done in the past two decades to achieve and retain good relationships between UHWI and Government doctors at Kingston Regional Hospital (KRH), which had hosted the first clinical year students, Oct., 1951 to Oct., 1952. The program was transferred then to the UCHWI, which was formally opened a year later, in Nov., 1953 by Winston Churchill. The teachers and their students had left KPH a bit hastily, without properly saying thanks, and a few older heads still remembered that piece of bad manners, so they were justifiably cool to our overtures to establish formal teaching there.

But we admitted the error, with apologies, and good relations had been restored in the specialties of Surgery, Internal Medicine, Pathology and O&G. In 1971, the Director of the Victoria Jubilee (Maternity) Hospital (VJH), Dr. Leslie Williams, an arrogant man at the best of times, but highly skilled, did not have a good working relationship with his more reserved University counterpart, Dr. Mavis Anderson. We needed access to the patient base at the VJH for the training of obstetricians and gynaecologists. Things improved when she left, and Dr. Hugh Wynter took over, bringing a low key approach to managing the department's activities. He allowed me to deal with Dr. Williams, whose concerns I discussed frankly and settled, to his satisfaction, so that the VJH could join us, in the same way that a year or so earlier, the Chest Hospital, Kingston Psychiatric Hospital and the Bustamante Children's Hospital had done. All consultants were given UWI academic Associate status.

Each had also agreed to host Lesser Antilleans for 3-6 month clinical upgrades, sponsored by their Governments, which would be arranged through the Dean's office and the Ministry of Health.

Paediatrics then was ably directed by Professor Eric Back, a good-humoured Englishman, with whom I had done a six-month internship, and who had endeared himself further by never failing to perform a hilarious skit at the annual medical "smoker," parodying Faculty personalities in ribald pub style. He left in 1972, when the first episodes of violence affected the campus housing area and scared his wife, as it did others. He had served for nineteen years, and had been popular and highly admired. He left hurriedly before we could give him a proper memento. I corrected this on a conference visit to Denmark via England, in September 1972, and presented him the Faculty's gift at his home in Yarmouth, where he had established a consulting practice, and his wife was at ease. He was succeeded by his student, the ebullient Colin Miller, a good friend, who was an SHO (first year resident) when I was an intern.

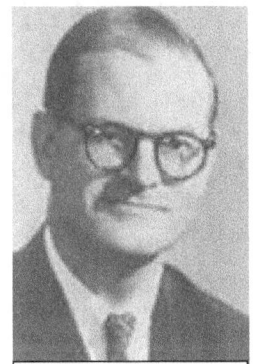

Fig 22-1: Prof E. Back

The Paediatrics liaison with Government was smooth and exemplary, and recommended to all specialties. It was started by Dr Back and his Government counterpart, Dr Leila Wynter-Wedderburn, head, and Drs Keith McKenzie and Barbara Johnson, with clerks at each hospital. They held alternate rounds, the first of their kind, and were a huge success. It also helped that Drs. McKenzie and Johnson were early UCWI graduates, 1954 and 1955 respectively, and had both worked with Dr Back.

He was undoubtedly one of the most effective clinical teachers and his untimely departure sincerely regretted. He was an original supporter of Community Medicine, based at, and extending out from the UHWI, the Divisional plan and the curriculum changes to enable them, and would have been a strong and level head to keep them afloat. But as violence reached the campus, it brought back memories of the 1968 Walter Rodney riots and revived intense fears in Mrs. Back, hurrying their departure. The riots were downtown, six miles away, but the main agitators had been UWI students, led by sociology student Ralph Gonsalves, President of the students Guild, with such verbal venom that she felt that the fear generated among residents would fracture the campus, and she did not want to see it happen. It did not help that even WIGUT, the teachers union, struck twice, each time for a week of harsh words.

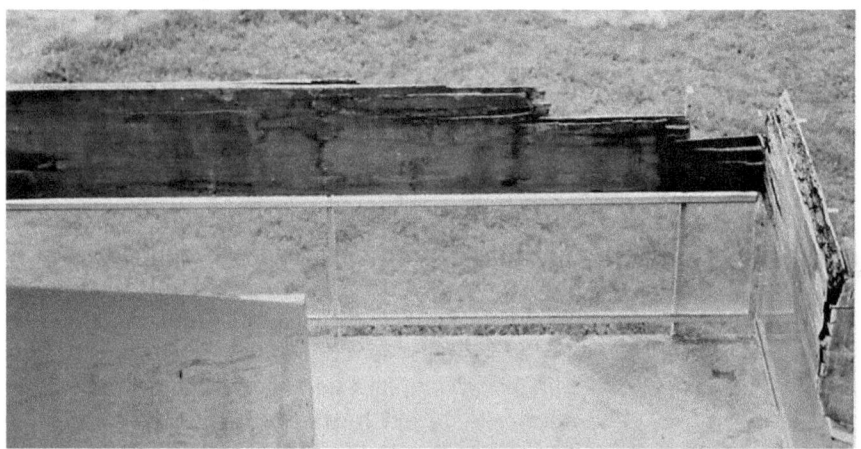

Fig 22-2: Mount Hope Hospital, Rotting railings. 1985; the buildings lay idle for over 4 years.

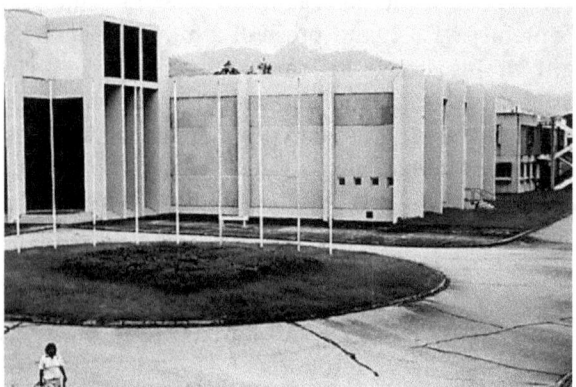

Fig 22-3: Left: EWMC, Mount Hope, 1985, a lone visitor passes beside forlorn buildings.

Below: Fig. 22-4: EWMC 2016; the Hospital finally opened in 1989, and is the clinical centre of the T&T campus; other photos are on p.217.

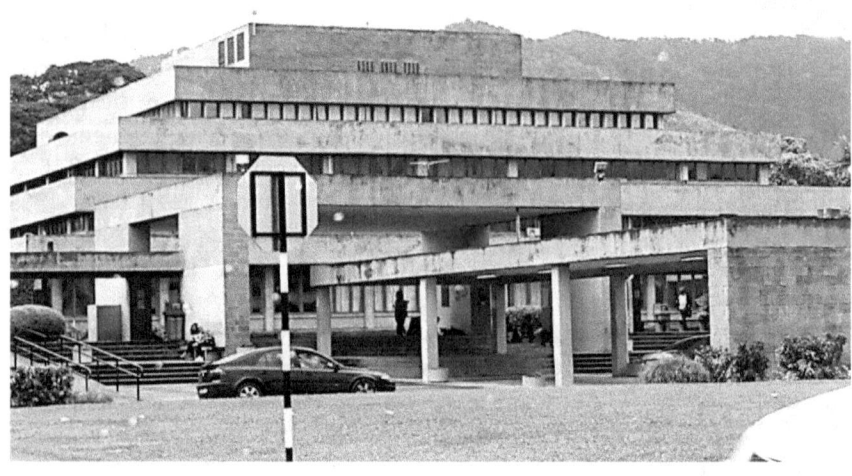

Chapter 23
Strikes on Campus; turmoil in the city

Among the tasks undertaken for CHMC was the design of a model of Health care delivery, which the Medical Research Council had suggested, but it had fallen to my office. Karl Smith, KL Stuart, D. Picou, G Alleyne and A. Davies contributed briefly, and at the second of two meetings, agreed that the principles and plan were covered in my Community Medicine and Family Medicine proposals. We decided to merge the two and add notes of general organisation and methods and the need for CHMC-UWI collaboration. My memo to CHMC in Oct 1971 and the paper by Mr. Burton and me in 1972 stated the principles of "collaboration." CHMC Resolution 27/1974 urged us to pursue a means to fund this model. The diagram below summarises some aspects.

University Collaboration with governments

Faculty   ⟶   Joint Ventures ⟵——— Governments
Planning (CHMC)

Education and Manpower:
MBBS program
PGME & CME
ANE/Admin
Paramedical Training
Medical Ancillaries

Organisation, Management, Services and Funding Model
Central and Local Administration
Primary Care and Community Medicine
Specialty Care and Hospital Medicine
Other Programs in defined Areas e.g. Research

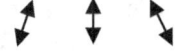

Individual Health, Education & Research Programs

Dean and Deputies   MOHs;   Adv. Comm. of Faculty and CHMC
Educ. Committees   Policy; Curriculum;   Hospital Boards
COPMED   Conduct of Educ. Activities;   Local Health agencies
Academic units,   Transport, Communications etc.   Govt. Hospitals

(MSR. Ref. CHMC 17/74 1974, annex)

Fig 23-1: a model for Government-UWI collaboration

Violence had simmered in Jamaica for years, and had surfaced in union riots before WWII. It tended to recur before each election, especially among working-class partisans of the PNP and JLP in the crowded sections of West Kingston. The country had never been able to provide full employment for its young; up to 1962, large numbers had migrated to the UK, where they, Barbadians and other colonials, found work in transportation, factories, offices, construction, and in domestic and social services. They generally adapted to British society, having been conditioned to it. Some upgraded their education and improved their status, taking advantage of opportunity. (Braithwaite, *Bibliography*)

Jamaica and several colonies became independent in 1962, and within a year, the British passed a Commonwealth Immigration Act that curtailed manpower traffic from former colonies. In the following years, unemployment in Jamaica nearly doubled from 12%, as the economy had no cushion for this growth. Youngsters gravitated to the political gangs they had grown up with, PNP and JLP, depending on geography; they became part of the smouldering tensions in those areas and the violent clashes that periodically erupted.

The relaxation of North American immigration laws did not help this poorly-educated class, tending rather to lure away the skilled and professional worker, with negative effects on the economy, and increasing the plight of youth. Add to this the expansion of drug trafficking, and for the peasant farmer, sales of marijuana for his family's upkeep, against both of which the security forces — Constabulary (Police), and Defence Forces (Army) — were relentlessly campaigning; thus an intractable social evil had destabilised the state, shrinking the middle class and deterring small business operations. By the late sixties, the JLP government had been unable to improve the lot of the masses; they lost to the PNP under Michael Manley in February, 1972.

For the Faculty of Medicine and the UWI, nationalistic statements from Prime Minister Manley and his senior colleagues caused EC partners to suspend capital expenditures in Jamaica, prompting the UWI Council to accept the principle that each government may fully fund a capital project in its own territory. Manley's association with Cuba, growing after the elections, in the face of US opposition, affected the Faculty in a way that violence alone did not. It threatened the concept and reality of the UWI as a regional institution. Fears of campus nationalisation led to changes in the financing of campus structures, and Trinidad under Eric Williams actively explored the feasibility of establishing its own university.

Alan Butler had agreed to become Vice-Dean, EC Scheme, in 1972, after we had reorganised the administration of the Faculty Board and Dean's office, with the invaluable support of VC Marshall, Carl Jackman,

Registrar, Zach Preston, PVC Finance and Hugh Holness, Bursar, and their staffs. That made it possible, with a dedicated staff, to function when conditions were getting really rough, especially during the violent years, compounded by the bitter strike of subordinate staff at Mona, in early February 1973, called by the University and Allied Workers Union, which was formed in 1971, and had the security guards as its members! We were caught between the strikers and non-striking hospital staff. The strikers took to bullying hospital staff to join them, used force and threatened lethal force, adding to the general unrest. Staff became jittery and wary of even a slight variation in routine.

Early one day, I had attended a meeting of the Committee set up to negotiate an end to the strike; I was one of the University negotiators. The union leader was Trevor Munroe, a social scientist on the University staff. On my way back to the hospital, I was stopped by a burly student I did not know, who refused to let me through, and began to berate doctors and people at the hospital who had *"no feeling for the sufferers, exploit subordinate workers and deny them a pay increase."* I asked him whether he knew that Dr Munroe had agreed to instruct strikers not to obstruct free passage by staff along that road. He didn't, but further hassle was prevented when an older man who had been silent so far, lifted the bar and waved me on. Earlier, a lecturer had tried to drive through the main gate barricade, and was beaten. The VC called police; students were charged, and later suspended.

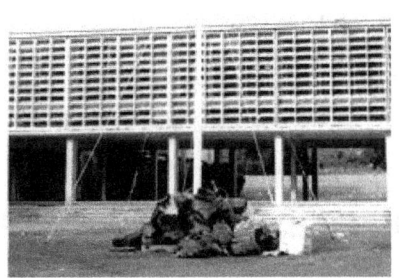

> Fig 23-2: *Strikers hoisted garbage bag on flagpole at Registry and pile others at base,*

That same day, the Medical Students Association, after an intense debate, turned down a request for support, a decision that was wrongly ascribed to pressure from my office, and was quickly followed by two death threats to me, delivered personally, with guns to my head, and attacks on staff. That evening, I accosted two men who were trespassing in the O&G offices and had just terrorised two late-working secretaries. I had responded to their screams, which were startling enough to carry to my office in the next building; I met the men on the broad open landing two steps up from the driveway that gave to the office complex. When I asked who they were, they quickly came up to me, one on each side and boldly pulled pistols, the younger one holding his to my right temple, barking, "*...ih no tek much fe me to pull dis triggah!*" The older man, thirtyish, asked me to explain my objection to the strike and why staff were still working.

"Simple; we're not in your union! This is a hospital; we look after your children and your parents; and we save your lives when the other side shoot you. Why d'you want these poor people to go without bread? If you want them to strike, you should talk to their union." He looked at me quizzically, while the cold steel of the other's gun still played on my head; it had moved to the right mastoid. The older man said, "*Awright, busha, we let you go dis time.*" With that, they pocketed the guns and quickly moved off, jumped on bicycles and pedalled furiously down grade towards the University and the barricade they had put up across the connecting road. The upper photo on p. 214 shows the area.

Although I made every effort to keep news of these incidents from spreading, others had seen them, and threats had occurred elsewhere; the entire hospital soon knew of them; staff became more jittery. The result was that very few remained after work, as many had done before. The dangers further stymied our efforts to fill vacancies at Mona, slowed HOPE recruitment, and scuttled our plans for a series of after-hours activities in education (p. 250); several permanent staff requested transfer to the Eastern Caribbean (EC), as the program developed there.

Next day, after a negotiation session at the Registry offices, at which the sides had locked horns, I was leaving, when Munroe accosted me, complaining that I had "harassed" a student and two workers. Hardly had the word "harassed" left his lips than one of his goons grabbed my shoulder and pressed a gun against my right occiput. This happened in plain sight of two women leaving the building, who hurried away, and of others at windows overhead, who had stopped to look. I said to Munroe, "I don't think you have to stoop to this. Is this how you settle differences? Find out the facts first, man, if you call yourself a scientist." I felt the increased pressure of the gun. How uncanny, the image that flashed across my mind; this was a replay of the 1963 incident at the Georgetown Laboratory, except at far closer quarters! "So you shoot me; that hangs you both, my friend." I said. The incident discredited Munroe, weakened his position at the negotiating table, and set him up for prosecution for threatening murder. Even some of his Faculty colleagues censured him, and called me to commiserate. I decided not to press charges. The strike soon ended.

CHAPTER 24
Housing the programs: PGME Building at Mona, and Mount Hope Hospital

For the initial phase of capital needs at Mona, I needed J$140,000, then worth US$154,000. With Jamaica granting J$70,000, her share, according to the funding formula, we would have the funds if the three major partners contributed, leaving the junior territories to finance improvements in their services at home, adding teaching space, and getting ready to develop special programs and take electives. But, with the two major Eastern Caribbean islands reneging, we had a difficulty.

I lived on the campus in an old sprawling war-time bungalow with a large yard, next to the Nunnery and the University Clinic. One morning, as I was leaving for work, I saw an excavator rolling into the Clinic parking lot, went over and found out that the crew had begun to prepare the site for an extension of the Clinic to house Karl Smith's Family Planning service and research. I introduced myself to the foreman and asked that he suspend work for a few hours to allow me to contact a few persons. He was, naturally, sceptical, but agreed when I told him that he may be at the wrong site! Since he had no way of checking then, and digging at the wrong site was a serious mistake, he gave me till noon.

USAID had provided US$60,000 to put a second storey over the clinic, requiring new foundations along the perimeter of the existing building, and erecting concrete stilts to support an upper floor. I called Karl Smith, who agreed that the location of his unit was not critical and the PGME building would be suitable, in fact superior, as it would spare the Clinic months of disruption, and be near to the O&G department and Hospital clinics. So I contacted USAID and proposed the merger of their grant with the Jamaica Government's and approval of the new site.

The idea of merging US funds with another agency's was unknown to the USAID officer, just then waiting confirmation of an office visit from a Washington supervisor, who had arrived in Jamaica the previous evening. VC Preston had earlier encouraged my seeking funds from likely sources and readily agreed, offering to meet them. I left a message for Mr. Goldson of the Ministry of Health, who called back with no objections, requiring, in due course, a formal note from us and USAID.

The USAID officer called and wished to meet at my convenience. "I could be down in half an hour," I said. "No, we'll come up. Your office?" I called the architect, Lascelles Dixon, who was anxious to get started on the building, and he came up to join me. And so, the USAID officers,

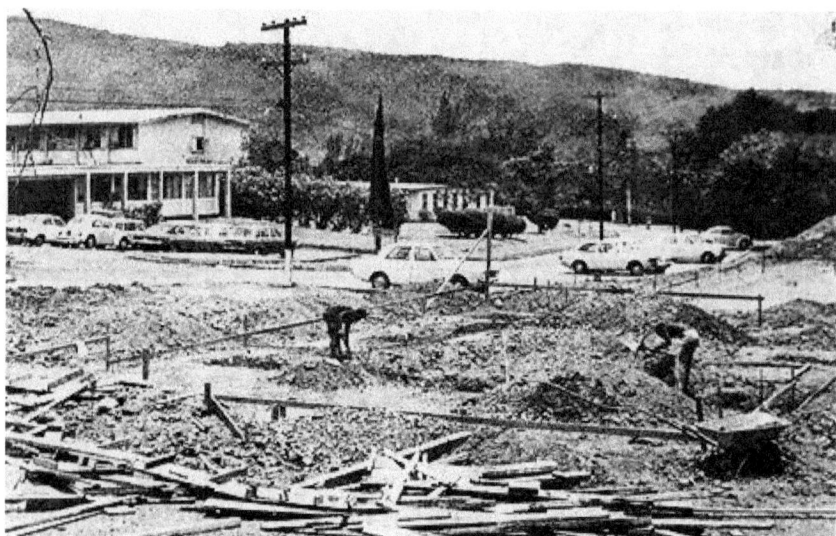

Fig 24-1: *PGME Building: location and site preparation, 1975. The Dean's and Surgery Offices at left where gunmen greeted me, the road on right was their escape route to the campus beyond the trees; TMRU is low building, far left; Long Mountain is in background (Photo ©by author)*

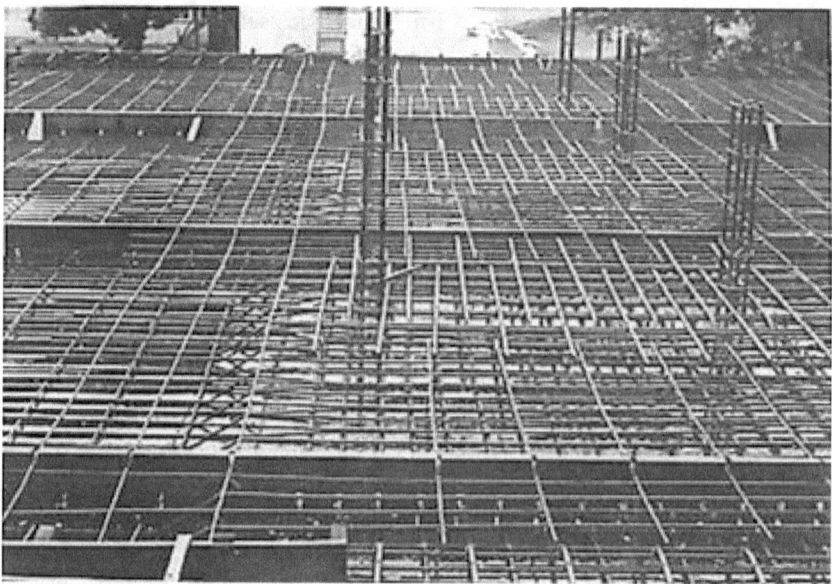

Fig 24-2: *Postgraduate building: steel girders for first floor plus skeletons for posts (author©)*

after visiting the Clinic site, and speaking to Karl and the work foreman, came with Karl to my office, met Mr. Dixon, briefly reviewed the plan, visited the site and approved the change. The supervisor commended our unusual initiative to merge the two grants to achieve a superior outcome; his only condition was an exterior wall plaque recognising the gift, the giver and its purpose, and notification of the official opening. He did say that this was a first for USAID, not only in amalgamating their grant with another's — it helped that the other was a Government — but in the speed with which it was conceived and concluded. The VC was pleased, as the act removed one source of carping between Jamaica and T&T. A formal confirmation and exchange of notes followed among the parties. When the building was opened a year later, Sam, who had just started as Dean, did not invite Karl Smith or me, but at least had the good manners to invite Dick Meltzer. It amazed me that high officials had also forgotten this basic courtesy: the VC, Architect Dixon; Manley West; Heads of Faculty departments, etc., while inviting others, who had no knowledge of the background of the building or its purpose. How quickly had the new entrants removed traces of their forerunners and had forgotten the "fund-seekers" and the nice little drama of how they had gotten the building funded. At least, the USAID official referred to it, and wanted to know what had become of that "unusual Dean!"

In Trinidad and Tobago, we faced poverty in the midst of plenty, the opposite of the situation in Jamaica, which was under "heavy manners" (restrictions), in Manley's socialist haven, matched in the Caribbean then only by Burnham's oppressive dictatorship in Guyana, even surpassing the egotism of T&T's PM Williams. It was a formidable sight to see these three side by side with Errol Barrow, the only level head among them, at the launching of CAREC. It was a replay of the pre-federation meeting of the previous generation in that same city, when Norman Manley, Albert Gomes, Grantley Adams and Cheddi Jagan banged heads together over federation. Only this time, Eric Williams had stared at me, and bluntly and suddenly said, for no real reason, "You don't belong here!"

We were in a Port-of-Spain Holiday Inn elevator on the way to lunch. Later on, I pondered what his peeve could be. At the morning session just ended, I had upheld the Faculty's position against claims he was making, and unfair charges. He was wrong, and contradicted the position of his own Minister, siding with a criticism Burnham had made of the UWI, which others had corrected. Besides, it was a small point and could not possibly provoke such an expression of peeve; yet one knew that a megalomaniac does not want to be corrected, especially, in Williams case, by an Indian, a trait he shared with Burnham. But that did not justify his bad manners in public. The look on the others' faces showed that too; light-heartedly, Manley said, "Come on, Eric, you must be joking; you have the wrong man!" Williams sulked. Manley added, "We'll keep him in Jamaica," and to me, "Don't mind him."

We had looked forward to the CAREC opening to have a chance to advance the EC scheme. We had discussed at length with Hon. Francis

Prevatt, Minister of Health, an initial addition of 120 beds to the Mount Hope Hospital, to create four teaching units of 30 beds each, in Medicine, Surgery, Paediatrics and Psychiatry. He had admitted that the government had to build a general hospital somewhere east of Port of Spain, in view of the increasing density of population along the Eastern Main Road, and the impossible traffic on that narrow artery. The argument see-sawed over the next two years, in an incredible dance among professionals, with the Ministry staff seeming to enjoy the exchanges ((*buhbul*) in the spirit of a carnival. Educators were seen as intruders, and the Port of Spain (POS) Hospital professionals painted as feeling threatened, though there was no reason for this, except that our staff insisted on academic control of teaching programs, and UWI autonomy, which Williams did not like, and preferred to dictate—as Burnham did in Guyana, much to UG's Vice-Chancellor Irvine's dismay.

The clash of personalities was the very stuff of calypso; mercifully, it escaped the satirist's attention, but remained a persistent hindrance for us. Personality problems soon began to fade, as assurances and example worked in our favour. Allan Butler, the Vice Dean, EC, working with Courtney Bartholomew and Harold Forde, and later Frank Ramsay, as Associate Deans, T&T and Barbados respectively, joined with those already on side: Drs. Ratan, Ince, Adam, Thesiger (POS), Poon King and Ramdial (San Fernando), and others, to improve working relationships. By 1974, Trinidad was mentally prepared for postgraduate medical education. However, the big hurdle remained: the bickering between T&T and Jamaica on growth and expansion of the UWI.

We were assisted in understanding some of this coolness by the Permanent Secretary in the Ministry of Finance, Mr. Frank Rampersaud, who had alerted us in 1972 to the real possibility of Trinidad's "going it alone," in reaction to Michael Manley's political bravado in Jamaica. T&T had wasted enough money dithering on programs on its own soil, and it did not want to do that in Jamaica as well; thus, at the last minute in 1974, it had cancelled its commitment to support the PGME building. Barbados did the same, for the same reason.

That was the time that the UWI Council decided on the principle that member countries were free to finance projects on its own soil (p. 210). The cancellation of funds for the building slowed PGME but did not stop it, as EC staff were not affected, and in fact the EC undergraduate program gained staff wishing to escape Jamaica's political shenanigans. This was a different scene from two years earlier. The differences of opinion, attitudes and vision stalled UWI development in the EC for *fifteen years*. Eventually, the building of the Medical Sciences complex was started in 1981, after the death of Eric Williams. It was completed by

1985, but not commissioned, standing idle, with exposed timber rotting (p. 208), until it was finally opened in 1989!

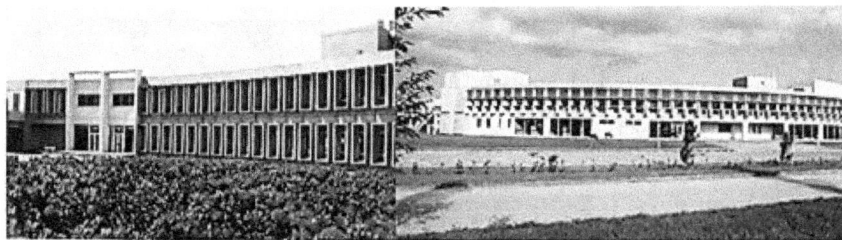

The Medical Sciences Library   Dental Hospital

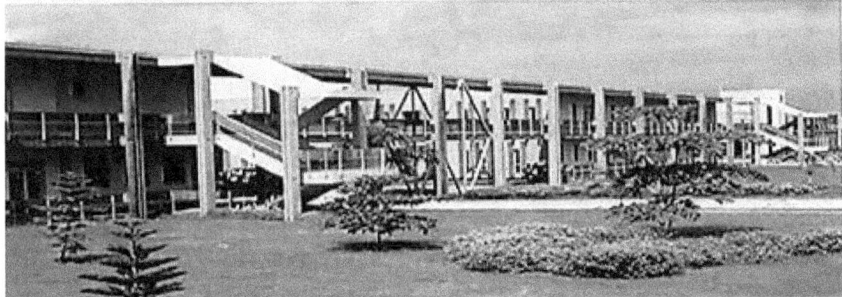

Fig 24-3: *Impressive Buildings at Mount Hope for the Trinidad Faculty of Medicine, Dentistry, and Veterinary Science: Library and Dental Hospital, above, General Adult Hospital, below, 1985. The buildings were completed during PM Chambers' tenure, and remained unoccupied for years as the PM pondered their use! Railings rotted and junctions separated; fungi thrived in the cracks and spiders celebrated in every corner and hidden place (p.208). Offices and function rooms looked as desolate as a scene from Neville Shute's "On the Beach," after radiation had taken all life! Finally, the hospital opened in 1989 as the Eric Williams Medical Sciences Complex (EWMSC), and the home of the Trinidad Campus of the UWI Medical Faculty.* (Dean's collection)

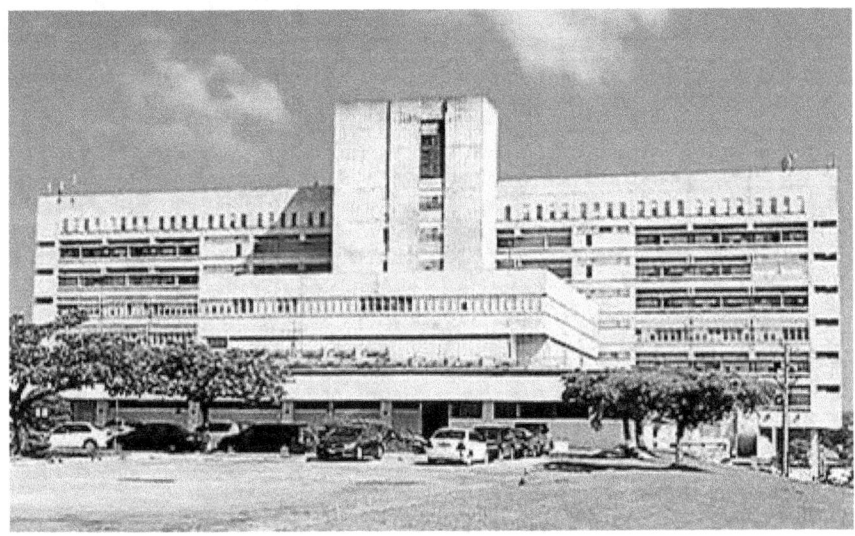

Fig 24-4:The Cornwall Regional Hospital (MOH), Montego Bay, Jamaica

JAMAICA- NEED FOR MEDICAL SPECIALISTS
DOCTOR: POPULATION RATIO (Com. Carib.): 1:1,000 – 1:30,000

Specialties	Present Establishment	Estimated Additional Needs in 10 years	%increase
Medicine	011	17	155
Surgery (including	047	56	120
"Super/Specialties", the organ specialists)			
E.N.T.	003	4	133
Ophthal.	008	2	25
O & G	009	12	133
Path/Micro	009	12	133
Public Health	021	21	0
Paed.	003	12	400
Radiology	013	2	15
Radiotherapy	001	5	500
Anaesthesia	010	21	210
Psychiatry	008	12	150
Community Medicine	000	20	∞
Administration	002	5	250
Dermatology	001	4	400
Urology	001	3	300
Nuclear Medicine	001	2	200
Orthopaedic Surgery	002	4	200
TOTALS	**144**	**233**	--

Table 24-1: *Estimated needs of Jamaica Health Services for specialists. Note the inclusion of Community Medicine specialists as endorsed by Ministry of Health and CHMC, and the corresponding restriction in numbers of Public Health specialists. It was felt that this group could concentrate on population health and carrying out general measures to achieve that, while their CM colleagues would integrate PH and clinical practices in general health care, from their proposed directorships of district hospitals and clinics, following a coordinated plan by MOH, aided by an extended health care team. The CM Division at UWI would include S&P Medicine and be responsible for student clerkships, training CM specialists and Family physicians, and liaison with MOH and PH services. For results of specialty training, see p. 261, Table E-1.*

Burnham visited Jamaica in Dec., 1973. In *The Indelible Red Stain*, I had written, *"In the years between 1967 and 1976, I made frequent trips to the country (Guyana) and saw the steady decline of a once beautiful capital city (Georgetown), where renegade gangs now roamed, under a regime that devastated education and healthcare infrastructure…,and failed to replace lost professionals. By the mid-seventies, health, social and education services had declined to a level inconceivable in 1950, in facilities, personnel, range and quality, and remain a major problem...*

"*In December 1973, ignoring criticisms of blatant self-promotion and jibes at his electioneering frauds, Burnham had come to Jamaica, presumably to discuss politics with Michael Manley: a plan to bring the island nations closer, the future CARICOM. He had used the occasion to get Manley to arrange a meeting with me and any Guyanese and other doctors I could muster, to discuss solutions to Guyana's many health problems, primarily staffing: the flight of physicians, recruitment failures, the growing reliance on Cuba – which had changed from a pariah in his early years to an ally and rescuer, especially in health worker training – and the need to train more Guyanese physicians... The (Health) service was increasingly staffed by Cubans and Chinese, and by locals trained in Cuba. The language gap obstructed effective care and reduced it to dispensing symptomatic remedies to large crowds at national centres, including the Georgetown Hospital.*

"*We met at Manley's residence where I briefed Burnham about training requirements for various levels of staffing, from aides to specialist doctors. He, like Jagan before, was particularly keen on* **feldshers** *and* **barefoot doctors.** *I explained their use and limits, and methods of training. Our meeting was followed by a gathering of physicians, about 20, interested in his aim to 'transform the Guyana health services'. Most were Guyanese or Antillean, to whom Guyana was still a land of promise. Manley came in and introduced Burnham to them, turned the meeting over to me, then left, giving us two hours, when he would be back to socialise for an hour and 'wipe up the blood!'*

"*Burnham explained his situation and his perceptions of need to which I contributed the results of our 1971 enquiry into specialist needs. He deflected criticisms, excusing his staff who 'have to cope with rapid changes to implement socialist practices and bring fairness and justice after deadening colonialism.' He ended up dealing with some flak from a few who had wanted to return a few years ago, but were ignored by his Health Ministry, with not even a show of politeness by acknowledging the enquiries. He apologised and magnanimously invited the 'justifiably disgruntled,' and anyone else interested, to visit at his expense. He joked about his earlier encounter with pickets at PM Manley's office – several Christian groups protesting his legalising of obeah, a West African practice, Igbo of Niger delta, Ashanti of Ghana, etc. – with mystical and religious overtones. It was widely believed to have benefits, if correctly understood and practised, and was carried on by the descendants of ex-slaves in Caribbean islands, until outlawed by pressure of Christian proselytes and the banning of native practices. Obeah is allied to voodoo (Haiti), shango (Trinidad), santeria (Cuba), juju (Bahamas) and candoblé (Brazil). He humoured the picketers and was able to complete his agenda there. One doctor quipped, 'With your need, sir, for funds for Health Services, you would be wise to keep Obeah!'*

"*In the end, he undertook to send information and solicit applications. We have yet to hear from him or from his Ministry of Health! I wasn't surprised, having met with various people in Georgetown, and hearing of his self-aggrandising priorities, which then was the pending CARICOM agreement with Barbados and resumption of diplomatic relations with Cuba, which he planned to pursue with Manley, against US wishes. That was the real purpose of the Jamaica visit; medical staffing was raised to distract the press, which gave him good publicity in Georgetown for his efforts... Several of the doctors had stated an interest in going to Guyana, had he acted promptly. But he had achieved his purpose when Jamaica joined the new CARICOM."*

On Manley's return, Burnham became more affable, teased a few doctors and said to Manley, "You're right, this crowd shoot straight; glad it's only words." He reminded me of a postponed trial for which he had wanted my testimony. I had said I would attend, once I received a return ticket, a safe conduct pass signed by him and a *sub poena*, as advised by VC Roy Marshall, to whom Burnham had spoken at some length. But the papers never came. So I wasn't surprised when none of the doctors there that night ever heard from him. His bravado was classic Burnham.

We bade farewell, earlier in 1973, to Prof. Hoyte, a reliable, open and engaging supporter, honest to a fault. A man of fine principles, as noted, and his behaviour re the vice-deanship the stuff of chivalry (p. 100). He helped me for two years after that, and at CHMC meetings; when I had to present something, I tried to sit where I could see his face, as it told me perfectly how I was doing. His students and colleagues had the highest opinion of him, and he was relied on for help and advice. He was the most missed of all the teachers who fled Jamaica's anarchy in the 1970s.

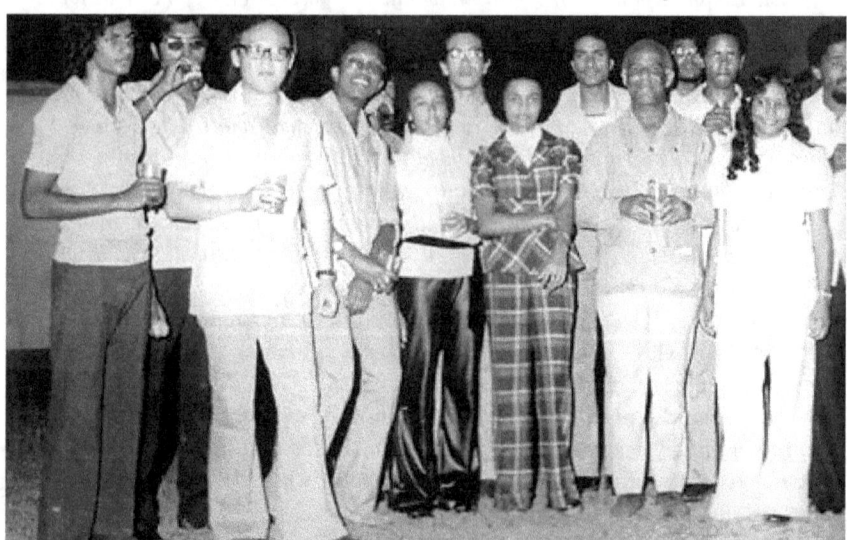

Fig 24-5: Professor. Hoyte (second from right, front row) at his farewell, with some of his students.

CHAPTER 25
A "crisis" meeting

In April 1974, amid the unrest of political gangsterism, robberies, home invasions, rape, shootings and murder, the Jamaica Medical Association joined with its British and Canadian counterparts to hold a gala medical meeting at the Kingston Pegasus Hotel, then quite new. Its star attraction was American cardiac surgeon, Michael De Bakey, who made an ostentatious entrance by helicopter from Palisadoes Airport to the roof of the hotel, was greeted on that fine day by an enthusiastic crowd of doctors, and other medical staff, feted mightily, led like royalty to the podium, from which he gave the keynote address, lunched with officials, among whom I was somehow included, and just as dramatically sent off, the throbbing of the helicopter blades lingering in the air, hours after the great man had gone. I was glad I did not have to give my address on *Teamwork for Developing Countries* that day. We welcomed the meeting, its social functions, and the tightened security, as a respite from the tension of our daily lives. But the violence and terror soon resumed.

Michael Manley had taken over the PNP from his father, Norman, in 1969, and announced his policy of "democratic socialism," sounding rather like Hungary's Janos Kadar's "democratic centralism". Seaga replied with his "social democrat" stance, a mere reversal of words, it seemed to many; people were justifiably bewildered.

The growing violence killed several businessmen and lawyers. One of my friends was browsing in a small grocery store, owned by Chinese, when two men came in, waving pistols; one killed the old cashier, for no reason, and the other shot my friend, also Chinese, as he dived for cover. He was hit in the head and apparently fell dead. The killers escaped on motorcycles with the contents of the till, less than $10.00! My friend slowly woke up as rescuers arrived and found that the bullet had parted his hair neatly from front to crown. Within a week he and his brother, both electronic engineers, were escaping to Canada.

Manley was moved enough by the rash of armed robbery and random killings of civilians to plan a harsh response, even though he knew that many of the gunmen were his enforcers, gone wild. He created "gun courts" where an accused was instantly tried and found guilty on a policeman's evidence alone—like the British Raj's disposal of anyone called a thug, guilty or not—and sentenced to life imprisonment in a high security jail. Morris Cargill (Thomas Wright, p. 200-4), one of the lawyers and Gleaner columnists who had criticised the political leadership, was stalked by gunmen at his St Andrew home and shot in the buttocks as he too dived for cover. The shooter was said to be the notorious PNP enforcer, *Feathermop* (George Spence), one of a motorcycle gang of several dozen, based in Arnett Gardens, Kingston, that he led, with *Burry Boy* (Winston Blake) and Tony Welch. They terrorised the city and environs, and on 1, Jan '75, trashed the JLP HQ on Retirement Road, causing a furore in the Legislature. The JLP protested by staying away.

The attackers were alleged protégées of the housing minister, Tony Spaulding, and had unusual privileges. They had a contract to clean a major concrete gully, at an exorbitant fee, but did not pay workers. A civil servant was killed for probing the anomaly. The gang often invaded the parish offices and extorted money from those present. The Prime Minister was embarrassed, but the crimes went unpunished. So close were they to the PNP brass that Manley took Blake and Spence to Cuba where they are said to have embarrassed him at a dinner party given by Fidel Castro, where pork, Cuba's national dish, was served. *Feathermop*, a Ras Tafarian, shunning pork, upset the tables with the offending dish.

By the time Manley was forced to discipline or rein in his enforcers, they had become unruly, flushed with the power and freedom to terrorise and rob at will, and to pick fights with opposing JLP gangs, the Police and the Jamaica Defence Force (JDF), as if it were a game. Manley realised that its continuance beyond 1975, with an election due in 1976, would jeopardise the support of moderates and cause his Party to lose the election.

Burry Boy was killed in March 1975, while travelling in a car, by men in another car, and some months later, Spence was shot to death by a lone gunman, probably from Massop's group (JLP) or by an executioner from his own mortified PNP. Massop headed the Phoenix or *"shower posse"* gang, which had grown under Curly Locks and Carl Mitchell (*Byah*), in the JLP strongholds of Tivoli, Rema and Wilton Gardens. A brief respite followed, until new leaders took control (*footnote 28, p. 142*).

Other incidents, including several bank robberies, home invasions, assaults and rape regularly reached the fringes of the campus, and occasionally female student halls of residence and staff homes. One raid occurred into Mary Seacole Hall, next door to my home. The intruders were driven off by campus security guards. From my window, with all house lights off, I could see two men running up the lane (Shed Lane), which led to a campus entrance near Irvine Hall, where it met Gibraltar Camp Road, and another pair ran off in the opposite direction, hotly pursued by guards, with occasional bullets flying. They escaped on motorcycles. In an ironic incident, unionist Munroe of UWI was chopped to near death in Kingston as he tried to lure strikers away from the National Workers Union, the PNP's Union affiliate.

The fears were city-wide and spreading; when complaints blamed Manley and his Ministers, he stunned his critics, telling them that there were *"five flights every day from Jamaica to America!"*

The regular meeting of the UWI Council in early June had discussed the severe social unrest that had terrified the campus and was depleting the UWI of staff, from all Faculties, affecting all programs, eliminating evening events, slowing reforms, and even discouraging HOPE. I had summarised, for Council, the Medical Faculty problems, as shown in the graphics below, approved by the Faculty Board (those shown here were from the set used for the ACPJ's *Jeff Wilson Memorial Lecture* in 2004).

Sir Hugh Wooding, a retired Chief Justice of Trinidad &Tobago, had succeeded Princess Alice as Chancellor of UWI and Chair of Council. He was alarmed by the picture of unrest at the Hospital, the fears among staff, the possibility of campus invasion by armed thugs, the anecdotes and discussion provided by University officers, and by the data shown on the slides, prints of which had been given to him. He concluded that a crisis was threatening to disrupt the Hospital and "throttle infant programs." He noted that the problem was Jamaican, and political; there were radical voices on other campuses, but no movement towards armed rebellion, not even in Jamaica, where the violence seemed to be an expression of political exuberance that had become uncontrolled. He suggested an emergency meeting with PM Manley, to which the latter agreed. We met on 6 June, 1974, with the following present:

```
Sir Hugh Wooding, Chancellor, U.W.I.
Hon. Michael Manley, Prime Minister of Jamaica
Hon. David Coore, Minister of Finance and
                    Deputy Prime Minister of Jamaica
Hon. K. McNeil, Minister of Health & Environmental
                    Control, Jamaica
Hon. Howard Cooke, Minister of Education, Jamaica
Mr. Robert Mason, Permanent Secretary, Prime
                    Minister Office, Jamaica
Mr. A.Z. Preston, Vice Chancellor, U.W.I.
Prof. L.R. Robinson, Pro Vice Chancellor, U.W.I.
Mr. C.E. Jackman, Registrar, U.W.I.
Dr. M.S. Ragbeer, Dean, Faculty of Medicine, U.W.I.
Dr. K.A. Smith, Vice Dean, Clinical Affairs,
                    Faculty of Medicine, U.W.I.
Prof. K.L. Stuart, Department of Medicine, U.W.I.
```

e Chancellor thanked the Prime Minister for agreeing to see him and his legation on what was a most important matter concerning the education of lth personnel in the Commonwealth Caribbean region. The Chancellor iefly outlined the objectives and functions of the University Hospital

6, June 1974

223

At the meeting, Sir Hugh, after thanking the Prime minister, and other courtesies, focussed on the dysfunctional state of the UHWI and its academic responsibility to its Caribbean partners, increasingly affected by events of the past two years. He highlighted the steady decline in academic capacity, staff losses, and the increased workload on those remaining, all apparently due to a state of terrorism caused by *"gangland-style thuggery, related to partisan political conflicts,"* in which guns played a fearsome part. He summarised the problems and possible solutions, above all, the pressing need for a return of peace and safety on campus, if we were to save any staff, uphold the noble aims and vital role of the University, and preserve its educational activities, especially the new programs, which, *"like tender buds, were most vulnerable."*

The Prime Minister claimed that external anti-socialist forces (read CIA) were *"stirring the political pot"* nationally, and keeping the gangs busy with fighting over control of the drug trade. He mentioned friendship with Cuba, and its freedom from the drug problem. He expected that beefed-up Police and Defence Forces should soon make a difference, by assisting UWI and Hospital Security, increasing patrols along UWI accesses and residential areas, with guards at each gate and housing entrance, and fences in good repair, to maintain law and order.

With respect to the service problems, the Minister was planning to introduce several measures to re-balance workloads of the major hospitals: "The number of house officers has increased, which should reduce clinical workload per person. Other measures will be taken to Cabinet, where discussions have already begun on provisions to ensure a proper service to all people, regardless of their ability to pay."

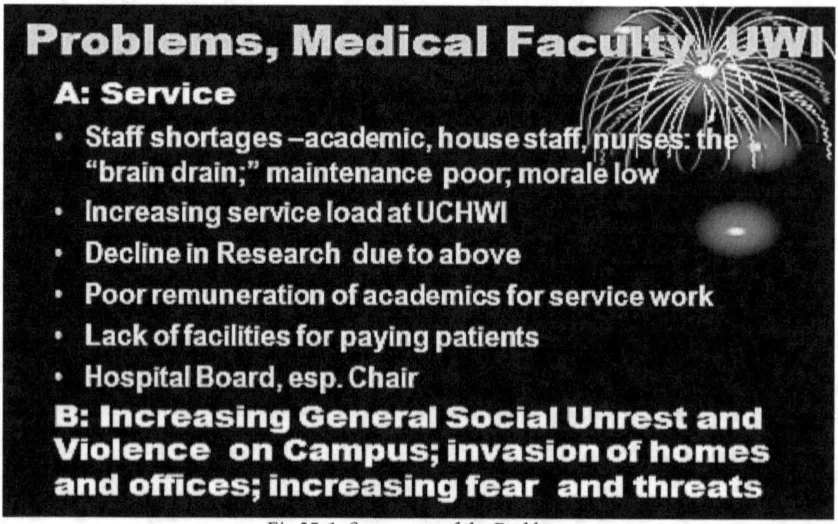

Problems, Medical Faculty, UWI

A: Service

- Staff shortages –academic, house staff, nurses: the "brain drain;" maintenance poor; morale low
- Increasing service load at UCHWI
- Decline in Research due to above
- Poor remuneration of academics for service work
- Lack of facilities for paying patients
- Hospital Board, esp. Chair

B: Increasing General Social Unrest and Violence on Campus; invasion of homes and offices; increasing fear and threats

Fig 25-1: Summary of the Problems

Workloads KPH vs UHWI

KPH 1972	UHWI 1972	Hospital	KPH 1973	UHWI 1973
11,891	12,344	Total Admissions	10,279	12,800
82,581	105,343	Total OP	78,119	108,723
93,644	61,225	Total Casualty	80,518	54,088
4,107	12,536	Operations	4,838	12,727
-	204	Overseas		189

Fig 25-2: *A comparison of workloads of the Kingston Public and University hospitals*

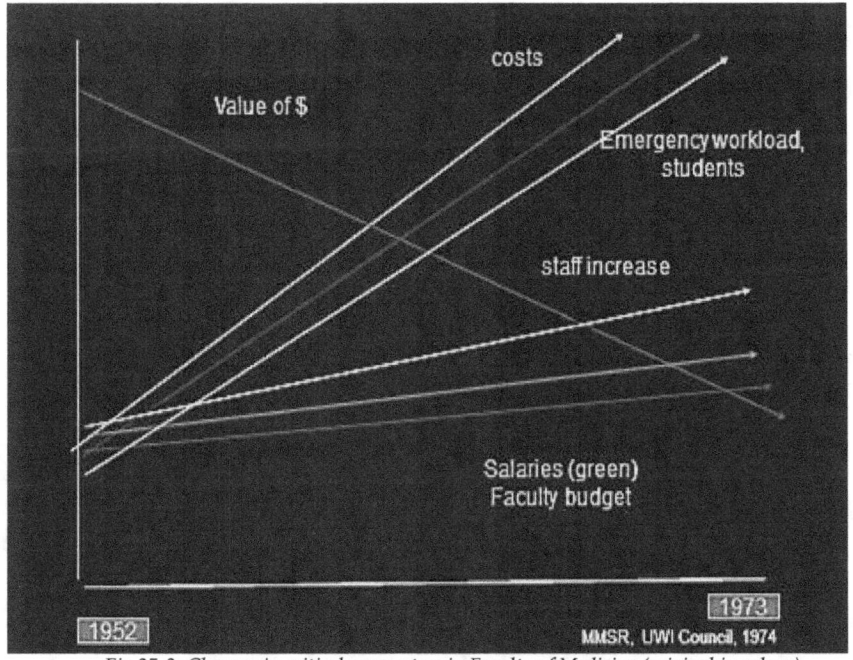

Fig 25-3: *Changes in critical parameters in Faculty of Medicine (original in colour)*

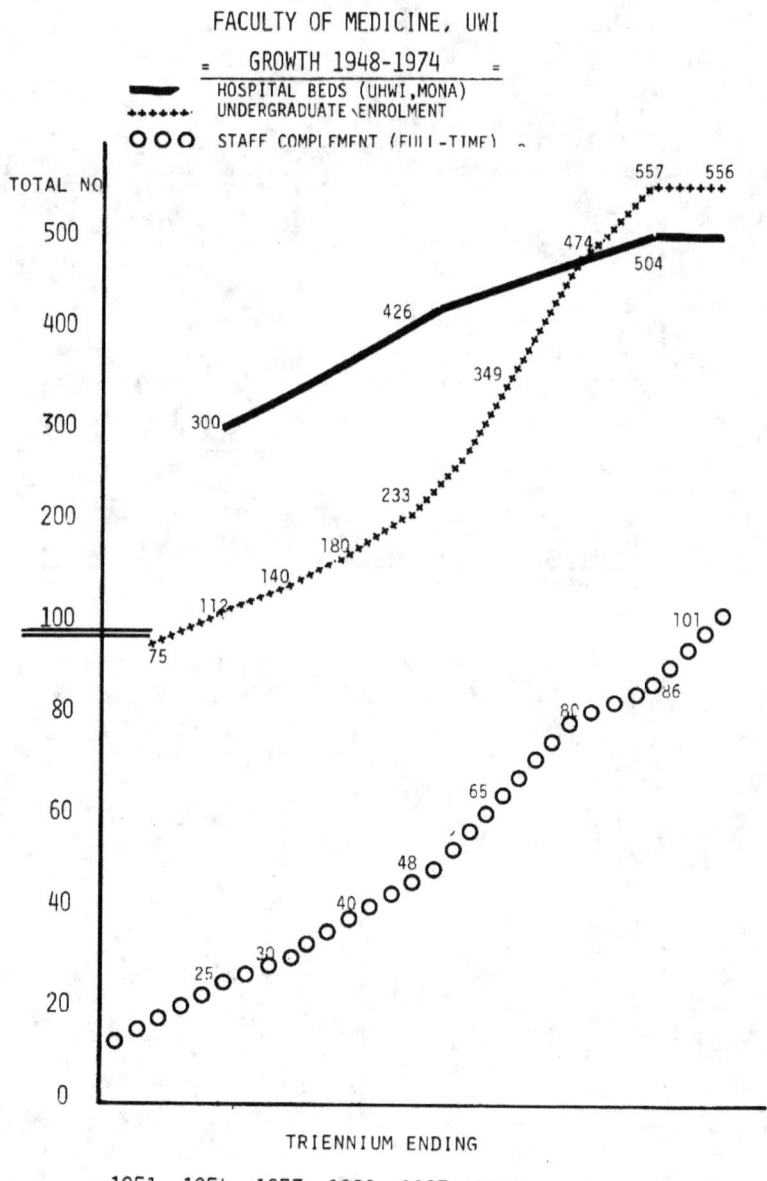

Fig 25-4: Data re status of Faculty of Medicine, 1974

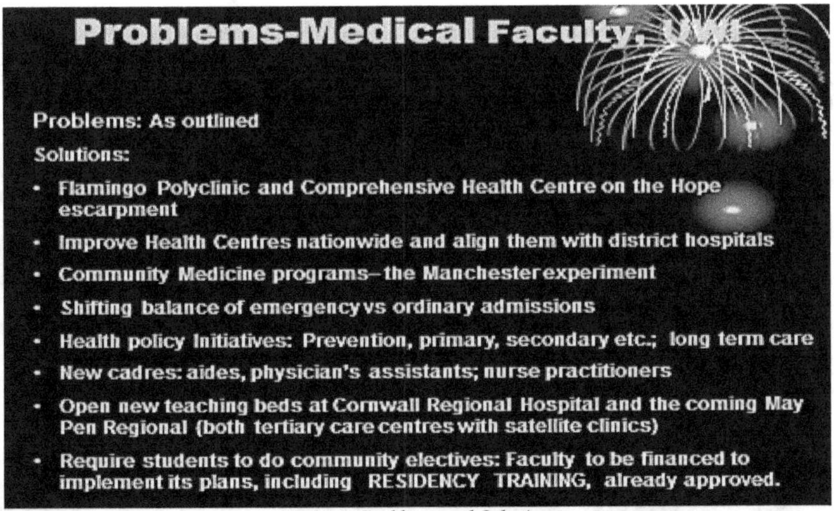

Problems-Medical Faculty, UWI

Problems: As outlined

Solutions:

- Flamingo Polyclinic and Comprehensive Health Centre on the Hope escarpment
- Improve Health Centres nationwide and align them with district hospitals
- Community Medicine programs—the Manchester experiment
- Shifting balance of emergency vs ordinary admissions
- Health policy Initiatives: Prevention, primary, secondary etc.; long term care
- New cadres: aides, physician's assistants; nurse practitioners
- Open new teaching beds at Cornwall Regional Hospital and the coming May Pen Regional (both tertiary care centres with satellite clinics)
- Require students to do community electives: Faculty to be financed to implement its plans, including RESIDENCY TRAINING, already approved.

Fig 25-5: Problems and Solutions

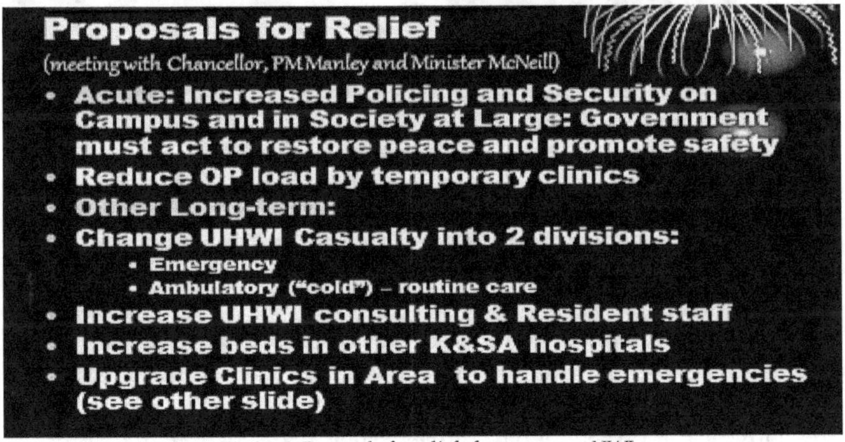

Proposals for Relief

(meeting with Chancellor, PM Manley and Minister McNeill)

- **Acute: Increased Policing and Security on Campus and in Society at Large: Government must act to restore peace and promote safety**
- **Reduce OP load by temporary clinics**
- **Other Long-term:**
- **Change UHWI Casualty into 2 divisions:**
  - Emergency
  - Ambulatory ("cold") – routine care
- **Increase UHWI consulting & Resident staff**
- **Increase beds in other K&SA hospitals**
- **Upgrade Clinics in Area to handle emergencies (see other slide)**

Fig 25-6: Proposals for relief of pressures on UWI

Those of us resolving to stay, soldiered on; for me, the situation was nothing as dangerous or widespread as Guiana of 1962-63. After the meeting, we could do little more than place trust in the PM and Police, or get armed and become vigilantes. Privately, an officer of the JDF had offered to assist, incognito, and I was, with a few others, given a tour of Up Park Camp, but we chose to trust in law and order, and carried on.

My 1973 paper on *Training of Ancillaries* had triggered an offer from the Commonwealth Fund of a travelling Fellowship to study projects on that topic in the Commonwealth. Earlier that year, I had met Professor Satya Gupta, an Indian paediatrician, who was on a WHO-sponsored tour of the UWI and the Caribbean, reviewing our clinical and educational approaches to child health problems, and we had also discussed Community Medicine and team training. She had invited me to New Delhi to review their approach to providing comprehensive paediatric care to a mainly poor clientele.

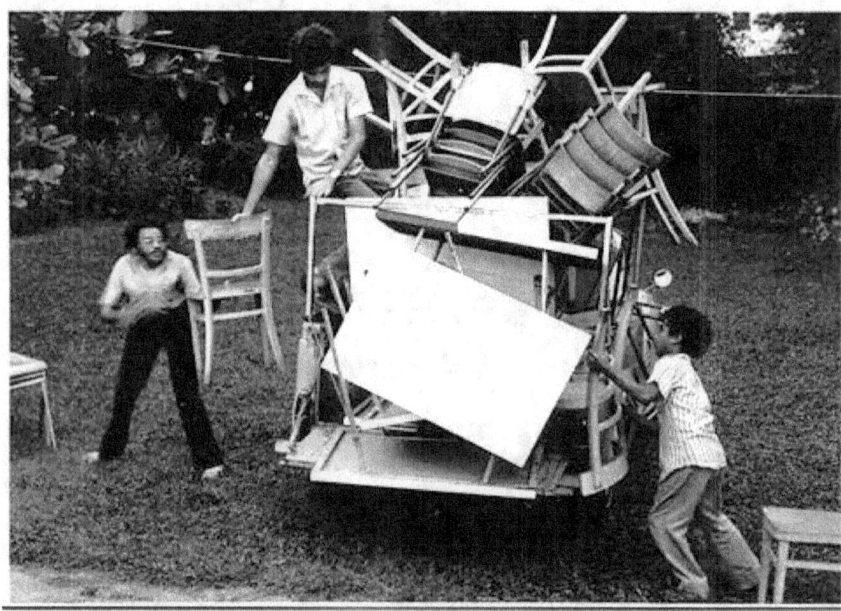

Fig 25-7 *"Instead of the requested solutions, we got to this, a handicapped man directing a teenager and a child; we still have them and thank God, because they do the work of many, while we try to deal with a bad situation." A light-hearted look at how we've drifted by Jan '74. Mr. Manley was amused, and commented, "Not that bad, is it? I should have that little one in my office!"*

Subsequent enquiries had led to a choice of five countries: India, Bangladesh, Tanzania, Kenya and Nigeria, all actively engaged in the effort to reach large needy populations with timely curative and preventive care, on slender resources. They realised that this could be done by training care-givers for specific tasks, from the simplest skills to the most complex "(aides" to "physicians"), as portrayed in the diagrams on pp 55-7. I chose to devote my study leave, due in the second half of 1974, to learn more from examples in the field.

The countries chosen were all tropical, which North Americans — with their ignorance of geography and history — tend to lump together in discussions, the adjective "tropical" triggering a belief that they were, in every way, identical. Even Latin Americans were guilty of this. Increased travel, commerce and other interchanges have mitigated this, but TV commentators continue to confuse Ghana, Guyana, Guinea and New Guinea as the same place somewhere in the African "tropics." Despite similarities among these four of latitude, climate and to some extent of flora and fauna, (largely by colonial transference), there were major differences, which must be recognised, if only so that one could avoid the clear error of concluding that what was true of, say, Nigeria, might therefore be true of Kenya or Bangladesh or Malaysia, or of the Caribbean. This is so obvious that it seems silly to have to write it, but I have repeatedly, both in my travels and in other contacts with persons from and in North America and Europe, heard this erroneous conclusion reached, and repeated with authority, by people who ought to have known much better, including coloured and Indian Americans.

I spent my 1974 leave studying field training of ancillaries, and in December, served on a WHO renal tumour panel. I missed a conference on population, held in Sweden, which included us as recipients of a Ford Foundation grant for family planning; but I went to an *International Academy of Pathology* conference in Hamburg, on September 16-21, and took part in spirited discussions on classification of malignant lymphomas, a long-time interest. After this conference, I visited Berlin, West and East, and obtained a flavour of Communism in practice, as I expected to meet it in my tour, and was facing it in Jamaica, the Antilles and Guyana. A comparison between the two Berlins explained the risk of death that many accepted in escaping to the west. Earlier, in London, I had reviewed my plans and arrangements with an officer of the Commonwealth Fund, and picked up my ticket from Air India.

From Berlin, I flew to Rome via Zurich, and then on to New Delhi, India, a whole new world that instantly swallowed me culturally; everything was so familiar, it seemed as if I had always been there. But the language was different, the ambient sounds and the varied smells in the misty dawn, and the mass of people filling the streets. My visit with Dr Gupta took place as planned, and I saw a positive work atmosphere in a deprived setting relieved by Dr Gupta's charisma. They were, like Guyana, short of everything, depleted by the costly 1971 Pakistan war, which had led to the founding of Bangladesh, as East Pakistan seceded and changed its name. India faced the high cost of improved defences, having met, with USSR aid, naval threats from the US and UK. In May, India had tested its first nuclear bomb. Pakistan did the same soon after.

Indian cities were congested, their problems aggravated by lack of affordable healthcare, while advertising sophisticated private and public facilities, like the All-India Institute of Medical Sciences (AIIMS) in New Delhi, where postgraduate training was similar to ours. At the time, malnutrition, malaria, tuberculosis, leprosy and smallpox were endemic. The country was part of the global immunisation effort to eradicate small pox (achieved by 1979). Yet regular immunisations did not reach many of those most in need. National spending on education fell short of the population increase (high birth rate and falling death rate). Family planning was difficult, despite incentives offered to males and females for ligation procedures; but the basic need for education of the poor hampered many well-conceived plans. The Johns Hopkins rural project at Ludhiana, which I had hoped to examine, had closed, illustrating the fragility of schemes based on foreign research and welfare grants, once the grant ended, and there was no provision for, or local gain from continuance. Researchers took their data and moved on, leaving a community wondering why they had bothered to come.

I was rescued, however, by being allowed to join, for two weeks, the invaluable sessions of the *National Institute of Health Administration and Education (NIHAE)*, founded in 1964 to train Government health workers, military and voluntary groups, in management, and provide consultant services to domestic and overseas agencies. Workers were taught as a team and maintained contact thereafter through an Alumnus Association and the NIHAE Bulletin. About 20,000 workers had already been trained, at various levels, to manage health initiatives for rural populations at different and corresponding levels of need. Some were similar to the Jamaican areas chosen for Community Medicine clerkships; many lacked pure water and sanitary facilities. Defaecation in the open was common, as in Bangladesh, and gave opportunities for sexual assaults on women. Caste, although unconstitutional, was a heavy burden, especially for untouchables (Dalits), people with menial jobs linked to disposal of excreta, and thus shunned by others.

Mr. Thimapayya, the head of NIHAE, had recently learned of the work of a most unusual Brahmin named Bindeshwar Pathak, who had invented a cheap pour-flush toilet—not the thing one would expect of a Brahmin—that could be installed in a very small space, and had been demonstrated in Bihar, shown to be efficient, odour-free, aesthetic, used minimal water, 1-2 litres per flush, and produced biogas and fertiliser. The initiative would spare workers, mainly women, the obloquy for a degrading livelihood, and allow him to retrain them for better and more rewarding occupations, and to improve their health.[36] Other positive influences on healthcare included the expansion of allopathic and traditional (*Ayurvaidic*) medical schools, the use of birth attendants— often illiterate—and their incorporation into the care team after further training. The use of a variety of ancillary workers, trained in health education, early case finding, first aid, supported by nurses and other skilled ancillaries, enabled villages, such as Jamkhed, near Bombay, to receive comprehensive primary, and some secondary care, with only two doctors. I visited the Hindu University at Varanasi (Ayurvaida), where

---

[36] Its success and adoption won for Dr Pathak the 2009 Stockholm Water Prize. (see *India, under siege*, Amazon, 2015, 370-2, Bibliography), and Commonwealth Foundation *Report on Bangladesh, India, Kenya, Nigeria and Tanzania*, 1975, for details on others.

scientific medicine is also taught, and an Ayurvaidic course is offered to allopathic doctors. The country then had some 400,000 Ayurvaidic physicians, who were the main rural primary caregivers. (In 1977, NIHAE became the *National Institute of Health and Family Planning*.)

Bangladesh was three years old and still seething in the aftermath of revolution, ultra-cautious of light brown strangers who looked remotely North-Western, like Pakistanis, until reassured by my Hindu name, which one official suggested I wear on my pocket. They were submerged in red tape, so near to drowning that I almost understood why Pakistan had abandoned them! Like the Caribbean and India, they slavishly continued using British methods, without realising — so brain-washed were all ex-colonial civil servants — that colonial systems were devised to subdue populations, not to provide them good or efficient service.

Many of the checks and re-checks, and layers of authority for the meanest approvals, could have been simplified. I had the opportunity to discuss this at the end of a long frustrating day in a Dhaka Government bank, when I finally got to someone able to authorise my payment of bills in local currency, as London had assured me. He was attentive, sympathised with my frustration, over-rode a junior, who had refused my request until I threatened a report to the CFTC, whose cheque, in *takas* (1T=0.12US), I was trying to change, and demanded to see his boss.

He kept me waiting for two hours, with many excuses, until I told him I was leaving to cable my complaint to London, and walked off. Five minutes later, I was in the manager's office. He gave me hot sweet tea, and heard my story, heard the man's reason for refusing, in rapid Bengali, to be told next time to bring him the papers, and not waste a visitor's time. The junior looked balefully at me, as he left to complete the authorisation. The manager apologised, blamed his excessive zeal, called in another official and generally entertained me while I waited; I was sufficiently calmed to comment on red tape, which they seemed to have adopted as a national emblem, and I suggested that three, certainly two of the five steps I had to take were unnecessary, that I had served in the Colonial Service as a youth, recognised their imprint, and that the first clerk was incompetent and needed a lot more training to act as a teller.

Later, I reported to Dr Sam Street (p. 52), the WHO representative, who undertook to call the bank, if needed, and gave me a full briefing on the country, and several papers to study; he also arranged a meeting next day with the Dean of the Medical Faculty at Dhaka University. Sam headed the UN Relief Operations, Dhaka, with primary emphasis on water control and sanitation. With 75 million people, expected to double in 15 years, in 64,000 villages in a flat, waterlogged delta, a GNP per head of US$70, Bangladesh had huge additional problems: education, health services, nutrition, high fertility, and personnel deficits in all categories. Plans existed to meet training needs. For health, there were eight medical schools, the newest at Rangpur, planned to train many categories of workers simultaneously, to work as teams, as was the mode elsewhere. But the current medical education leaders were steeped in tradition; when I defended reform, some faculty agreed, but even the advocates doubted that Rangpur would be the model for the future, and could not see medical teachers teaching health aides: "That's for the Ministry!"

Bangladeshis outside of the bureaucracy were enterprising and reform-minded, but would have a tough task to change entrenched habits and a crushing inefficiency in Government, and Islamic fatalism that had hardened even at the University, keen on preserving tradition. Hopefully, younger academics would in time begin to make changes.

Tanzania was the closest to Communism of the East African states, but by the time I visited, it was shifting toward the middle. Five large tribes and numerous small ones made up the population. Mount Kilimanjaro was its best-known site, although the Rift valley, Lake Victoria and the Serengeti were justly famous. Guianese Walter Rodney had been active in the country. Joshua Nyerere, whom I met and whose questions I had fielded about UWI, India and my project, asked me about him. I told him what was safe to say, and confirmed Rodney's Marxist beliefs, but had no idea whether he was in the Castro mould. He smiled at that, and said, "You're making a fine distinction. And Jagan?"

Nyerere was aware of the significance of training an entire health team and hoped I would be able to see and comment on the initiatives at Muhimbili, the main teaching hospital, and in rural clinics. Their projects were similar in concept to ours, India and Bangladesh, but their facilities, resources and educational material were far fewer, matched by lower expectations, but with more zeal and unity to improve—as shown by students at a workshop on Community Medicine and teamwork that I conducted—and eager to pursue issues. Several students were Marxist and curious about Castro and other Caribbean Marxists, including Jagan. I met Dr Chagula, former anatomist at UWI, who had joined the MOH as a planner and educator, and was impressed with his work.

Tanzania is a fairly dry elevated plateau, with about 14 million people, 90% or more rural, and GDP of US$75 p.c., same as Bangladesh, and problems of outreach into rural villages, some located in difficult areas with poor transportation. Infrastructure was poor, as in all British colonies I visited! In 1973, the Government decided to move the capital to Dodoma, a crossroads town near the centre of the country, as a stimulus to development. That move had not yet begun, and probably would take a few years of planning and improving infrastructure. Dar es Salaam was an important commercial hub and port, and would remain so. It had the main teaching centres; its medical school trained doctors and pharmacists, adhering to a list of performance objectives that included administration and leadership in the health services, promotion of health, providing emergency, curative and preventive care, individual and community, like CHMC Community Medicine plans. Colonial practices however would delay changes; it was hoped that a joint University-Government working group would suggest coping measures.

I visited a Māsai region north of the capital, and two clinics in that area, and discussed nutrition with officials. Agriculture was cattle-based and croplands were marginal. But heart disease was rare, despite a diet of dairy and meat, credited by the district physician to a bitter seasoning used in Māsai cuisine, but the active life-style and lean habitus of the tribe must contribute considerably to their physical fitness.

Kenya had potential, with 13 million people, a good agricultural base and GNP of US$247p.c. in 1970. Rural services were poorly developed, as expected, and tribal rivalries strong. Kikuyus formed about a quarter of the population and dominated society; the three next largest tribes: Luo, Kalenjin and Luhya, made up about 50-60%; a dozen or more small tribes made up the rest. President Jomo Kenyatta, (Kikuyu, of *Mau Mau* fame), former Vice President Oginga Odinga and the late Tom Mboya (Luo) and Vice president Daniel Arap Moi (Kalenjin) united to form the Kenya African National Union (KANU), a centre-right party that allied with the US in the Cold War. The most influential public figure, it seemed, was not Jomo Kenyatta, but his young wife, Mama Ngina, 44 years his junior, said to be busy acquiring large acreages of the country and amassing great wealth. There were several scandals affecting high government officials; and in Nairobi society in general, one was warned to be alert to avoid being scammed.

In Health and Education, the Government planned to increase by hundreds the number of health centres and rural clinics, train a variety of health workers in the field, and increase spending on health care. New medical schools were planned — with innovative curricula to train a variety of health workers suited to Kenyan realities — as were changes to existing training programs. I was able to discuss Community Medicine and delivery of primary care to all sectors of society; the concepts were already accepted as was multidisciplinary training of doctors, nurses and paramedicals. I met with a paediatrician, originally from Antigua, who had developed a popular teaching and service project but feared that his origins affected his chances of continuation. I suggested he apply to the UWI CM program, which he liked, but heard no more from him!

Although in a better economic position, Nigeria shared health care and other problems with Kenya and Tanzania, e.g. tribal rivalries, crime, social instability, inefficiency, mismanagement and poor infrastructure. With 80 million people in 1974, and considerable resources in energy and agriculture, Nigeria could be a leader in the emerging nations of sub-Saharan Africa; it even influenced Caribbean states where links were being forged with African and Asian countries since independence, and growing feelings of pride in history, culture and ethnicity. As this feeling of kinship grew, Universities and Governments must respond to the potentially uniting forces of shared political history, and recent membership, as equals, of international trade, financial and social clubs: the World Bank, the United Nations, the Commonwealth, and others.

The teaching hospitals, which were established before independence, contributed, paradoxically, to deterioration in the general state of public hospitals and health centres, as money was often preferentially spent on the new academic medical centres. These began rapidly to develop as tertiary care centres, needing specialists. Thus, though teaching facilities were provided, doctors being trained and research being done, no impact was made on primary care; instead, the need increased, while resources either declined, or in the best circumstances, remained unchanged.

Unmet needs had begun to receive attention, as in the remote northwest, with 7 million people scattered over a wide rural area; there, an NGO started a flying doctor service, while the state provided dispensary services, for 130 villages, each staffed by a trained male medical auxiliary and two untrained persons; they provided curative services, supervised by local health officials. Communications were poor; telephones few, and electric power lacking. In one area, expensive pedal-operated 2-way radios provided contact with central facilities, improving patient care and communications. The scheme was taken over by Government. Rural health care must for a long time rely on specially-trained rural health workers and multidisciplinary teams.

For tertiary care, new medical schools were planned, similar to those for Kenya. Some, like the one at Ife, would train multidisciplinary teams and function as "health science centres" rather than as purely medical faculties, and comparable to the UWI's forthcoming expansion in Trinidad. The curricula would be designed to provide conjoint learning for dentists, veterinarians, nursing, and ancillary health care providers. It was thus hoped that these new schools would be better able to meet regional and national needs than the more traditional institutions, such as the University at Ibadan, which had begun to focus more closely on national needs and the plans of Health Ministries, while jealously protecting its autonomy.

CHAPTER 26
Community Medicine

It was difficult, at UWI, to maintain the integrity of programs, and make extra demands on staff, when most were distracted by the terror around them, adding to the unsettling effects of student unrest since the late sixties. Schools were not exempt, and many had taken to installing iron grilles across entrances, especially at girls' schools, with their assemblies of blossoming young women. Yet we had programs to carry out, and deadlines to meet. In this demanding atmosphere, we debated the effects of the multinational nature of the UWI on the ability of the Medical Faculty to grow and respond to its multiple owners, while having tight funding, little control and limited flexibility.

I believed and advocated that we should be allowed some form of autonomy to ensure progress as a regional institution, to grow and be responsive to health care needs, as the Saudis had chosen for their new schools of health sciences. The political and social conditions were becoming increasingly menacing in Jamaica, and the resulting tensions and instability threatening our educational and research roles, placing heavy demands on the service functions of the UHWI.

In 1971, in reviewing the IADB Committee report, I had proposed to VC Marshall a scheme that would allow the Faculty to relate directly to the Joint Committee of Council and Senate, and to substitute the intermediate steps at the University level with similar controls at the Faculty level. A semi-autonomous medical school would thus develop, of which the UHWI and the regional teaching hospitals in Jamaica: Kingston, Spanish Town, Cornwall, and May Pen, when built, would become primary facilities in the West, and the Trinidad (POS General, Mount Hope, San Fernando), and Barbados (QE) Hospitals in the East, and others, as identified, with associated rural and urban clinics and health centres in all regions, for primary care and Community Medicine.

Adoption of a *divisional* structure, with fewer administrative parts — which the IADB Committee advocated, and most staff supported — should facilitate this. Autonomy would allow the Faculty to collaborate more easily with technical colleges, nursing schools, other universities and research institutes, e.g. Miami, Guyana, Suriname, and PAFAMS, in research, and to train manpower, as needed, at all levels. This design would be cost-effective as some 36% of Faculty funding was withheld centrally for administration and accounting services. However, several department heads were sceptical, but had not yet examined the issue, and wished it deferred to a "more settled" time *(pp. 42-3, and Ch. 11).*

This was especially important for Nursing, the most developed and expansive of the services, where the Faculty collaborated in Advanced Nursing Education and Administration courses, under the general direction of Nurse-educator, Syringa Marshall-Burnett. We supported Dr Mary Sievewright in her campaign to establish a degree program in Nursing (B.Sc.N). We could more easily sponsor training of ancillaries as I had proposed to the Commonwealth Foundation in September, 1973, and acclaimed by Eric Cruickshank, Dean of Graduate Studies, Glasgow former Head of Medicine, UWI, (p. 151), and by Jamaica's Minister of Health Hon. Ken McNeill, *(Appendix 15.4, p. 359).*

The new Division of Community Medicine should have begun in the 1972-5 triennium when the Professorship was approved, but coincident social unrest in Kingston had caused staff losses and reduced our success rate in staff recruitment. The early seventies were a period of growth in tertiary institutions, not only in North America,

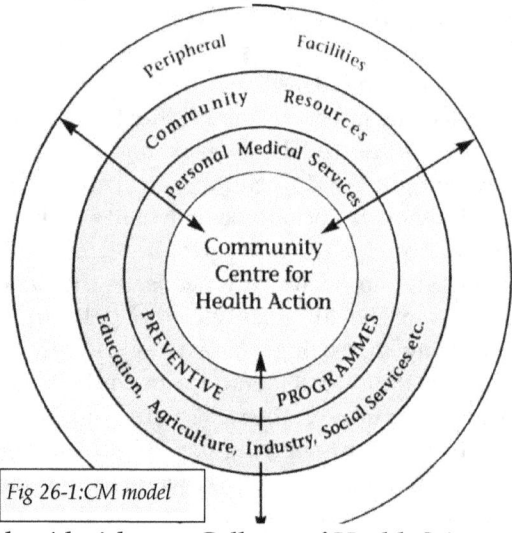

Fig 26-1:CM model

but in Saudi Arabia, as noted, with rich new Colleges of Health Sciences allied to the University of London, and enticing the very people we were hoping to attract, luring at times entire departments, in the fashion of the Americans after WWII. To keep programs afloat and to get new ones, I had to hold down three professorships for four years and was thankful to get support of dedicated talents like Colin Miller, Eric Cruickshank, Karl Smith, David Hoyte, Andrew Masson, Harry Annamunthodo, Ken Stuart, Gerrit Bras, Rabin Sahoy, Rolf Richards, Ken Standard, Mickey Walrond, Molly Thorburn, John Sandison, Siva, Gene Burkett, and others, from the start, and later, Reg Carpenter, UF Amin, Hugh Wynter, B. Sen Gupta, Herb McDonald, Manley West, David Atkinson, Louis Grant, Owen James and others, including many residents and students who were eager to launch Community Medicine (CM), Family Medicine (FM) and PGME. Dr Thorburn was qualified for the directorship of Community Medicine, and would have applied, but for the requirement to travel, which clashed with her commitments to a young family.

In 1973-4, I was elected to the Administrative body of PAFAMS as representative for Mexico, Central America and the Caribbean. It had stated principles for Community Medicine, and obtained from the Kellogg Foundation, of Battle Creek, Michigan, up to ten 3-year grants for Latin America and the Caribbean, to develop experiments and models to educate students in Community Medicine. An *ad hoc* Committee approved by the Medical Faculty Board: Profs C. Miller and K. Standard, Drs. K. Smith, H. Wynter, O. Minott, and myself, selected five clinics in Manchester, the test parish favoured by Minister Ken Mc Neill: at Lincoln, Cross Keys and Prattville as intervention sites, Mile Gully and Harmons as controls; the Mandeville Hospital for referrals, and UHWI for tertiary care. As Dean, I would serve as interim Director—a role I filled until mid-1975—while the Committee would supply technical and clinical expertise, and conduct periodic evaluations. This would provide the continuum of care required of the model. The figure on the next page (Fig. 26-2) shows the cover of our proposal to Kellogg, following the curriculum outlined on page 58.

Our application was a model for several others. The ideas for it, the curricular changes and the approved plans had been debated since 1971 with Department Heads, EC staff, CHMC, the PAHO director, the IADB Committee, students, and sociologists; it was approved by PAFAMS officers; and the principles, arguments and conditions set out in several, widely-circulated Faculty documents *(see Appendices 9-11, pp. 335-40).*

Our proposed start was the 1973-4 academic year, while others in LA had begun a year or more earlier, but events in Jamaica delayed us to 1975. The first phase of our plan was voluntary, and involved a five-week elective in the Manchester project for final year students. In 1974-5, several students opted for CM electives in Jamaica and in the EC, the latter supported by a travel grant from my office, obtained from PAHO. In Jamaica and in the EC, they followed the experimental plan as detailed in the document, which I explained to all supervisors: Dr H. Hanoman, our Lecturer in CM in Trinidad & Tobago, Dr H. Shennan in Barbados, and others, selected with the assistance of the CMOs in those countries, and accepted by the Faculty.

This new program was contentious to some in the Faculty, who saw threats to their authority, since direction was in the Dean's office, a convenience, due to the multi-specialty nature of inputs, and secondly, some teaching would be done by community physicians and other non-departmental health workers, who had no "formal academic degree," that is, through completion of a graduate degree by residency or thesis, and whose supervision could not be guaranteed, but we felt that those we had interviewed could train field assistants (ancillaries), and guide students; in fact it would be to students' advantage to take part in this.

FACULTY OF MEDICINE
UNIVERSITY OF THE WEST INDIES

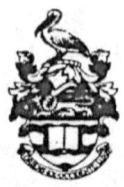

PROJECT FOR TEACHING OF COMMUNITY MEDICINE
MANCHESTER, JAMAICA

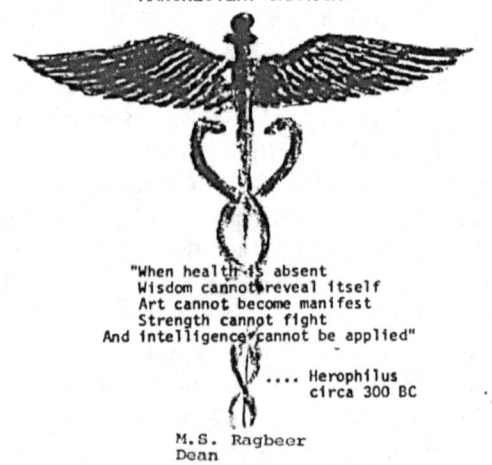

"When health is absent
Wisdom cannot reveal itself
Art cannot become manifest
Strength cannot fight
And intelligence cannot be applied"

.... Herophilus
circa 300 BC

M.S. Ragbeer
Dean

In Cooperation with the Panamerican Federation of Associations
of Medical Schools (FEPAFEM), Bogota, Columbia;
Funded by the Kellog Foundation, U.S.A.

Fig 26-2: Cover page of application to PAFAMS and the Kellogg Foundation for support of the project to teach Community Medicine in the parish of Manchester, Jamaica.

At Mona we had stressed to the Heads Committee and to the Board that CM should not be perceived as a threat and competition for scarce funds, but was, in reality, a proper complement to their activities, and would add to their funds since the training of community physicians would involve nearly every medical specialty, clinical and pre-clinical. It would also force us to embed principles of health promotion and disease prevention in *all* clinical practice, a feature lacking in current hospital medical education, and which each discipline had undertaken to rectify. Rich entities got away with the neglect, by doubling staff, which we could not afford, nor procure. We were thus cautious, recalling the 1969 triennial funding shortfall of 6%, £600,000, by the UGC, while student intake had increased by 100 students, prompting Roy Marshall, the new VC then, to request a review, or approval of a novel deficit financing.

My arguments to meetings of the Faculty Board remained simple. Our supporting governments were clamouring for multi-skilled doctors for clinical and preventive work in the community, and in promotion of health. Few graduates from western medical schools had any training in health promotion, and very little, if any, in Nutrition, as I had confirmed, directly, at several NA medical schools, and from work done for HOPE by Amy Meltzer, wife of Dick Meltzer, and a great resource person. These topics: health promotion, disease prevention and nutrition were key components of a strategy, agreed by CMOs, to improve the health of Caribbean communities, and reduce illness and hospitalisation. We could deliver that; and any training needs of local associate physicians could be met by short courses funded by Governments and/or PAHO.

In a presentation to the Commonwealth Foundation on Sept 1, 1973, *(Commonwealth Foundation, 1973, Occ. Paper XIX, 75)*, I had argued, *"In any society, medical education can no longer take place in isolation from community needs. This means that the University must be in close contact with the main providers of health care, the Governments, and with the consumers, the communities. Only in this way can the university obtain all the information it needs for rational planning of training schemes, or gear itself to educate these groups on particular themes. The role of the new university then, in the training of medical ancillaries, must be critical and all-pervading. While the University does not have to do the actual training of ancillaries, it must be a major participant, contributor, indeed the prime mover, in schemes for such training, by supervising, stimulating, and carrying out the groundwork required for such schemes, and by suitably rewarding staff for their contributions to this work."*

Later, I had said, *"The new University should ... aim at a flexible plan for its medical school, and avoid the rigid systems which hinder rather than promote its purpose. It might, therefore, be preferable for the new university to establish a School or College or Institute of Health Sciences, with autonomy in deciding programs in consonance with needs, resources and the desire for the highest standards of training, whatever the level to which it is done."*

I had further suggested, *"The University, particularly the new university, must be an agent of this social and educational change. Its programs must reflect concern for national goals; its products must be aimed to meet the nation's needs; and it should create conditions wherein all members of the team can be trained together, rather than as now, where each is trained in isolation from the rest."* (Ten days later, Carlisle Burton of Barbados said something similar at the *PAHO Conference on Manpower*, Ottawa (p. 187).

At that time, we relied on Public Health doctors and departments to attend to community needs, but their training stressed epidemiology and statistics, and little clinical medicine. Some of the non-medical professors that I had to convince, understood our aims better when I cited their own medical needs, with the question: "to whom would you go when you fall ill?" It was, often, only by this approach that our positions eventually became understood. It helped, too, that government leaders, the CHMC, were grappling with the problems, and favoured our plans, and that the IADB Committee had strongly endorsed the development of capacity to train primary care and community physicians.

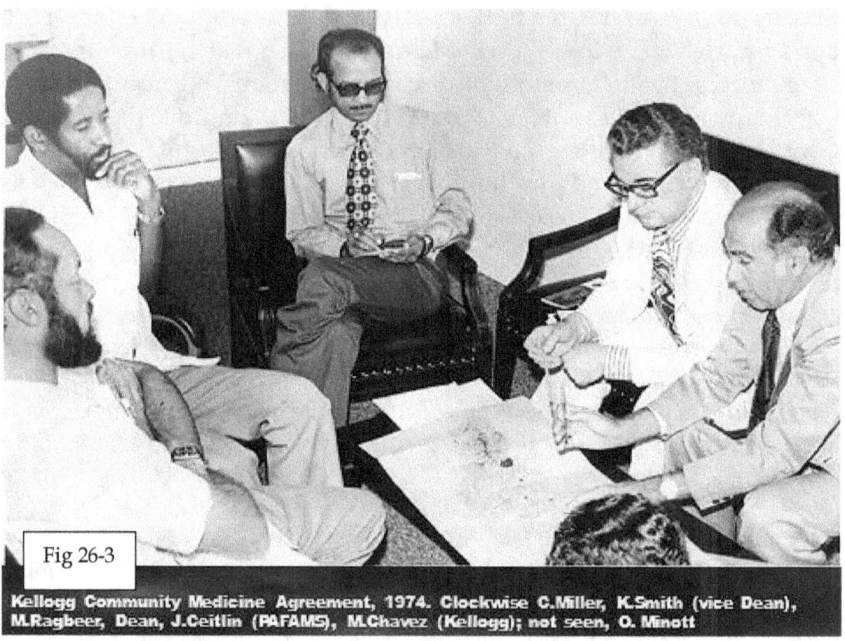

Fig 26-3

Kellogg Community Medicine Agreement, 1974. Clockwise C.Miller, K.Smith (vice Dean), M.Ragbeer, Dean, J.Ceitlin (PAFAMS), M.Chavez (Kellogg); not seen, O. Minott

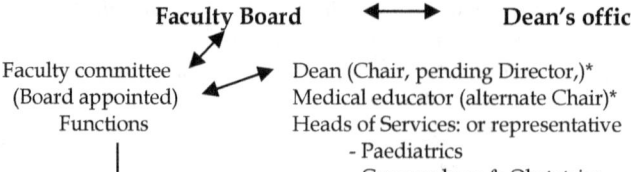

Faculty Board ⟷ **Dean's office**

Faculty committee
(Board appointed)
Functions

Dean (Chair, pending Director,)*
Medical educator (alternate Chair)*
Heads of Services: or representative
  - Paediatrics
  - Gynaecology & Obstetrics
  - Family Medicine (when approved)
  - Social & Preventive Medicine
  - Co-opted Members (Govt. CMOs or delegates)

Planning and Development of Projects in Jamaica, T & T, Barbados, and others*
Curriculum;
Program Implementation and Evaluation
Supervision of Students
Training of Health Personnel other than Medical Students
Liaison with Collaborators in University, Government, Communities, Industry and
  Others

*Director of Community Medicine to replace these as Chair; they would thereafter serve as ex-officio members.

Fig 26-4: Faculty-supported organisation for program in Community Medicine

The Kellogg Foundation award persuaded the University Grants Committee to approve funds for senior staff, including a professor to head a Division of Community Medicine, as argued elsewhere (p. 43). Until then, CM had started as part of the Dean's Office, as explained. Faculty had agreed to this and to the organisation plan, without dissent, as did the CMOs at their regular planning meeting for CHMC (Fig 26-4).

A sister to the Manchester project, located in the mountain village of Chimaltenango in Guatemala (Fig 26-5), exemplified what the projects could achieve. There, the dental segment of the project had intervened to solve a widespread community problem of tooth decay and the digestive diseases that followed, starting in the very young. In Guyana and the Caribbean, I had seen the same condition in children chewing sugarcane, and neglecting, or unable to afford dental prophylaxis. The causes in these secluded mountain villages were more varied, and part of the investigative aspect of the project. Senior dental students, nutritionists, nurses, physicians, and other workers were teamed to conduct research, treat, advise, show and tell, and do follow-up care and prophylaxis. The community responded and within a year had shown improvements in individual dental health, along with higher rates of immunisations, improved nutrition and more timely illness care, including prevention.

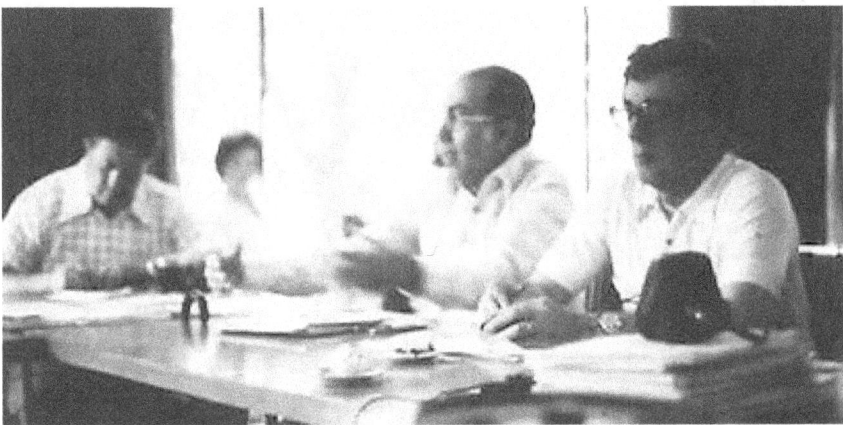

Fig 26:5: From right, Drs Julio Ceitlin and Mario Chavez, with a Guatemalan project dentist (left) and a secretary in background, at Chimaltenango, 1975

We often quoted this and the earlier Cali experience of eradicating hookworm disease in a part of Colombia — stretching west from the Cauca valley over the Andes to the Pacific shores — by the simple gift to each one of a pair of slippers made from discarded motor vehicle tyres.

Similarly maternal health was improved, and the new clinics were able to advise and pay for, or subsidise prescriptions, which turned a dejected look, which one saw often at the clinic (see Fig 26-6) to one of hope. This shared experience among Latin American neighbours was often ignored by anglophone West Indians, who copied the British and European biases against the indigenous peoples of the Americas, and for whom nothing "less" than American fare was worth copying.

A related difficulty that we shared was how to change bad habits. The poorest Latin American and Caribbean mother had been convinced of the "superiority" of powdered milk over breast milk, by seeing, in all media, advertisements with healthy, well-fed babies next to cans of brand-name milk powder, some given as free samples to new mothers; large colourful posters decorated ante-natal and other maternity clinics!

Members of *La Leche League* — founded in 1957 in the Chicago suburb of Franklin, twelve years before we met them in Cali, Colombia — toured Latin America, and other developing countries, advocating breast milk as the natural food for infants! So powerfully and completely had US corporations convinced Americans and the rest of the world — by predatory trade agreements and persuasive advertising — that American industry and ingenuity had bettered Nature, that women came to believe that babies were better fed by US bottles than by their mothers' breasts! As a measure of desperation, we even showed them that the English word *"advertisement"* may have derived from the French *"avertissement,"* which meant *"warning!'*

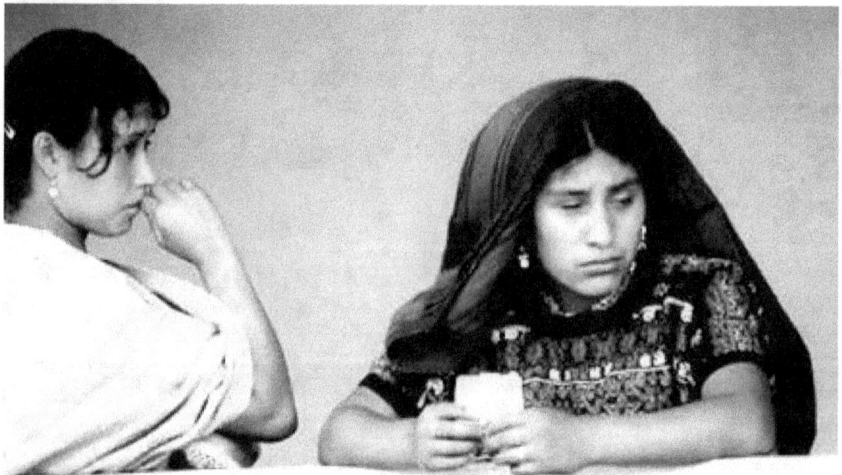

Fig 26-6: Chimaltenango: Community Medicine clients, worried re possible bad news at a clinic visit

La Leche League was well-intentioned, but had no way of neutralising the gifts of free commercial milk powder, which was rarely used by the poor as directed, and often so diluted as to be useless and harmful. This was a common cause of infant malnutrition among the poor, and a major problem in Jamaica, where sweetened condensed milk was often the cheaper choice than milk powder, and served diluted down to a weak sugar solution. As an intern, I had spent many frustrating hours with poor mothers explaining the difference, and handing out skimmed milk powder. For every success, there were half a dozen failures, as the powder was shared among other children, or sold to buy other needs, often to satisfy the mother's partner.

The Manchester project had full support of politicians, parish officials, and the Ministry of Health. Drs Julio Ceitlin of PAFAMS and Mario Chavez of Kellogg had visited and approved our plan (Fig 26-3). I assisted in vetting various drafts, visiting sites and assessing problems. For the implementation, we were careful to specify the actions to be taken at every stage of the process, that students were fully briefed, and that each understood the aims. We had stressed the importance of maintaining links between the UHWI, the Mandeville Hospital and the health centres, and that students must become expert at using this link, and must understand the role of each to achieve total care. Local doctors, nurses and other health workers, and politicians, confirmed their belief in, and support for the project, and looked forward to helping students.

For research, students would select from a range of community issues of epidemiologic, social and medical value, as in Guatemala, to enhance their learning, and to see how simple actions in caring for its members, along with inputs from others in the team, affected the health of communities; accurate records would enhance their work. The manual gave details, including the need for self- and peer-evaluation.

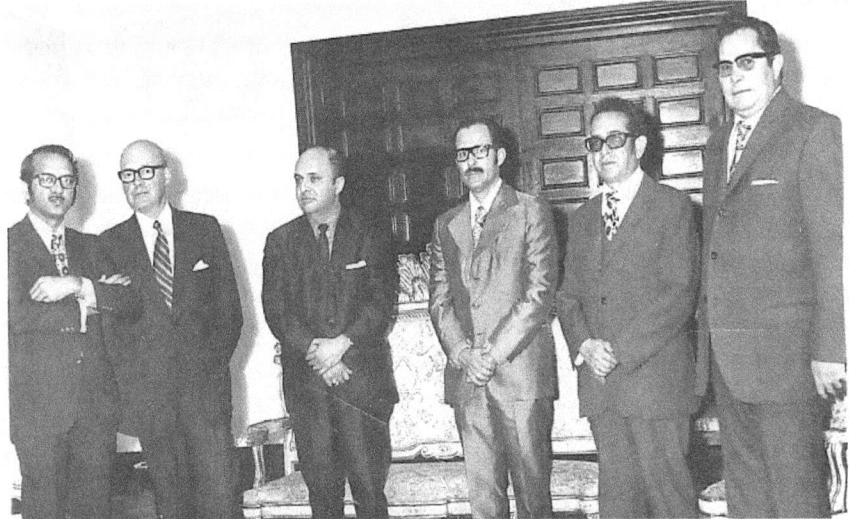

Fig 26-7: Dean Ragbeer (L) with Kellogg (2nd left) and PAFAMS executives re Community Medicine Grants for Latin American and Caribbean Projects, 1974, and talks on Family Medicine

In 1974-5, as Director, I visited the clinics on weekends, and met with the students, examined their work, and gave feedback. Dr Minott joined me a few times, but he had preferred to visit on week-days. I had several meetings with Mr. Mason, the Mandeville Hospital Secretary (Director), twice jointly with Public health officers and Dr Minott, shared project documents, explained details of our grant, the role of the MOH, and dealt with questions and concerns. Close supervision of students allowed refinements, and the discussions cleared doubts and suggested further work. I gave students medico-legal advice and defined boundaries, often having to curb the urge to prescribe without approval from the supervising District Medical Officer (DMO). Problems arose when (s)he did not come on time, leading to delays in treatment; appropriate OTC preparations were given in such cases. I discussed with the DMO and Dr Wilson the compilation of a list of medications, indications and dosage limits that students could dispense, to be reviewed at each supervisor visit. Dr Minott would follow-up and monitor use of the list. Students and Nurses agreed that this would help to relieve prescription anxieties.

The Manchester project document and the Commonwealth Foundation Paper on *"Ancillaries"* had also been discussed in 1974 with Vice Dean Butler and Associate Deans in the EC, as a programming guide. In Feb 1975, Minister McNeill and I discussed it with "Black educators," when we spoke at the conference on *Health Problems of Black Populations* at Howard University, Washington DC. Minister McNeill also repeated his endorsement of my ideas on training ancillaries, as did others from West Africa, several of whom I had met the previous year. He also described our CM project, and thanked the Kellogg Foundation. A group of us had a lively session — on closed circuit TV, and recorded — on the place of medical schools in training *all* levels of health workers. Discussants were impressed that our S&P Dept. was already geared to train aides, once resources were provided (Fig 26-9).

In 1975, at the height of the social disruption in Kingston, Queen Elizabeth II and her husband, Prince Philip, visited Jamaica from 26th to 30th April, and came to Mona on the 28th to open the professional Law School and meet people. She also wanted a capsule of "work on hand, and what made the UWI distinct." The UWI Royal Charter granted her visiting rights; article 6 of the 1972 Charter stating that *"the Monarch, her heirs and successors, had 'Visitorial Authority', and shall be regarded as Visitor of the University. In exercising this authority, the monarch, her heirs and successors, can inspect the University, its buildings, laboratories and general work, equipment and also the examination, teaching and other activities of the University, from time to time."* This was such a time. The security was tight, mindful of social unrest in Jamaica, and militant student protests of recent years, in 1970 against "attendant" services to Chancellor Princess Alice, at the opening of the campus' Library in St Augustine, and later, at dinner. At Mona, they protested at the Creative Arts Centre, and soon after, at Easter, in the Chapel, among others. These probably caused her resignation, and that of Pro-Chancellor Eric Williams, in February 1971.

Some social scientists and student acolytes had been hostile to VC Marshall, from the start of his tenure, perhaps for his prompt use of legal tools to quell what he called needless disruption of campus activities, for political, not academic reasons. I saw him as always fair, and agreed with his views on the gullibility of most protesting sociology students, and their unwillingness to consider issues less emotionally than they did. Their actions may have prompted his resignation in March, 1974.

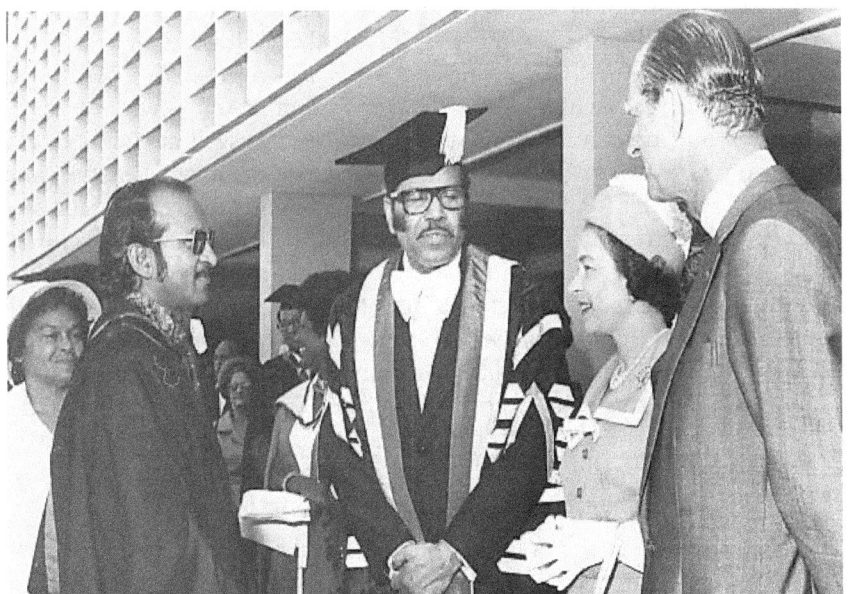

Fig 26-8: Explaining UWI Medical Faculty and PGME to QEII, April 28, 1975, in one sentence! VC Preston and Prince Philip are on either side.

For the visit, politicians cooperated by reining in the hounds. By then, several of the toughest hoodlums had either been killed or jailed, leaving several score on their best behaviour. VC Preston presented dignitaries, then the Deans, having asked each one to give a one sentence 30-second capsule of his Faculty. I said my piece, *"Our Faculty of Medicine has sole responsibility for training medical doctors for 14 small countries; this is a unique situation and a huge challenge! We've started to train specialists and have just graduated three."* She actually asked a question, *"How many students do you have?"* *"550. We take in 110 each year for five years, and will be starting a new school in Trinidad in the next three years, if all goes well, and there we'll also train dentists, veterinarians and others."*

She smiled and looked as if she wanted to say more, but time was up, and we moved on. A day later, she opened the fifth meeting of the *Commonwealth Heads of Government,* which ran from April 29th to May 6th. Of this Conference, Hansard (UK) reported comments from a number of lords. One said, *"Thirty-three Commonwealth Governments were represented and the meeting was one of the most important and successful Commonwealth meetings ever held. Much of the time was spent on economic matters and on the problems of Southern Africa, and on both, a substantial measure of agreement was reached."* It's worth noting that the group then numbered 34 and is now 52. The reference to South Africa had to do with the coming independence of Namibia, a protectorate, and whether South Africa would peacefully relinquish its mandate.

At the mid-June 1975 meeting of Health Ministers in Kingston (styled *Meeting of CARICOM Ministers responsible for Health – CARICOM, MRH*), Dr Hector Acuña, the new Director of PAHO, wished to be briefed on our ideas re manpower; I did so, and gave him copies of my papers on *Community Medicine,* the *Manchester project, Teamwork,* and *Ancillaries.* Minister McNeill reviewed Government's plans in health care to reach all sectors of society, promote healthy living and prevention, taking full advantage of vaccines and biological advances then available, in nutrition, heart disease, infections etc., (but for the public health failure re Polio immunisation coverage: *see Footnote 13, p. 72*). He outlined their manpower initiatives, and explained the role of the Community Physician as conceived in our PGME plans, stressing the *integration of public health* with *clinical specialties* to match the budgets of smaller countries, as Finance Minister Coore had presented in May (Fig. 26-9). He had anticipated some resistance among Public Health officers to the proposed changes, but was optimistic as several younger officers were in favour; older ones would retain their current duties until retirement. Barbados, Trinidad, and the Associated States were on-side. He had met with Dr Acuña and hoped for PAHO's continuing support.

He had repeated to *The Daily Gleaner* his concern that Jamaica's hospital services needed much improvement to fulfil their role in PGME. But, by then, specialty training had started in Jamaica, and had already produced full specialists in Medicine and Paediatrics, and diplomates in Child Health, Anaesthesia, Pathology, O&G, and Public Health. In my report to the Health Ministers, I noted these, described our elective start of CM education, the end of my deanship, and introduced Manley West, Vice-Dean, Preclinical Studies, who would act as Dean, on my departure, until one was appointed. The Ministers confirmed their intent to recognise our DM and MS for specialist appointments at Senior Registrar and consultant levels, and seemed more attuned to the spirit of a regional university, even though the two major heads of governments continued to lock horns on future development and capital spending.

Despite the strained atmosphere of high alert, existing for six years, we had ploughed on and completed plans to include the new Cornwall Regional Hospital, Montego Bay, for teaching, first explored in 1972. Dr Monty Burke, the chief — an internist and one of the original 1954 UCWI graduates — and most consultants in Montego Bay, supported the new role for the CRH, which, the Minister hinted, could develop into a safer western base for medical education. We had identified sites in St Thomas and St James as suitable for teaching projects in CM. Drs. Lampart of Morant Bay and Hagley of Spanish Town were willing to participate, and had regularly accepted elective students, and the latter interns.

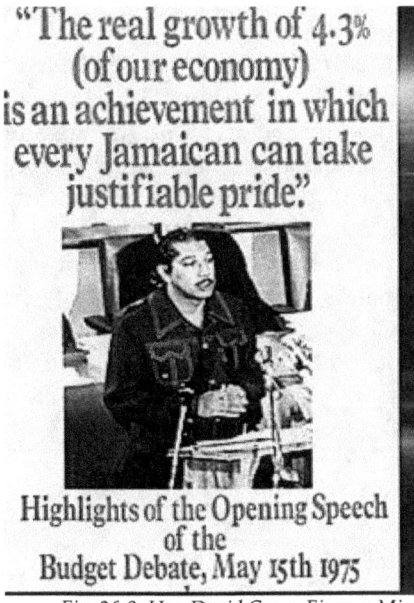

"The real growth of 4.3% (of our economy) is an achievement in which every Jamaican can take justifiable pride."

Highlights of the Opening Speech of the Budget Debate, May 15th 1975

HEALTH

"A number of new initiatives are either being started or expanded this year. Considerable attention will be paid to clinics and health centres. The amounts for this are being increased from $150,000 to $2.1 million.

The programme of Community Health Aides, started in 1972, will be expanded from 350 to 1,200 Aides at a cost of $2.1 million.

A nutritional programme, aimed at the pregnant women and children under four years old, will be launched. The programme will be started with a provision of $1 million. It will stretch over five years and by 1980 will provide pre-natal services for 90% of the nation's pregnant women, one post-natal visit to 70% of mothers and surveillance to 90% of mal-nourished children."

SPECIAL EMPLOYMENT PROGRAMME

"This programme is provided with $53.2 million, an increase of 53% over last year. This provision will provide 24,500 jobs of one year's duration. 51% of the expenditure will be on projects of capital

Fig 26-9 Hon David Coore, Finance Minister, opening Budget Speech, Kingston, 1975

We had submitted to T&T and Barbados our ideas on expansion for the 1975-78 triennium. The curriculum had been revamped to allow the final year clerkship in Community Medicine, from 1975, postponed a year to accommodate students. Social, behavioural, environmental and organisational topics pertinent to Community Medicine, Primary Care, and Family Medicine, would be covered in the first year, and the principles incorporated in each clinical clerkship to enhance the social and behavioural aspects of clinical medicine, in and out of hospitals.

The students who had done electives with me in the Manchester project, gave positive feedback. CM had also started in Trinidad as an elective, under Dr Hanoman, as noted, in association with the MOH. A draft curriculum for Family Practice was left with the Faculty Board, which Dr West would pilot, with Dr Dyer's guidance. The loss of staff due to the social disruptions in Jamaica was threatening, and the security measures that PM Manley had outlined had not yet reduced the extent, frequency or viciousness of the gang violence in Kingston.

We expected the Antilles to develop a capacity for clinical electives as hospital standards improved. We were aware of fiscal constraints and that several CHMC resolutions from 1973 remained to be addressed.

Dr Comissiong reported that several Antillean governments were being wooed by a group of businessmen from New York for approval to set up "for-profit" medical schools, the first in Grenada. A lawyer heading the group had contacted me in 1974, explaining the plan and offered a "bribe" for support. In rejecting, I had promised to warn the CHMC to decline, unless we had many more details. I informed Dr Philip Boyd, Secretary, but his agenda was "full" and he would "have to play it by ear," and he too had heard from the Americans. I had urged, and he had agreed that the Caribbean should wake up to the strengths in their own institutions before allowing American carpetbaggers to buy the islands for a few dollars, which islanders could earn honestly otherwise. I told him of my suggestion to UWI to reserve 50 of the new places for private foreign students, to pay for the expansion, but it had not gone over well among UWI's dominating socialists (p. 118). Dr Boyd would discuss this further in executive session with the Ministers.

But, surprisingly, the matter did not come up for discussion in 1975, and *"St George's University Medical School"* became a reality by law passed in 1978, with the support of Grenada's flamboyant PM Eric Gairy. Such schools had all but disappeared in the USA, and seemed a recall of pre-Flexnerian "medical schools," not attached to Universities, and operated unregulated by doctors who were themselves poorly trained, following capricious curricula, some requiring no more than three months apprenticeship, and ignoring such science as was already widely known. They had existed all over the United States, without regulation or

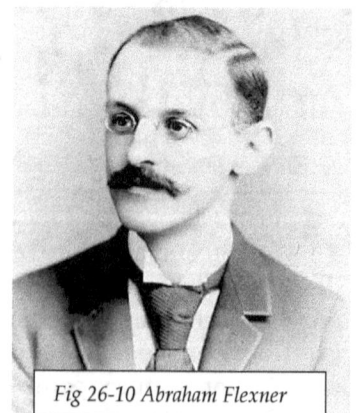

Fig 26-10 Abraham Flexner

official scrutiny, until Abraham Flexner's 1910 study of all 155 US and Canadian schools on behalf of the Carnegie Corporation. His famous Report changed the face of medical education, and set it on a sound base of research, clinical, teaching and service, naming the 17 year-old Johns

Hopkins Medical School as a model. It admitted both genders, already had an enviable reputation and was widely regarded for quality and the excellence of its achievements. Flexner's recommendations dominated every NA medical school, but did not include the "physician as a social instrument," an aim we advocated and hoped to achieve with our Community Medicine program. For interest, one should know that Flexner was not a physician, nor scientist, but an educator, and had included the "negro schools" in his recommendations, which they too were persuaded to follow.

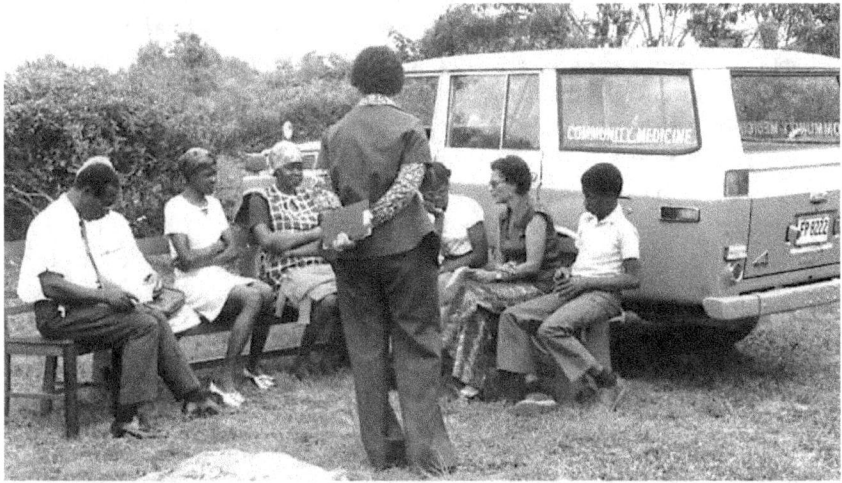

Fig 26-11 Manchester CM project: education session at Lincoln Clinic (Dean's collection)

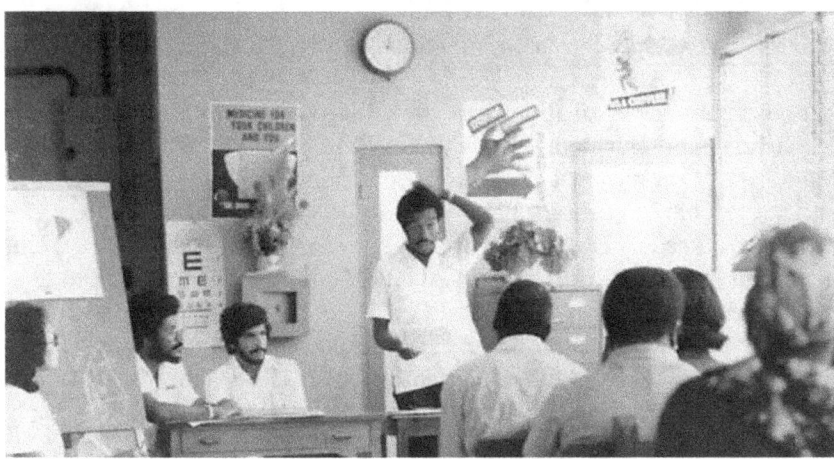

Fig 26-12 Manchester CM project: education session at Ptatville, Clinic (Dean's Collection)

The violence and threats to the Mona campus scuttled plans for several events to discuss Curriculum, Community Medicine, and medical education, using as a start the papers I had already circulated:

Curriculum plans on pp. 56-8; Appendices 9-11, pp. 335-40; PGME papers; Kurt Deuschle and IADB reports; resolutions of the CHMC between 1969 and 1974; UWI Council decisions for the triennia 1969-72 and 1972-75; my report on the ways other developing countries tackled the same issues; several bulletins from the WHO; staff papers, and so on.

The format envisaged was a series of informal evening sessions, 5-7 pm daily, or at any other preferred time e.g. 7-9 pm, for five days, with pre-circulated papers, open attendance by students, residents, faculty, university administrators, associates, guests, with a moderator for each, and a lead speaker (10 minutes) to introduce the theme for that session. A rapporteur would summarise each session. The overall aim would be to describe current Faculty status, get feedback, and review outstanding needs and future outlook. The Friday (fifth) session would be a cocktail party, followed on Saturday with an inaugural meeting of alumni, with the VC present, to launch an *Alumnus Association,* for which Mrs. Jung and Ann Costa had begun to assemble addresses and draft invitations.

Besides this, we would begin a monthly lecture, as a Faculty highlight, perhaps on Saturdays 9-11 am, to inspire students to excel, by exposure to fine role models: researchers, clinicians, basic scientists, teachers, external examiners, administrators, Ministers of Health, CMOs and SMOs. We would begin with CMOs, distinguished graduates, current faculty, residents, and students. They would be given time after speaking to meet and discourse with the audience. A roster would be drawn up in consultation with campus research units. The annual MRC meeting was a Caribbean-wide event, but attracted few students.

I had also planned a gala conference on medical education, with themes like: *Challenges for new medical schools*: *old rum and wine in new bottles?* Or, *A single servant for fourteen masters?*). I would invite well-known regional personalities e.g. from the UWI campuses, Universities of Guyana and Surinam, PAHO, PAFAMS, HOPE, ACURI, Kellogg, Macy and Commonwealth Foundations, among others, to join with Faculty teachers to present papers for audience discussion, focussing on Caribbean needs. The work of UWI researchers, past and current, including students and residents, would be highlighted. UWI Students had little contact with Latin America, and had probably never met dynamic educators like Alberto Cristoffanini, Gabriel Velasquez Palau, Julio Ceitlin, Andreas Santas, or Mario Chavez. All had agreed to take part, and assist with organisation and fund-raising. Kellogg, Macy, PAHO and HOPE were considering support.

But with all after-hours and discretionary activities scuttled by social unrest, I had hoped at least to get an hour at the joint JMA-BMA-CMA meeting, in April 1974, to launch our Alumnus Association and fund-raising, but the organisers could find no time for this.

CHAPTER 27
Swansong

My last official duty for the Faculty was a presentation to the UGC of estimates for the 1975-78 triennium, which had been vetted by the Heads of Departments Committee, chaired by Sir Harry Annamunthodo, and by the Finance Committee. We were warned not to ask for too much, even though a Council decision had been made to support expansion in this budget. In presenting my case to the Grants Committee, I regretted the unsettled state of the University and country, and stressed that we had remained optimistic, and were merely seeking to complete the package we had presented three years ago, provided only skeletally, and even so, with a few limbs missing, chopped by the "evil hand of political dissension!" The chair was the sympathetic Hon. Errol Barrow, Prime Minister of Barbados, who respected our position, but in the end, we lost by a thin margin. Some administrators were almost hostile, including a new PVC, Mona, Dr Gerald Lalor, one of the first chemistry graduates of UCWI, and a friend of VC Preston, who had added him recently to his team of PVCs.

An incident in April, 1975 illustrated the *personal* hurdles we faced, and the sourness in the atmosphere. Did stress stemming from the general unrest cause this? Possibly. After initial meetings with USAID in November 1974 on issues re "social development," I had done for the VC a paper on the role of the medical faculty in this; I had heard no more until April, 1975, when the administration was finally drafting an application, collated by the new PVC, G C Lalor. The theme was relevant to our starting program in Community Medicine, about which he was ill-informed. He had, nevertheless, said to me, "you have enough," adding that the application concerned social sciences and humanities, and had "nothing to do with Medicine." I had disagreed, arguing that health was a key factor in social and economic advancement in any community, and was included in our new curriculum as an important early addition, and a timely inclusion in the proposal.[37] He had frowned at this, and summoned at short notice a conference of Deans, program heads and PVCs that overlapped with a 4 pm meeting of the Medical Faculty Board. No one was available to chair our Board meeting, so, on attending

---

[37] In 1977, the third meeting of CARICOM Ministers responsible for Health (previously CHMC) would state this as a fact in its Resolution 4/77, a "Declaration on Health for the Caribbean Community" I had given PVC Lalor several references, including the WHO.

PVC Lalor's, which started at 3 pm, I asked for an early hearing, explaining why. No one objected, but Lalor stuck to his agenda, and at 3.50 pm, I rose, nodded to him and departed. His secretary had my written submission, already sent to the VC.

The application went forward without our input, Lalor reporting to the VC that I had left his meeting without excuse, hence the omission. I wrote to VC Preston, contradicting Lalor, and recalling prior discussions with VC Marshall, of which Preston was aware, re taking steps to obtain some autonomy for our Faculty, and particularly now, to recognise the added pressures we faced, due to the social turmoil, the staffing difficulties, the lingering hostility of some senior staff, and the extra burden on each one: *"Some consideration must be allowed members of the clinical Medical Faculty, the nature of whose day to day commitments often*

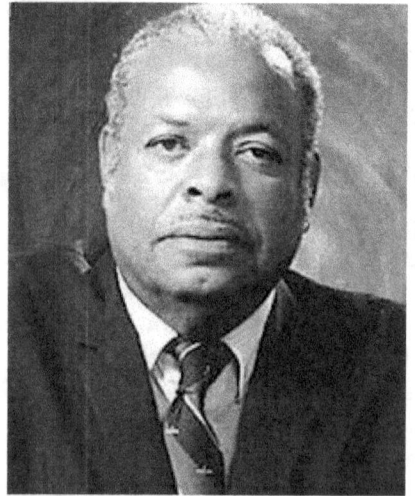

precludes dropping everything and rushing to an administrative get-together. Repeated failure ... to take account of the nature and demands of medical practice and medical education, and their many incompatibilities with the structure of this university, will do the institution no good. The feelings of frustration running high in the Medical Faculty at this time are a direct result of this ... Leaving it (the Faculty) underprovided in the face of grave wants will only reflect on the quality of your stewardship." The application failed.

Fig 27-1: Hon. PM Errol Barrow, Barbados, cropped photo, (from The Archives) www.nationnews.com/lMG/380/53380/barrow

Late in June, the UGC met to discuss the UHWI requests, a few days after completing those from the University. I had no time to consult anyone, so I promptly reinserted in our Hospital requests items denied us — which I had previously removed to avoid duplicate submissions — and sent the requests to the Hospital Administrator. In the mid-morning, PM Barrow called and wished to visit the Hospital to get a closer look at our situation, prior to a meeting with the Hospital Board. He had time then. We met in my office; Anne arranged a light lunch, according to his wishes.

We toured the teaching facilities; I showed him the changes made since the last budget, the areas of need, and the PGME building site where the foundation had been laid (p. 214). He was pleased to hear of its financing, and had deplored his own forced withdrawal.

The conversation was unexpected, but welcomed, and exhilarating to me; he requested confidentiality. But I wrote it down soon after it had ended, almost verbatim, with his permission, provided I kept it to myself for 25 years. I have only now revealed it:

"You've upset a few people; one or two are even fuming, and they can hurt you."

"I'm sorry; whatever I did, I did in good faith, and for a long-term cause."

"I know, but they don't see it that way. They think you're grandstanding; but what I see is you have a better case than the rest; they are too accustomed to get their share without arguing for it; you came prepared and caught them sleeping. Marshall, Preston, Holness and Jackman liked that; made their decision easier. Now, they see you as already favoured and yet you want more; realistically you should get it, as part of a package; they think they should make that decision, they don't think it should come from you; they see you as an upstart, and if I may say so, not one of them. *Their decision is not logical, not academic."*

I felt their misunderstanding, saw the faces of those for, like Reg Murray, Education, Marshall Hall, Management Studies, and those against, like Lalor of Chemistry. I felt resentful, but controlled myself, impressed with his kindness.

"But sir, my job is to serve this Faculty; it's been my life, almost as if by destiny. I've put heart and soul into it. Our task is to plan sensibly, get approvals, and do the best we can. If we're ahead of them, they should graciously accept that. If it's credit they want, I'll give them that; they can remove my name from the papers, insert their own, as long as we get a fair deal. We don't want favours; we want judgements based on merit."

He laughed, and sipped his juice.

"You're passionate about this; good. I too think they're making a mistake. You can come to Barbados and work for us, if you wish. But I suspect that's if we win the next election, and if we get a medical campus there. Nita thinks highly of you, and your wife, by the bye."

"Great lady, sir; the hospital lost heavily when they lost her; Sievewright is OK, but nowhere near her in style; too aggressive."

"Good word, heavily; she is still overweight, like me."

Embarrassed, I apologised.

"No, no, I'm only teasing; good pun, even if unconscious. Now, tell me about your position, and the Faculty. If you get what you want from the University, can you recruit the bodies?"

"That I can't say, sir; a couple years ago, I tried hard to get Massiah and his wife..."

"Tough one; neither White nor Dos Santos would budge on the lab position for a while; but agreed. What happened?"

"I sat with each in turn, I've known Errol since 1960; and Harold and I have been friends for years. Harold does the tissue work and firmly believed that a university appointee would erode his private practice. I assured him that our

contracts were different, and would protect him. I spoke to Harold Forde, to James Williams and Carlyle Burton. White agreed."
"Why didn't the Massiahs come?"
"I really don't know; he was so positive until the post for the wife was cleared. I believe he never expected that I could get the post, so he put that as a condition. We surprised him. I suspect the money pull in Toronto was too strong; the job he took is in private practice, not academic, which he had said was his goal."
"Pity, we could have used both."
"If it was here, I would understand, but not Barbados; they don't terrorise."
"At least, not yet, and not as long as I'm PM. So what happens now?"
"We've advertised the post; there are a few leads, and HOPE will fill the gap until then. But even if that's slow, we need the assurance of an established post to show commitment, especially to PGME, and to base our search."
"You have many sceptics; I read that Canadian article last year; but already you've given a strong answer. Preston was amazed at the building deal, and told me how you pulled it off; and there it is, all started. I believe that is your drawing card. An investment in the future. If you get an increase at the hospital base, would that bother you?"
"Not really. The University base would give us more flexibility between here and EC, but a hospital increase would free existing staff for tours of duty there, as needed, as we expand there."
"You will probably get most of what we can afford through the Hospital. The University will not like that. They'll see through it. They'll blame you for double-dealing and plotting. Can you take that?"

I didn't tell him about the letter exchange between me and the VC. Nor the verbals with PVCs Lalor (hostile, Brooks' ally) and Augier (benign), nor my letter re heads of Pathology and Medicine (& oral to Augier). If any of these circulated, I'd be fried by other heads, but I could stand that heat: anger, not fire. It was after lunch, and we were walking along the covered way to the Hospital Board Room. I said simply,
"Can I tell you a little story, sir, to answer?" (I was talking to a man I greatly respected, if only for his courage in two things: he had flown 45 WWII missions as an RAF tail gunner; and he had switched from Communism to pragmatism, a move that had saved Barbados, and one that Jagan should have made in BG.)
"Yes, of course."
"Champ Alleyne said to me the other day, after a debate on priorities, 'I wouldn't want to be Dean; you're just a pissing post!' To which I replied, without thinking, 'That's because of all the sons of bitches I have to deal with!'"
The PM laughed and slapped my back, *"I've always noted that you liked to play with words. Good answer; it's just like being PM: I can use that, may I?"*
"Of course; but you're very good at puns yourself, sir."
He changed the subject.
"How long will you be in Canada?"

"*A year, sir, probably two, if I can get the funding.*"

"*What will you do in Canada?*"

"*Last year, CHMC wished for information and an analysis of insurance-based health care delivery. I've been studying Ontario's and Alberta's systems. One of my good friends in Hospital Administration is a consultant to Ontario's Health Ministry on this very thing, and deals with academic hospitals. He'll help me.*"

"*Good; you have finance?*"

"*Not yet, I'm applying to Foundations. Kellogg might help; I have a grant from them for Community Medicine; or maybe CIDA. My experience in Chicago tells me not to be hopeful; they don't know Indians and have a very warped view of us; they follow Churchill's declamations and think we're all naked fakirs, and were stunned when I gave a talk with improvised visual aids. Or else, I'll have to find a job. Hector Acuña, the new PAHO director, suggested I join them, and PAFAMS supported me; my wife visited Washington, but wouldn't live there.*"

"*Be careful, no one goes to Canada and comes back; you told me about Massiah; I know some more. The money's too good, even if race relations aren't.*"

"*Well, if I were moved by money alone, I would have taken the Columbia offer ten years ago; I go for children and wife; two of the boys were assaulted at school last year, and she took them away soon after. But I look on this place as mine; I liked its motto from the start. I'll leave it only if it pushes me out.*"

"*Not if I have any say.*" I was so moved, I almost choked. "*I'll tell you confidentially,*" he continued, "*Harold Forde is proud that he once taught you, and even Ken praises you. Carlyle too. Will you come back as Dean?*"

"*I'd prefer Co-ordinator of PGME or Director of Community Medicine. They're bigger challenges. They could collapse if not handled tactfully or competently; Postgrad seems safe now, but Community Medicine is fragile. A jigsaw puzzle, with missing pieces. That's why I'm so worried about the research project in Manchester. I'm not confident in those who will run it, especially at this time.*"

"*I see,*" he paused. "*I'll keep that in mind. Now, who will do the Postgrad work when you go? You're doing that now, as well as Community Medicine, from what I hear? That must please Preston, with two Professors' wages and benefits saved for three years!*" He chuckled in good humour.

"*Yes, sir, and I can't let go; we're trying to recruit a Director for Community Medicine; so few available; PAHO will help, but we may have to grow our own; already we lost a year from CM because the person who will run it misinformed students re the scheme, because he didn't fully understand the issues; we've gone over the ground several times since, and on site, and with the Committee, which is still new and unstable. I'm putting trust in the working document and on the briefing visits we've made. We've had excellent results from elective students, so far. I hope their comments are used to the full. I've offered to help by six monthly visits, which Kellogg will cover; I've checked with Mario Chavez, the Director.*"

"*And Postgrad is safe, you say; how so?*"

"*It's better positioned; it's way is clear; all departments are on side, Minister McNeill and CMO Wilson. Dr Carpenter knows the issues; he will chair the*

Coordinating Committee and manage the daily stuff until a Coordinator is hired, or I return. By the way politics is happening here, it might come to that."
"So you've already laid all this out; everyone here knows what to do?"
"Yes, and in EC too. Three years ago, we agreed to curriculum changes and Community Medicine; the new one is yet to be implemented; not everyone is cooperative; some see loss of territory; so I spend a lot of time explaining why not. I was sorry to lose Prof. Hoyte, but he, Profs Cruickshank and Bras got offers they could not delay. Here, I've had to cajole, and you know we had to let go of Manchester; that was a heartache; it made me enemies. But we're over that. The violence affected HOPE. Meltzer, who was like a twin, left two years ago, but has continued the support, and is now in Barbados as well, and my friend Hughley Hanoman has fled Burnham, and took our CM job in Trinidad. His family is quite rich in Guyana, and at risk to Burnham's 'fund-raising'; he took to politics and got threatened for criticising Burnham. Here, recently, Sir Harry's daughter and wife were assaulted in their Hope Pastures home, a community we had thought safe. And Rolf Richards wanted me to approve his transfer to EC, once the second year clinical is approved; his wife was also assaulted in College Common. Even Mickey Walrond wants to go home. Those will be big losses. I'd hoped he would stay and become Dean."
"I see your dilemma. But Walrond is not on your side, is he?"
"Everybody and nobody is on my side, sir; it depends on the time of day. But I know what you mean. I respect his ability; he backed the new curriculum."
"He didn't think you should have opposed Ken for the Deanship; he thinks you let ambition win, instead of good sense."
"Everyone with an opinion on that thinks the same. But I'll tell you what I've said only to Ken Standard and Karl Smith, the ones who got me into this, David Hoyte and my wife. I worked for over 2 years to get the PGME program organised, and expected Ken to continue as Dean. But he told us things about the VC's position, which Roy denied had been discussed. Walrond was part of our protest, and signed the Action Group report. After that, enough people felt that Ken had too many activities, and would continue the status quo as full-time Dean, and so I listened to the arguments. After the announcement, I had second thoughts. I really wanted to remain Coordinator of PGME, which I had been from the beginning, so much to do, and I knew the ground and the players. So I planned to tell Ken that I would turn down the deanship, and apply instead for the PGME or Community Medicine job, or do both. But before I could go over, he charged into my office, tore me to shreds, called me dreadful names and finally consigned me, my ancestors and progeny to hell. His face looked murderous. I couldn't believe it. I know I'm not a coward and have walked away from a rifleman in a mob. So I took a deep breath and told him what I wanted to say, but because of his damning tirade, I'm going to show him I'm none of those things, at least not yet, and was afraid of neither workload nor responsibility, even if the entire squad of professors ranged itself against me. It would be their reputation on the line, not mine. I try to play fair, not favourites; my friends

know that, that's what Karl Smith said when he and Ken Standard approached me; they knew how much and how long their persuasion was, and that I was backing Ken, but I could not ignore their evidence, and argument."

"I heard some of this from Ken Standard, but not those details. I'm glad you told me about that. It had troubled me, and seemed out of character, as I got to know you; it falls in more with Nita's estimation. She's very insightful."

His relaxed and friendly manner emboldened me to mention the negative effect caused by Munroe's union activity, and whether a poor young country could afford such extravagance. His eyebrows lifted and I quickly added, *"He stood beside me outside the Registry, while one of his men held a gun to my head."* I told him the context. He frowned, and expressed concern re "overzealous socialism" on the Mona campus, and Marshall's first attempt at a code of professional conduct, for staff and students, which neither liked. He was concerned re leftist unrest at Cave Hill. *"I've been there, so know the exuberance, but we're not Cuba; we must be more objective and cautious. Munroe is like a spoilt child playing with trouble. Ralph Gonsalves at Cave Hill and Walter Rodney in Guyana are the same extreme left, and a problem. If Tom Adams wins next year, he will cleanse Cave Hill."*

I told him that I had met many radicals on my India-Africa trip, including Julius Nyerere, who asked me about Rodney, whom he had gotten to know well, and whose 1972 book *How Europe Underdeveloped Africa* was causing quite a stir. But even Nyerere was pulling away to the centre, as I was later informed by Dr W. Makene, the Dean of Health Sciences; Dr Abdullah Mamujee, a University surgeon; and by a Swedish Aid volunteer in their Health Services. So Rodney had left. Not that he risked expulsion, unless he crossed the line and meddled in local politics.

We were then in the Hospital Board Room. The PM's attitude was so convivial, I risked asking him a burning question: how did he manage to skirt, or ignore or confront the power of Barbadian whites, notorious throughout the Caribbean for racism and heavy-handed militarism, whose forebears did not regard Africans as humans, classified races as white, brown and black in that order, and denied any rights to the last, exiling many excellent cricketers to Trinidad or BG or the UK, starting from the turn of the century. I had been sensitised to the issue by Cameron Tudor at Queens, and had seen residues of racism at UCWI in the fifties, how domineering and aloof white Barbadians could be, and how at the Students Union few socialised with Blacks, and most avoided mixed groups. This was hardly a problem for Jamaicans and the others. I had wondered whether Walrond's style had any connection with the 17th century governor of Barbados, also critiqued by Mr Tudor, among others. He had also told us of the early colonists and slavers, the Harewoods, and their dominance, both there and in Jamaica, where their Barbadian colonists developed plantation farming *(also p. 122).*

He smiled, *"That's a whole different story, but yet at the core of our social system, and we must deal with it. So far, whites respect their place; they have the financial clout and maintain large land holdings. They own major businesses, but leave the politicking to us, and that's our fight. I avoided a referendum for independence because many Barbadians feared their power to block it. I suspect that we haven't trod on their exposed toes, but if we do, the banks will tell us. It's almost certain though that the Harewoods will leave by year-end. They're astute moneymen. They cashed out in Jamaica when prices were high in the 18th century, after a hundred years trading slaves and sugar. With 300 years of looting they built a handsome castle in Yorkshire, which I've seen. It's the same as the Indians tell us how thoroughly generations of British aristocrats have bled them; same for Africans. But they hardly talk about it."*

"At UCWI, some Barbadian Blacks avoided their white countrymen; a few behaved deferentially to them, and at first were wary of white Jamaicans, as in my class, until the Jamaicans showed no overt prejudice, greeted them like everyone else or started conversations. I would have been puzzled had Mr Tudor and our deputy principal at QC, Mr. HAM Beckles, not talked of these things."

"Those are names prominent in Barbadian scholarship; several have already passed through this place. It's good to know that Cammy taught you; he has a long history in our party and is now High Commissioner in the UK."

"It's ironic, isn't it sir, that those who were treated so harshly by whites, returned such selfless service to them. You, sir, are a legend for courage and achievement, in the war, and luck, surviving so many missions; you became one of my heroes when I first heard of it nearly twenty years ago, from Ernest Peart, now one of PM Manley's Ministers. I wish that Burnham had possessed even a tiny bit of your values, or your character, and respect for people."

He looked sharply at me, so that I felt that I had gone too far. But then his gaze relaxed; he smiled and said,

"You speak with feeling; we must preserve our history, and you seem to have an interest in that. I wish you well, and hope to see you back in two years."

"I cannot thank you enough, sir; my prayers will be for you next year."

Our talk ended as others came in for the Board meeting.

Sir Harry had joined us at the start of our meeting, but had had to leave abruptly to do an emergency operation. Afterwards, when I told him that we would get our main requests, his doubtful reception of this news was natural enough, as he had been at the University meeting that had denied our requests. Ann Costa later wrote of his stunned reaction when it was confirmed. I was thus able to pass on to Reg Carpenter and Manley West positive functional and structural resources, at Mona and in the EC.

"They will hate him for this!" Sir Harry had said to Anne, "and yet what he did was smart; many wouldn't have thought of it."

I had hoped that Alan Butler in Trinidad, and Frank Ramsay, who had taken over from Harold Forde as Associate Dean in Barbados, would push the T&T government to make a decision on the expansion plans, suggesting to Dr West, and VC Preston, that I would be prepared to take over the implementation, on return from leave. We had sent rough drafts for Mount Hope to Port-of-Spain, which UWI architect Dixon and I had made, with inputs from T&T colleagues, and I had, at a recent meeting of Council in St Augustine, shown them to Engineering professors Ken Julien and Max Richards, whose department was close to Government; they promised to track the PM's decisions. VC Preston had okayed the move, and would follow-up. I had wanted to ask PVC Braithwaite privately to explain the apparent animosity between the MOH and St. Augustine, whether it was part of the "feud" with Jamaica, but the opportunity didn't arise as he had hurried away that last evening.

At the Health Ministers' Meeting in June 1975, in Kingston, Dr Comissiong told me more about the rumblings in St Vincent, stirred by sociologist Ralph Gonsalves, a Communist pupil of the Munroe school of agitation, active in Barbados, and steeped in the Jaganite belief in a pan-Caribbean communist *nirvana*. PM Barrow believed that he would be expelled, once he had acquired a long enough rope. Maurice Bishop of Grenada was a UK-trained lawyer and communist agitator, attractive to the masses, and shared ideas with Gonsalves, Munroe, Walter Rodney, and the older communists, Cheddi Jagan and Jamaican Richard Hart.

The unrest and concerns shown by Health Ministers in 1975 reminded me of 1968, a turbulent year worldwide, with deadly outcomes for the people in the war zones of Vietnam and its neighbours, for protesters in the USA, whether youth for peace, or blacks for civil rights, with the murders of ML King on April 4 and Robert Kennedy on June 3; the shooting of Andy Warhol, and the opposition to Hubert Humphrey's nomination, with Muskie, at the Democratic National Convention in Chicago, as that Party's candidates for the White House. Mayor Richard Daley, a doyen of US Democrats, had assembled 11,900 Police and riot squads, 7,500 men from the National Guard, while President Johnson had sent him 7,500 soldiers and 1000 Secret Service agents to counter the protests at the convention in the last days of August.

That same month, Soviet armour had rolled into Czechoslovakia, to quell dissent, restore the Union, and remove any threat of secession by moderates, led by Alexander Dubcek, during the Prague spring of 1968. I was on the fringe of both events, having been on a train in Austria that was halted at the border, en route to Prague for a week. Ten days later, I was about to board a flight in Toronto for Chicago, when it was cancelled because of the "Police riots" in the latter city (p. 26).

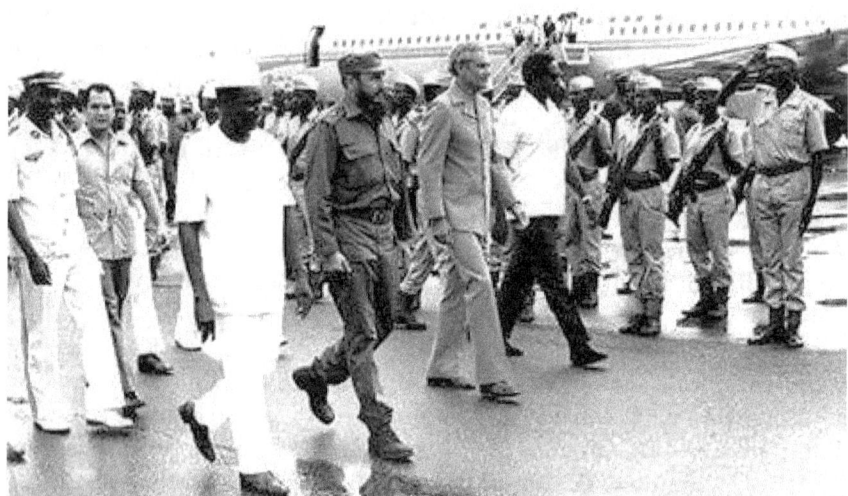

Fig 27-2: In front row, unidentified man, Fidel Castro, Michael Manley, Forbes Burnham, in Cuba (courtesy M.Manley)

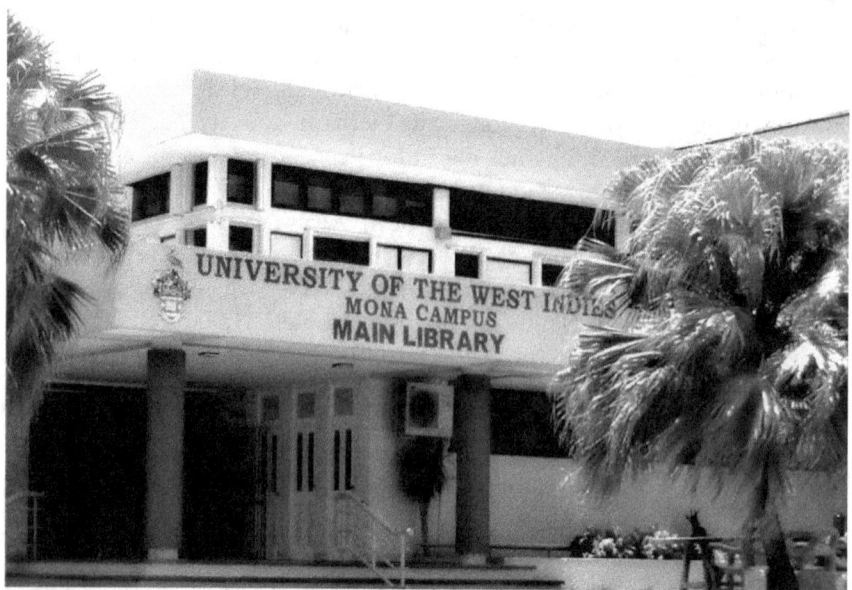

Fig 27-3; Mona Library, 2017

EPILOGUE

Perhaps the most satisfying outcome of our efforts between 1966 and 1976 was the success of the specialty training schemes. The output of the program, started on a shoestring, and in desperation, to stem a crippling brain drain, is shown in Table E-1 below, to 2008, that should make people like Korcok choke on their biases (pp. 190-1). How often had I heard myself dismissed in those years as a dreamer, and the whole scheme as a fantasy, even by eminent colleagues! I had tried to steer Canada's RCPSC towards an international role in specialty education (pp. 5-6), but even they had doubts that the UWI was *really* producing high-class specialists, and marvelled at "your boldness to try such a thing." "Why do you doubt?" I asked these sceptics, "when you've been stealing our graduates for thirty years!"

| Specialty | Number Graduating 1968-96 | | | | | DMs + |
	Dip	DM	M.Phil.	PhD.	MSc	1999-2008
Anaesthetics	151	22	0	0	0	32 (30)
Anatomy	0	0	0	1	0	0
Biochemistry	0	0	14	16	2	0
Child Health	110	55	0	0	0	37 (24)
Community Nutrition	51	0	0	0	0	0
Community Medicine	0	1	0	0	0	0
Family Medicine	0	13	21	--	--	2 (2)
Haematology (Clin)	0	3	0	0	0	4 (4)
Lab Medicine (Pathology)	1	23	--	--	2	13 (11)
Medicine (Internal)	0	38	0	0	0	39 (32)
Microbiology	0	1	1	4	8	6 (5)
Nutrition	47	0	0	10	59	0
Obstet. & Gynae.	95	66*	--	0	0	43 (42)
Ophthalmology	13	0	0	0	0	0
Pharmacology	0	0	3	2	3	0
Physiology	0	0	4	4	0	0
Psychiatry	26	20	0	0	0	15 (15)
Psychology (Clin)	0	0	1	0	1	0
Public Health	34	0	0	0	141	0
Radiology	0	20	0	0	0	17 (15)
Surgery (9 specialties)**	3	30	0	0	0	61 (57)**
Emergency Surg	-	-	0	0	0	21 (20)
TOTALS	**531**	**292**	**44**	**37**	**216**	**290 (257)**
TOTAL DM+MS (1974-2008)						**582**

Table E-1; Postgraduates trained to 2008

*MS; **21 General Surgery, 12 Orthopaedics, 8 Urology, 7 ENT, 6 Neurosurgery, 5 Paediatric Surg., 2 Cardiothoracic, 21 Emergency. **Figures in Brackets = numbers in WI: 88% of 1999-2008 total.** *(+ column adapted from Eldemire-Shearer &Roberts, Bibliography)*

Yet many educators in Canada and the USA — whom I got to know through my work on testing the competence of practising physicians — remain astonished that the program thrives, and those of its products who have migrated there, have done so well. Many of them took the UK specialty examinations, as if for quality control, or to bolster confidence, or, for surgeons, to retain the traditional British title, "Mr." It was perhaps comforting also to the UWI, whose non-medical leaders wanted some way to measure our product, to justify the investment and trust in a "dreamer." By 2008, *582 full specialists and 531 diplomates had been trained*; the work of medical teaching staff, graduates, and students prevailed over sceptics, and satisfied Senate and Council. I take pride in knowing how it was all done, and seeing it begun. A typical example of its impact is on St. Kitts, which had 5 specialists (1 native) in 1972, and 17 in 2012, including 4 surgeons, 3 interns, 1 pathologist, 1 psychiatrist, 2 O&G specialists, 2 paediatricians and a radiologist. *Overall, 88% stayed.*

In July 1975, the outstanding Faculty target was our plan to launch a Division of Community Medicine, and establish it as a base for primary care within the UHWI, and in affiliated clinics in the community assigned to it in the government health plan. A successful project would become a model for the islands. The Division, already approved by UWI, would train the unique *Specialist in Community Medicine,* as described; family doctors; and ancillaries, in line with my paper; and adopting the plan that I had described, which PAFAMS and Dr Wilson had endorsed.

The CM projects in Latin America were progressing well, and all were looking forward to our production of CM specialists to take charge of Jamaica's district and regional hospitals, as bases for integrated health services. This would provide a model for the entire Caribbean and Latin America, struggling with the inefficient division of health care between "Public Health" and "Clinical Medicine." Integration would save large sums, which could be used to improve facilities and equipment, and, in the words of Dr Andres Santas, a PAFAMS past president, to close the gap between *"médicos verdaderos y sanitaristas burocratas."* (true doctors and public health bureaucrats — *Appendix 10, p. 338*).

Leaving Jamaica was traumatic. My term was over and my leave approved. My family was in Canada, and I had to get them settled. The leave would allow me to study Ontario's system of health care funding, to address CHMC Resolution 27/74. Once in Ontario, without licence or funds, I eventually found a job as Laboratory Director for the Canadian Medical Laboratories Ltd., (CML), a start-up company, at its main laboratory in Simcoe, ON, a pleasant town, a few miles north of Lake Erie, at the edge of the wealthy tobacco region of southern Ontario.

The Company ran nine other, smaller laboratories in the region, within a 100-mile radius of Simcoe, and I was on call to them for professional help. CML was started by Dr John Mull, a pathologist, with whom I made instant rapport. I worked there for 2½ years. The work was light for me, since the brunt of daily problems was competently borne by the technical staff, headed by a bright and cheerful chief technologist. I did the tissue and other diagnostic work for 20 odd private doctors, and two small hospitals, plus forensic autopsies for six coroners. A piece of cake, compared with three professorships at Mona!

One morning, some time later, my secretary gave me a message, to call a Dr Grant at the Norfolk County Health Office in Simcoe. When Dr Grant answered, in a distinctly Jamaican accent, I could only marvel at the irony that had brought me to the same small rural Ontario town — the size of Mandeville — as the erstwhile head of UWI Microbiology, one of my former teachers. He had left Jamaica abruptly in 1974, for parts unknown — Canada, some had said — fleeing political violence.

He had taken the long-vacant post of MOH for Haldimand, Norfolk and Oxford counties, based in Simcoe. He wanted me to do his Public Health referral work, and wondered whether I still had an interest in Community Medicine, as he felt my model would be suitable for the area, and could cover all its small towns and villages. I agreed, and sent him a proposal. Nothing came of it, as his superiors could not relate to the concept, as several activities were distinctly clinical and "would upset the GPs of the region, unless their practices were preserved or enhanced by it." So it was shelved, but I used it in developing the Chedoke Health Centre project *(App 16, p. 372.)*

The other surprise call was in early 1976 from Dr Dick Meltzer to join him as adviser on Medical Education on an unnamed delegation to Mc Master University! I was surprised to find a team from the UWI, led by its newly-appointed Dean, Sam Wray, a shock in itself, as I had known him at UWI, where his Chairman had painted him as a "useful plodder". With him were Ken Standard, Owen Minott, David Picou, and George Alleyne, all long known as undergraduates, and since 1965, as staff.

I was dismayed to discover that they had little real knowledge of what had transpired in medical education at UWI between 1966 and 1975. I was handed several papers written by them, with uncredited and verbatim copies of my work *(Appendices 1,2,4,7,9,10,11)* — not the first time — and behaving as if the papers had authored themselves. I asked Wray, a psychologist, and later wrote him, re academic ethics, and he said that proper citations were omitted in error! How so, I asked, on three separate occasions? I reminded him that I was still on UWI staff.

His team, including two of my staunch detractors, had come to study the McMaster education plan, then being proselytised worldwide. He had not told me, the recent ex-Dean, not even out of courtesy, although I was a stone's throw from the University. Was it a snub, or just to avoid embarrassing his new "right-hands" by my presence? But Dr Meltzer, leading the HOPE team, had acted to correct what he saw as a clumsy piece of bad manners, and had recruited me as an advisor to his delegation! As it turned out, they were poorly briefed, and stood corrected on several key issues, with Wray embarrassed and apologetic.

To begin the exercise, Dean Fraser Mustard gave his pitch, followed by the head of medical education, Dr John Hamilton, an evangelist of British origin, a true believer, full of jargon and canned answers. He and the others, all equally fervent — British, Canadian and one Indian, an anatomist, only he wasn't called that: he was a *morphologist*. They covered Dewey and Rogers' principles of adult learning; self-direction; use of tutorials and learning resources; a small group format; "modules" of learning in a phased curriculum; and "continuous evaluation."

They summarised the curriculum, conducted a tour of the facilities, then allowed each visitor to explore independently, with a student as guide. Finally, each was assigned to get a specialty "perspective." I met with a Dr Chris Walker, a chemical pathologist, styled *"laboratory physician"* (PhDs were called *"laboratory scientists"*). He was British, like most of the staff we had met. We quickly found common ground; his supercilious bluster moderated when I told him of my training at Hammersmith. "Oh, we have one of your colleagues here, Mike Brain; do you know him?" "Yes, I did. We were contemporaries there."

They avoided the word "pathology" in the curriculum, and used euphemisms to describe it. Students learned it on electives, horizontal or block, or from a resource person after running around to find one; or from group mates. It was touch and go, and a curious substitution.

At the end, he asked me, "Are you really thinking of taking this to Jamaica? Few places can afford what we do; and soon we won't either, as soon as Bill Davis (the Ontario Premier) wakes up!" "Not me," I said, "I left a perfectly appropriate curriculum for the region, so I'm more surprised than you are. UWI is suffering a staff crisis, and here they are, in dead of winter, looking at the most staff-intensive model there is. Saudi Arabia has tapped London for 600 teachers! We can't afford North Americans; so where do we get staff? Manley told me Cuba or China!"

Walker had worked in West Africa, at a place I had visited, with a far heftier budget than the UWI. They had looked at the McMaster plan and the costs, and had walked away. "Mc works because the majority of students are honours graduates, many with higher degrees; they are an arrogant lot; they teach themselves and one another; they know the terrain, the pitfalls; all they need is a *roadmap*, which they get; they like that word here. You've been to the library and seen the mounds of slide-tape shows, carousels, TV monitors and other A-V aids; thousands of packages; replicates of everything; mindboggling; must have cost millions. The librarian and her ample staff are real eager-beavers. Hamilton is a preacher; he's really sold on this and will take it with him wherever he goes, if he ever leaves here," he ended wistfully.

When my opinion was asked in the debriefing, I deferred to Dr Meltzer, but he suggested I speak, "You were the Dean there for five years, and I heard you speak on self-directed learning, problem-based, in small groups. And I've heard you tell students that UWI does that now."

I said, "Yes, we do. I share the principles, but this model is for sure not appropriate, if you wish to retain GMC accreditation; besides, it is far too pricey for the UWI, even with a windfall, even for Trinidad, if PM Williams decides to move. The theories are fine, and we've used them, as far as affordable, in the phased curriculum we discussed for two years, and approved in 1974. Regarding small groups, we teach that way at every ward round, by the bed-side, with live patients, not as cloistered groups with paper problems, which seem to be the heart of this method. With our expanded intake, we'll now have an unwieldy 22 groups of 5.

"The huge capital outlay here, the space and staff, and the plethora of resources cannot be matched at UWI. Our Curriculum Committee turned down a cheaper plan based on Case Western Reserve, because of scarce resources. But we do have that priceless resource you would envy: compliant patients, in and out of hospitals, in clinics and health centres; grateful patients, who are *real*, and far better starting points than paper-based or simulated patients; they're spontaneous; they talk back; paper doesn't. We get steady and direct calls from 14 governments re primary and community care. You're buffered from that. Besides, we don't know if this model produces better doctors, more people- or community-oriented; is it cost:efficient; is it worth the money? I like the integrated curriculum, which we can't have at Mona, but will have at the Trinidad campus. In '72, when we started collecting data on alumni, we found UWI graduates all over Canada. We can't be doing such a bad job! This is a pricey novelty; I doubt whether it will meet GMC requirements."

Sam frowned, and a look of hate covered Picou's face. The others were deadpan. I had hoped they would rebut; none did. Sam weakly confessed ignorance of the GMC, and that "we're looking at all options."

When the UWI group assembled for a tête-a-tête, I asked, with assent from Dick, "Who's paying for all this? Trinidad? Why do you need it anyway? We had a review by GMC three years ago; they're loth to accept any of the new US curricula, whether Chicago, Stanford, Mt Sinai or Case. Full electives are not their style. We have a good model, with CHMC Ministers agreeing, on three campuses, and GMC approval. Why jettison all that work, by so many people? Who's pushing this? Who gains? You were at CHMC meetings, Ken, Dave, Owen; these others weren't; enlighten them. If you guys had studied Faculty papers, Mona and EC, you wouldn't be here in the cold. McMaster may be great for Ontario, but no model for the Caribbean, nor for that matter, Canada. Don't forget that our pass entitles the student to a license. A degree here doesn't; it only qualifies them to take the LMCC. I hear Mc has the highest fail rate in Ontario at it. Calgary follows the same principles, and costs less, but even that we can't afford. I was raised to be frugal and self-reliant, to squeeze the most out of what we had, so as to get things done, and done well; this is profligate. Their grasp of Community Medicine is nowhere as enlightened as ours, and Louis Grant agrees with me there. This is more like the version given by the 1968 British *Royal Commission on Medical Education*, which I suspect John Hamilton must have used as a model. GMC liked *our* model, now being tested in the Manchester project, and in Trinidad; right, Owen?" Minott was deadpan, so I continued, "The Brits too called it Community Medicine, suggested training similar to ours, but won't allow graduates any clinical practice except in remote areas, where Public Health doctors don't go anyway. What Ken McNeill, Jeff Wilson, Elizabeth Quamina, Carlyle Burton, Vaughn Wells, Max Awon, and Ken Comissiong approved in the last few years is a CM specialist who can direct regional hospitals, and be okay with clinical *and* public health duties. I thought you would tell them this, Ken? Owen? The WHO recognises such a pairing. We can do this. You're not planning to abandon that, are you? That would be going backward."

Sam was too un-knowing to be properly alarmed by my frankness, and my fear, but Standard, Picou, Alleyne, Minott should have briefed him on the innovative principles we had pushed at UWI. Standard and Minott knew of Wilson's hopes for Jamaica, and had been part of several key delegations to CHMC, and had known how tough it was to get them — non-medical politicians, and UWI's Academic Committee — to understand and approve the changes. I had had several sessions with the two, along with Colin Miller, and members of the Dean's Advisory and Curriculum Committees, ensuring their full agreement. Sam had attended the meetings on curriculum, and must know our plans, plus what he may have learned from my assistant, Norma Rainford, whom he had plied almost daily "for inside news," and who later, I was told, coached him in his bid for the Deanship. The changed attitude and deferring to Sam by better informed and experienced men puzzled Dick and me, until Sir Harry in 1978 explained the Dean's use of project funds.

Alleyne was the surprise, though. I would not have expected him to agree with this charade. Yet, it was consistent with his aloofness in the early '70s, and later actions and omissions. For example, in 1978 or '79, he would conclude a review of examinations for a Faculty workshop by recommending adoption of MCQs, specifically 5-choice completion items! He wrote as one totally unaware of all the studies that we had done in the later 1960s on examinations, in far greater depth than his casual look, and that there was much more to MCQs than mere format, to get the best from them. Objective ones had been used in Part 1 Finals, and for some parts of pre-clinical tests, for *ten years*! His department had participated in workshops on the subject, in 1968 and 1969, hosted by Professors Cruickshank and Stuart—its consecutive heads—and Professor Bras, conducted by Peter Jutsum, computer physicist, and me, but he had not attended any. *(See Fn. 4, p. 20 and Ch. 3 pp. 19-30).*

I could not support the directions Sam and his men seemed set on taking, said so, and wondered whether the rest of the Faculty at Mona, and in the EC, had any inkling of their plan. I confirmed that PGME was not affected, and in fact it was taking root nicely, and its growth might well distract the Faculty Board from probing the activities of the Dean's office, at this time of staff loss due to the sustained social unrest.

Campus security was improving at Mona, and the EC build-up was proceeding slowly. A Director of Community Medicine was not yet recruited, and the process suspended amid confusion re roles of the Director, versus Dr Minott's, as Sam Wray and his advisers had ignored the job descriptions, veering towards the idea of a CM program that was a mere extension of S&P Medicine, against which our document had clearly warned. This change in direction violated the spirit and aims of the PAFAMS/Kellogg agreement—which promised the creation of a novel experience in medical education—and threatened our CM project.

So I resolved to return, but Jamaica's denial of foreign exchange for my household needs scuttled that choice. My wife's family in Jamaica discouraged return, and stressed that Manley's handsome victory in the 1976 elections did not lessen the prospect of violence. Later in 1976, Sam Wray wrote *advising me not to return, as that might cause him to lose several senior staff!* I didn't have to think hard to identify the likely ones. I had met some at McMaster, and refused to surrender too easily. But my children's safety and education were paramount then, so I decided to stay in my CML job, until I could consult VC Preston and PM Barrow.

To start working at CML, I had to get a special licence as an assistant to Dr Mull. That had made me his captive, even though he and his staff were quite welcoming, sympathetic and deferential. To escape the restrictions of special licensing, I sat the Canadian examinations, first the Licentiate of the Medical Council of Canada (LMCC), in 1976. Passing this, I obtained a general licence and freedom to practise. Two years later, at McMaster, I passed the Fellowship examination in Pathology of the Royal College of Physicians and Surgeons of Canada (FRCPC), releasing me from the specialty practice restrictions of the academic license, obtained through McMaster's acceptance of my British degrees.

A letter from PAFAMS confirmed that my term on the governing body was still active and notified me of a meeting in Rio de Janeiro in late 1976 (p. 191) I used this occasion to visit various South American countries: Argentina, Chile, Peru and Colombia, returning via Jamaica.

In Buenos Aires, Argentina, I witnessed a bombing incident, with clouds of smoke, screaming police cars and heavy-booted security forces descending from turbaned trucks, rifles raised forward at an angle. That evening I listened to Jorge Bergoglio, a Jesuit priest (later Pope Francis) speaking at a church on the crisis. This was a fearful time in Argentina's dirty war, when 30,000 leftists disappeared, under dictator Jorge Videla.

In Santiago, Chile, I walked a block from the hotel to a camera shop, bought a roll of film, and on stepping outside, was suddenly enveloped in screaming soldiers, rifles at the ready, and out of this crowd, came a jeep with a colonel in the front passenger seat; in a trice, he was at my side demanding to know who I was, and what I was doing there. Luckily, I had my Jamaican passport, and blurted, "*Soy professor en la Universidad del Indes Occidentales, aqui por el congresso Latino Americano en Microcopia Eletronica; yo he registrado en el hotel Intercontinental là,*" I finished, pointing up the street. (It was the Society's biennial meeting that year, organised by an unusual scientist, an engineer, Irena Dumler.)

The soldiers were uncomfortably close. The Colonel focussed on my camera, and asked me why I carried a telephoto lens. I told him that photography was my hobby, that I had just arrived, had taken no pictures, had no film, and was directed to this shop by the hotel staff; I offered to open the camera. He nodded. I did. He took it from me, looked through the open back while working the aperture control, then closed the back, raised it to his eyes and pressed the shutter button; it clicked. He handed it back to me, told me to take no pictures, and ordered two men to escort me to the hotel desk to verify my registration.

Later, at dinner, two Americans came in and sat at the table next to mine, overlooking a park; they looked like Steve, the CIA man I had known in Georgetown, 1962-3. They asked me about the incident, having been in the lobby when my escorts brought me in. Smelling CIA, I simply said, "Nothing much; asked about my camera." Recalling the Pinochet coup three years earlier, and its fearsome aftermath, and thinking of Alberto Cristoffanini's fate, I had no further conversation with them.

After visiting Peru (Lima, Cuzco and Machu Picchu), I flew to New York via Bogota and Kingston, where I met with the VC, discussed my wish to return and concerns re the direction of Faculty policies, the sad state of the project in Manchester, and that senior staff were ignoring approved Faculty plans, and trashing the Manchester project and other plans for Community Medicine. He knew of the McMaster visit, and we discussed my doubts. I reminded him too of our ties with PAFAMS, their role in our grant, and urged an audit of the Manchester project, to protect it and our reputation. (This reminded me of conditions that had led to the Action Group reviews in 1970; the irony now was that the two people at the head seemed to be Picou and Alleyne, who had stood aloof then, and had disagreed with the Action Group reforms!) He dismissed as rumours the idea that my return would somehow be prevented; and that a member of the Dean's group was overheard to say, "Now that he's out of here, we'll see he stays there!" Later, I sent him a copy of Sam's letter.

I was surprised that PAHO had funded two seminars or workshops for UWI staff, in Jamaica, the second styled "Community Health", a new usage for the UWI *(Fig E1)*. My work on examinations and curriculum was copied verbatim at these, as at McMaster, again without credit, from the extensive dossiers on Community Medicine, and other papers for the UWI, including that for the Manchester project, which had become a reference in the region. Karl Smith had helped to prepare these, pre-1975, with a few others. Standard, Stuart, Cruickshank, and Sir Harry had read them, and appropriate Faculty committees had given approval. Jose Teruel of PAHO informed PAFAMS of these workshops.

The lead role in medical education at UWI, taken by PAHO, reminded me of several conversations with Dr Abe Horwitz, the Director of PAHO until early 1975, whose long-standing wish, from 1962, had been to "take over" the organisation of medical education at the UWI, along American lines. He gave some financial support for the new department of Social and Preventive medicine, which had been carved out of the Department of Medicine, and shortly after, gave funds to the Faculty for a Senior Lecturer for the Diploma in Public Health course. Then, in 1969, I became Associate Dean, acted independently, and made various curricular changes, which Horwitz had earlier suggested, but had not been made; he was surprised and pleased at the launch of PGME, CM and the plan for Family Medicine—though not as he and his advisers had wished—and our support for, and from CHMC.

The Caribbean was becoming more important for PAHO, as each new country created a vote in its councils; by 1975, there were four, with more in the offing. These would, with Suriname, be crucial in the coming election for the Director, as it was known that LA was split on re-electing Horwitz, a Chilean. Acuña wasted no time visiting the anglophone islands and offering financial help, where Horwitz had been cautious. They remained sceptical of my summary version of Community Medicine: *"based in a hospital, integrating clinical with public health functions, linked intramurally with all departments, and extramurally with community centres related to the hospital. It would thus be the primary agency for all health care needs for that population. The teaching hospital(s) would network with other hospitals, their directors forming, with the Ministry, a national committee, to plan, oversee and evaluate all CM activities. These would be carried out by teams of workers – professionals and ancillaries – from the least to the most complex, and covering all levels of health promotion, individual and group care, to ensure continuity, comprehensiveness, and clear lines of two-way referral from primary to secondary and tertiary levels."* The Committee would report to a Joint UWI-Government Council on CM. Other details were discussed, and opposition was satisfied.

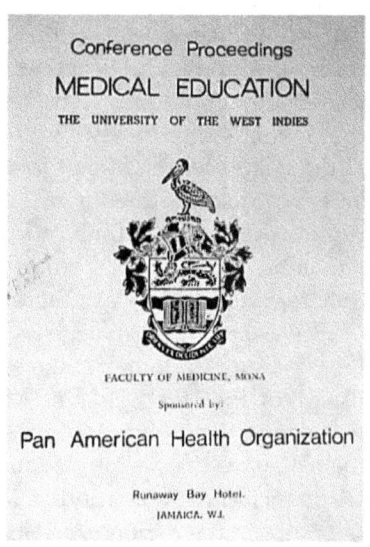

Conference Proceedings

MEDICAL EDUCATION

THE UNIVERSITY OF THE WEST INDIES

FACULTY OF MEDICINE, MONA

Sponsored by:

Pan American Health Organization

Runaway Bay Hotel.
JAMAICA, W.I.

Fig E1: Title Pages of PAHO-UWI Conference, above, and workshop, below, 1977-8

Report of Workshop in

Teaching of Community Health

to Medical Students at the University of the West Indies

held at

U.W.I   Mona

29th to 31st March 1978

What had concerned Dr Horwitz, and others at PAHO, was our plan to train a *"community specialist,"* who combined clinical skills of different specialties with preventive medicine and basic training in public health. No *developed* country did that! There was no model, but WHO had issued a Bulletin in the 1950s showing how! (see *Bibliography*). Yet current thinking at WHO, he had said, was veering away from integration towards a blitz to achieve global health in the next 25 years, by promoting *primary health care*. We shared that aim; but he had rather hoped to see us gain it from a Department of Community *Health*, combining S&P Medicine with Mental Health and Psychiatry.

He had missed the point, like some of his specialists at CHMC meetings. I reminded him that the UK Royal Commission on Medical Education had noted the charge of irrelevance against the DPH (1968), which many doctors did, as it was a quick specialty with prestige, which every colonial administrator had to have. As for "newness", there was no North American neurosurgeon, as such, prior to Harvey Cushing! The contributors to the UWI were undeveloped and poor in resources, and had to find innovative, non-doctrinaire and affordable ways of meeting needs, besides Public Health, and I acknowledged his great contributions to all the Americas. I told him that Minister McNeill, CMO Jeff Wilson, and others in CHMC favoured the home-grown Community Medicine model as it sought to extend clinical care beyond S&P Medicine, which many US educators liked, but some new schools preferred a concept like ours, e.g. Mount Sinai, NY, and Chicago's Abraham Lincoln University; Cuba practised it with stunning effect. Besides, Ken Standard had a distinct reluctance to move to the Hospital, when offered that choice in 1975 for the integrated clinical-preventive system we had in mind.

I told Dr Horwitz this, and that Jamaica had the luxury of eight or so extra Public Health specialists, who did no sickness care, and 22-25 community hospitals whose medical directors were ill-trained for their job. The cited WHO monograph covered training for the dual functions. Hospital directors had told us what their jobs entailed; we had simply translated that, with the help of UWI educators, into a curriculum, to provide training, and for periodic evaluation. Jamaica supported this plan. Thus we hoped to create a unique new specialist. Initially, district hospital directors would be "topped up" with missing skills, e.g. public health, paediatrics, ENT medicine, complex obstetrics, administration, dermatology, ophthalmology, and so on. Similarly, public health doctors could undergo specific clinical training, e.g. mental health or paediatrics, or dermatology etc. to become directors of district hospitals.[38]

For the new doctor, a four year program, eclectic in design, would provide rotations in emergency and general surgery, fractures, O&G, internal medicine, paediatrics, public health and preventive medicine, including health services organisation and administration, family medicine, and opportunity for an elective. The focus would be on holistic care, for individuals and their communities, including promotion of health and rehabilitation after illness. Conservative critics said it was "un-do-able." But CMOs and our team rebutted that and fully supported it. Of such controversies are medical (and other) advances made.

Like their colleagues in the WHO, Dr Horwitz and PAHO had favoured *"Community Health,"* described vaguely as community-based preventive and curative services, without specifying who or what

---

[38]In 1978, the World Health Assembly met at Alma Ata in the USSR (now Almaty, Kazakhstan), and issued the declaration *"Health for All by the year 2000"* to be achieved through a program of Primary Health Care (PHC). The term clashed with (and denied) Primary *Medical* Care. The definition however included all services, universal and effective coverage, with community involvement and inputs from various fields e.g. agriculture, and sees health care as *"integral to the social development of communities,"* the very point over which PVC Lalor had disagreed with me in 1975! In the details of implementation, the WHO planners agreed with us, except that they involved much larger teams to meet ends.

facility would be responsible; as a model it seemed, in wording at least, to be separate from the (teaching) hospital, whereas our model placed the base *in* the hospital, integrating with public health services. Teaching programs would be organised and administered from the Faculty's Division of CM. My fear was that a "Community Health" model would remain vague, and separate, physically and functionally, from other services and levels of care, clinical and pre-clinical, like S&P Medicine at UWI, risking loss of value, prestige, or funding, as politicians favoured technical advances in the more politically-rewarding specialties.

The Hospitals supported the CM plan when they saw that primary care for their communities would be part of each teaching department's duties, coordinated by the Head of Community Medicine, who would have an equal voice in the halls of power, and ensure that assessments of progress in care, research and training were regularly updated to maintain currency, and expand activities. We were too poor to afford the separation of services; and, with training, integration became not only palatable, but necessary. With this explanation and other elaboration over the years, Dr Horwitz had accepted our vision, and undertook to assist, monitor and even support it. It was likely that a statement of aim will be released soon, a part of which would back our initiative.

In spring 1975, Horwitz lost the elections to Hector Acuña, a traditional PH specialist from Mexico, whom I had met in Mexico City and on his campaign tour. He was cordial, and had asked for and received details of our plans and progress in CM, especially the Kellogg grant, and the current principals; I was surprised that he didn't know, or maybe he was just checking how close I was to the project, or wanted a personal copy. He also wanted to know whether I supported Professor Alleyne's renewal on a PAHO Research Committee; this I did.

The social unrest in Kingston was similar in its effects to the 1968-70 turmoil in Trinidad, when "Black Power" activity had invaded the island. A strike in 1970 had led to a state of emergency on April 21, during which two army officers, Raffique Khan and Rex Lasalle had mutinied at Chaguaramas; they were subdued four days later. T&T society was disrupted and travel to Port of Spain had become risky. The unrest had coincided with, or provoked student protests at St Augustine that led to the resignation of the Chancellor and Pro-Chancellor.

Minott was no Khan or Lasalle. He was Standard's peaceful classmate and Lodge-mate. He too was a Gibraltar Hall neighbour and friend. He had taught me photography (B&W), and had been the "best man" at my wedding. Standard and I had taken him from a dead end at the UHWI Casualty department, and given him an opportunity in academic medicine, with a Leverhulme fellowship, over the objections of others in the Departments of Medicine and Surgery, who had judged him "unscientific" in his approach to problems, woolly, and somewhat "messianic." In Laurence J. Peter's lexicon, they said, he had reached and comfortably settled at his "level of incompetence"! (Peter, *Bibliography*)

The societal turmoil of the sixties and seventies at Mona had unsettled many; we lost both young and older staff, including original members, like David Stewart, Gerrit Bras, Eric Cruickshank, Eric Back and Louis Grant. Ed Belle, Andrew Masson, UN Pathak and others also left. We neared desperation and any pair of hands, however shackled, had become indispensable; we were thus forced to spend more time in shaping new appointees to our curricular purpose. Ken Standard's positive appraisal of Minott's work in his department as a supervisor and advisor of students in field projects, and his clinical experience in the Casualty department (primary and emergency care), plus his pledge to complete courses in education theory, justified the offer of a three-year contract as Senior Lecturer in Medical Education. We hoped that this focused training plus his knowledge of Manchester, his home parish, and its people, would prepare him to carry out the CM activities as detailed in the Project documents; these points had reduced much opposition to his appointment. But his performance after two years, despite coaching, had been a failure, and thus embarrassing. While I was away on leave completing Commonwealth projects on manpower, he had misinformed students about the 1975 start date of the CM clerkship, did not give them the CM plan, and missed other essentials; the start date was postponed. His errors were serious, and I went over each one with him.

I had reviewed the CM concept once more with him, Professors Standard and Miller, who supported the fusion of health promotion, prevention of disease, and illness care for individuals and communities, as basic to *our* model, not the USA's or UK's, and a proper use of scarce resources. Each community health centre or clinic would deliver primary care, where students would learn to deal with individual issues, supervised by district physicians and assistants. Care would be available to all, equitably and sensitively delivered, as a human right, and organised in cooperation with all sectors of the community, including politicians. Students would treat patients holistically and learn the best use of facilities and techniques, whether available directly, or by referral, and thus become familiar with the structure and function of the health services, and the role therein of all caregivers.

But the pressures of a troubled society took a toll on senior faculty, and heavy workloads reduced the time available and ability to oversee functions outside their departments. It was not surprising, then, to hear that Colin Miller, Sir Harry and Vice Dean West were displeased with the management of the project, which they had left to the new Dean, Sam

Wray, starting in early 1976. This was compounded by Wray's arbitrary and hasty changes in the use of funds. The staff was dismayed, as Ann Costa related to me later that year, when she visited us in Brantford, on a holiday in Canada. Despite coaching, both Wray and Minott had failed to grasp important features of the program, neglected its clinical and investigative aspects, and in letters to the Ministry of Health, seemed unaware of the activities that they should initiate, oversee and evaluate.

In 1977, Colin Miller left the UWI for England, and he, wife Helen, a senior nursing sister at UHWI, and their children, visited us, *en route*. I was so surprised that this son of Jamaica — who had amply proven his dedication to the UWI and Jamaica, through the worst years of campus terror, and looked forward to resuming our joint efforts — had become "an outcast," like me, as the new Dean and a cohort of friends were overly willing to change the plan and submit to foreign ways, lured with small grants that might have clouded the vision of the Minister also. Dr Wilson was the lone hold-out, but that voice was stilled when he retired.

Former colleagues in Community Medicine had abandoned key ideas and strayed from our "IADB"-and CHMC-backed PAFAMS model, and renamed it *Community Health*, together with Psychiatry, replacing clinical care with administration. Colin doubted whether we could ever regain the momentum or integration we had achieved at the start of the Manchester project as an elective. Keen students were disappointed, as were PAFAMS principals, whom Dr Minott had tried vainly to reassure at project review meetings in Bolivia and Venezuela.

I told Colin that I had applied for a year's extension of leave. "Yes, do that, and visit when you can, and see for yourself. Even Harry and Ken (Stuart) are grumbling, and may quit. I don't know details, but seems that Sam is fiddling with Community Medicine funds, and Owen and Standard are either with him, or more likely, helpless to stop it. As Standard's reward, the new Department of Community Health will merge Community Medicine with S&P Medicine — as PAHO seems to have advised — and all that integration with clinical work that we had planned, will be lost, as well as the CM specialist. I'm so disappointed."

Colin had expected that the elevator incident with PM Williams would have persuaded me to stay away, but he understood why I wished to go back, as there was much to be done, and I still had friends in Council; and perhaps, if I made it back, he might return too. But his pessimism and Helen's fears were infectious, especially for the children, and impressed my family.

My request to UWI in 1977 for leave extension was denied, and I had to resign, or else return and abandon family, as, under Jamaica's new Foreign Exchange rules, I would not be able to send them money for subsistence. My big regret is that this measure, added to social and family considerations, and my own "expulsion," prevented me from completing what my colleagues and I had started, and for ensuring continuity of policies. A costly *forgetting* then set in, with re-definition of programs that Wray's junket to Hamilton had predicted.

In Feb 1978, I visited Jamaica to evaluate the Manchester project, on a request by the Kellogg Foundation. I was disappointed to confirm Colin's fears that many mistakes had been made, from faulty and incomplete guidance of students, to neglect of key activities at sites of intervention at Lincoln and Prattville, and omission of any study at the control clinic at Harmons, Mile Gully having been withdrawn. Students were poorly supervised, and linkages with the parish hospital had not been made, nor were local doctors recruited to help with teaching and supervision, which they had agreed to do, and were still willing to help. Dr Minott had not contacted any of them, so they had concluded that the plan had been abandoned. To cap it all, Dean Wray had diverted funds from the project, and space in the Postgraduate Building to personal and irrelevant "psychological research", while Dr Minott, the project director, was left without money to purchase supplies or clinic help, the real purpose of the funds. This clearly should have been better audited, and in the circumstances might amount to malfeasance.

Dean Wray's meeting to discuss my review of the Manchester Project, took place just a month before a planned workshop sponsored by PAHO that would scuttle Community Medicine *(see Fig E1b, p. 270)*, almost at the same time as the Colombian medical schools were seeking ways to strengthen links between CM and General Practice. The Chair of the Faculty Committee on CM, Professor Harland of Paediatrics — appointed to succeed Colin Miller — claimed that he was new, and had not been given the project document, or informed of the requirements for test and control areas, or what funds there were, how to be used, or the work to be done and reported; yet all were standard components of any research project. He had naively agreed to chair the Committee, without knowing its purpose, budget or commitments, or anything about Wray, who, he would find out that day, held sole control of the funds!

I simply warned them, and Dean Wray in particular, that my findings could trigger an audit, with implications for refunding of any misdirected monies, as it had then seemed too late to correct the many errors and misjudgements. I was surprised by this finding, as on leaving the UWI, I had shared my misgivings with Drs Chavez and Ceitlin, had asked the UWI Bursary to be vigilant, and had warned the VC in 1976.

Drs Chavez and Ceitlin reviewed my report; clearly, a financial audit was needed, to explain the failures; but after review, they accepted the "errors," and ended the experiment most forgivingly. Later they funded a project in the EC; so did HOPE, as if to emphasise their displeasure with Mona. That final event eased somewhat the pain of my decision to resign, as I had looked forward to moving on from a successful Manchester project to the next phase of building a Community Medicine Division, and start training community specialists for the Jamaica Health Services, and for other Caribbean jurisdictions in need.

Community Medicine fell to the very forces of distraction, which Andrés Santas had warned against in 1973, in launching our application to Kellogg *(Appendices 9-11, pp. 335-40).* Community Medicine, as conceived by PAFAMS, died at UWI and was buried into Social and Preventive Medicine, and replaced by "Community Health" in 1979-80. That *volte-face* must have been behind the evasive behaviour of Minott and Standard, who declined my invitation to share a drink while waiting for a flight at Toronto airport in 1979, where I had seen them seated as I came in for a shuttle to Ottawa. They got up and left, "We have to make a connection." Later, a letter from Karl Smith told me of the "hijacking!"

I felt hurt, as Standard had been a close friend, and we had shared so many things in our University life: he had been my next- door neighbour when I started university, encouraged me to become a Christian and a University Lodge member, both of which I had politely declined, with explanations that he had accepted. We served together on the Gibraltar Hall Committee for its closing two years, 1952-4, and on the Faculty Board, 1967-75; we had lived as neighbours on Glendon Circle, Hope Pastures, from 1965 to 1969, where we had discussed the kinds of doctors needed in the Caribbean, and on the future of the Faculty and UWI, in changing times. I had allowed him to persuade me into the Deanship; we worked closely on developing the CM program, and on our ideas for the curriculum; he supported the training of entire health teams in the same milieu; he had been the first to critique my *Ancillaries* paper.

I would have appreciated some explanation for the regressive change, instead of having to piece it together from UWI workshop documents. It made me wonder whether lodge brotherhood had had any influence, and I recalled my brief note to the VC re this factor, in June 1975: *"The University is increasingly at risk to become a slave to the UWI Lodge. The University must honour its own, not reject talent, regardless of Lodge membership, if only so that history will credit it with objectivity and scholarship, even at a time of grave political stress. When Francis Bowen formed the University Lodge in 1952, there were 2 students: Al Walwyn, 4th year Medicine, and Vernon Smith, final year Arts. Several others quickly followed, including Standard, Minott, Stan Luck, and my classmates: Lee, Hagley, Alleyne, Ling, among others. What I see instead is chauvinism and favouritism, island vs island, and the same ancient curse of ruthless divisiveness that made a little temperate island, a century ago, conquer half the civilised world."*

My 1978 visit had been on the eve of the "Peace Concert" at the National Stadium between political thugs, the JLP's Claude Massop and PNP's Aston Thompson (Bushy Marshall), the gang leaders then. But I was sad when I found out that those other gangs, in academic garb, had destroyed a unique CM project that so many in the Americas, and elsewhere, had viewed with anticipation, and some were already trying e.g. at Ramathibodi in Bangkok, and Cuba had introduced. Dr Wilson had retired in 1976-7; the Hon Min. McNeill had been wooed with "gifts" by PAHO's Director, Dr Acuña; Dr Comissiong was not known at UWI, and I had been exiled; thus, the project had lost its strongest advocates.

Dr Patterson, the new CMO in Jamaica, was a novice at the meetings of the Conference of Ministers. Knowing little of the PAFAMS concept of CM, which Dr Wilson had endorsed, she fell to the PAHO advocacy of Public Health, with Professor Standard becoming PAHO's man-on-the-spot, enticed with an enhanced building and a new title. It is a great irony, then, to find that the renovated Faculty lecture theatre at UHWI has been named after him, who had hardly taught at the site, the heart of clinical medicine, which he had rejected, declining to consider a move to the hospital for central planning and clinical–public health integration. He had also declined the headship of Community Medicine, to be based at the UHWI, in a redesigned "Casualty" space, with separate primary care and emergency areas. Instead, he settled for *Community Health* in the S&P building, isolated from both clinical and pre-clinical areas.

I was not surprised, therefore, to hear that Professor Sir Kenneth Stuart had left in 1979 to join the Commonwealth Secretariat in London as Medical Adviser; Professor Sir Harry Annamunthodo had resigned in 1980, to join a new university in Malaya *(p. 104)*. Professor Alleyne was rewarded with a research position at PAHO in Washington DC; Malcolm Adam and Rolf Richards of Medicine transferred to Trinidad, and Errol Walrond to Barbados; Gene Burkett of O&G left for Florida.

In the seventies, PAFAMS had begun to conduct research for member schools, on training in Family Medicine (FM); it was an essential function in our Faculty's Community Medicine (CM) model. The Family Physician or Family Doctor styling was spreading in the USA and Canada, supplanting "General Practitioner"; PAFAMS members had accepted FM in the context of CM *(pp. 335-40)*. It would focus on family units, mindful that the North American concept of "family" may not be the same as that of Latin American (LA) and Caribbean cultures. Of note was that most LA doctors were organ specialists, but many practised as primary care-givers, and saw "family doctors" as an erosion of their income. However, the idea did meet with sympathetic listeners.

To understand this reluctance, one must recall that most Latin American medical schools still followed the French model; but they were inappropriately structured, with few departments, and little integration of teaching and research, rather like the US situation before the 1910 Flexner Report. There were many hospitals, but few *teaching* ones, with formal grades of house officers and registrars (or residents), as in the US, and few directed by medical schools. Thus, no one was sure how or where students would get reliable clinical training. LA doctors became subject "specialists" through local apprenticeships, or US or Spanish training. At the other end, many secondary schools could not produce students ready for medical school, like the Caribbean when the UCWI began. Health care delivery was organised separately by governments, by the Social Security Services (SSS), and privately. In Mexico, some SSS hospitals offered comprehensive integrated care similar to the model proposed for the Chedoke Hospital (*Appendix 16, p. 372*).

In 1953, Colombia had set up the Lapham Commission on medical services; its report makes good reading, and could apply equally to the Caribbean. Most of its recommendations have been followed; but it had omitted General Practice as an entity, like most jurisdictions then, and had not considered traditional holistic medicine and its practitioners, long known in India and China, and practised in tribal societies globally, including Latin America.

It is not surprising then that it was not until the 1970s that the continent was looking at Family Medicine as a discipline, and PAFAMS had begun to work to encourage its adoption. Leaders had discussed the ideas we had placed before our own Faculty authorities and the IADB Committee on Expansion, in 1971, drawing on several conferences on medical education and manpower training, supported by CHMC in the early 1970s, and supplemented in 1975 with examples from programs I had studied in various countries in 1974. (see *Bibliography*)

Dr Dyer, the head of the UWI Clinic, a former classmate, a general practitioner who had acquired an MPH degree, was the closest we had to lead a Family Practice Teaching unit. He was head of the student and staff health services. I had obtained medical inputs from as many as cared to supply them: paediatricians Colin Miller and Bob Gray; Karl` Smith, E. Garret and O. Minott of S&P Medicine, J. Hall and G. Burkett, O&G; several surgeons and physicians in Government services e.g., L. Williams (VJH), K. McKenzie (Children's Hospital) John Hall (KGH), and others. Opinions were received from many on the three campuses, including Drs. M. Adam, C. Bartholomew, W. Ince, G. Busby, M. Jorsling, R. Hoyte, V. Massiah, and others of POS General Hospital; Drs. H. Forde, F. Ramsay, A. Graham, C. Nelson, R. Haynes, T. Hassall, H. White, among those at the QE Hospital, and M. Hoyos, Barbados; Dr

Comissiong of Grenada; Dr Cecil Cyrus of St Vincent (a unique and inimitable doctor, as noted, who was part model for our Community physician specialist); Dr Matthew Beaubrun and other members of the Caribbean Medical Education Council (CMEC), a private group promoting primary care; and others in various general practice settings in Kingston. (Matthew Beaubrun had worked at the UHWI briefly, but could not get a UWI post as he had no specialist qualification; nevertheless, he was a reliable adviser and strong supporter). Interest was so high that I began to canvass possible sources of funds for a conference on our proposals, and found that Macy (p. 192) and HOPE were receptive. But in 1972, Dr Dyer was lukewarm to the idea of a 2-year postgraduate FM program, post-internship, following the revised curriculum (p. 58). He felt differently, and a year or so later, I received an outline for a *four-year* plan after internship. That was too long. I had just then completed a study of programs in primary care in a few developing countries (*pp. 229-34; and footnote 39 p. 372*). I suggested reducing the time to two and a half years, but he balked, and there the matter stalled, until he revived it, with Sam Wray, late in 1978.

In a report to PAFAMS then, I summarised family doctor training in Canada, Cuba, East Africa, and India, and wrote an essay, titled *"World Trends in the Training of Family Doctors,"* which formed the basis of discussions in New Orleans and Bogota, in 1978. The general ideas had been placed before the UWI Faculty, and the IADB Committee, in 1971, supported by CHMC, and amplified in 1975, with examples from the countries studied in 1974.

My paper, translated into Spanish, was read at the 1978 Bogota meeting of PAFAMS, hosted by ASCOFAME (the *Colombian Association of Medical Faculties*), and published, with three other essays, in a book, *El Medico Familiar, el Respuesto al Futuro*. It showed readers how universal and developed the practice of Family Medicine had become, the approaches adopted in various countries, and the place of ancillaries in health care. I showed that the Cuban organisation of primary care and method of training of workers were quite suitable for several LA and Caribbean countries, but the US embargo of things Cuban trumped that.

Sam Wray had attended both meetings, but missed the FM sessions, after persuading me to speak for the UWI, because he had "a cold". In 1984, I met him again, at a PAFAMS meeting in Bogota. He avoided the interactive sessions, and thus missed discussions and questions on FM, CM, and a new initiative, *the International Clinical Epidemiology Network (INCLEN)*, funded by the Rockefeller Foundation, to train academic researchers. I had once more filled in for him at his request, and with PAFAMS' approval. I urged him to pursue the INCLEN initiative, and was surprised that UWI was not enrolled until 30 years later! *(See p. 292)*

The increased intrusion of PAHO into UWI medical education, although in keeping with its mandate and Horwitz's urges, was a breach of his tacit undertaking to assist, at government level, but not to intrude into medical education at the UWI, except on request for project support. I was surprised that in the few months between the New Orleans and Bogota meetings of PAFAMS in 1978, PAHO under Acuña, had funded a retreat for UWI medical faculty to discuss *"the teaching of Community Health to medical students at UWI"*, of which Wray had not informed his PAFAMS colleagues; this was discourteous, as UWI had obtained its CM grant through them, and information-sharing was expected.

Following the Bogota meeting, a Kellogg grant enabled me to host a group of LA deans at McMaster University in 1979, to study various Family Practice models, including clinics run by nurse practitioners — in which several CHMC members had shown great interest — in Hamilton, Burlington, and London, Ontario. Curricula were explored and models reviewed, including the Cuban one, which most judged as suited to Latin American schools, but Kellogg did not invite Wray to participate.

Cuba's results by 1986 had shown what great gains can accrue from promoting health and excellent primary care under personnel trained for both clinical and public health work, when a small nation is allowed to pursue its goals, in its own way, without bowing to global corporations with their primary focus on wealth extraction. The cost of Cuban care is still one tenth of that of the US, and by the mid-eighties, Cuba could achieve vital statistics better than the USA, which would begin to envy Cuba its health status. While the huge US expenditure and its lavishly-endowed medical schools did increase knowledge, produce medical specialists and researchers, it neglected community care and limited accessibility by those most in need. Ronald Reagan's slashing of child nutrition and food stamps programs in his 1981-88 term produced some 20 million cases of malnutrition: marasmus, kwashiorkor, low birth weight babies, and other deficiency diseases, all but eradicated in Cuba; its incidence of 1% contrasts also with LA's 2-38% average in late eighties (PAHO). In the UK, Thatcher cancelled the children's milk ration, with a similar effect!

Cuba offered universal access, full health education, and advanced specialist and technological services to its public. The doctor: population ratio matched the USA and allowed Cuba to assist the world, even offering medical help to New Orleans at the time of hurricane *Katrina*, and was the first to help the Antilles, devastated by 2017 hurricanes *Irma* and *Maria*. Professional salaries were low in Cuba, but doctors were allowed to spend up to two years earning higher wages in countries that needed them. They are common in Guyana's Health Services.

For the WHO the goal of *"health for all by 2000"* was elusive, but it did eradicate smallpox, and introduce new vaccines, but lethal agents have emerged, some the result of unchecked corporatism that followed the end of the Cold War, and has enslaved the powerful US government enabling profiteers to short-change populations by seizing all sources of nutrition, so that survival itself becomes a source of untold profit.

By 1978, St George's *Medical School* in Grenada had admitted its first students, including a few local "scholarship" holders. At that time, the flamboyant and foppish Eric Gairy was still Premier of Grenada, and had maintained his rule for over two decades, like a grandee. Grenada gained independence in 1979 and he became PM, only to be displaced soon after, in a coup by leftist Maurice Bishop. By all accounts, Bishop was liked by the masses, visited Castro, forged links with other far-left Caribbean elements, and set about to restructure Grenada. That was the year Burnham in Guyana had declared himself a Marxist, which was not a secret to anyone, except to the Americans, who had kept him in power. He had been heavily criticised by University of Guyana sociologist, Walter Rodney, who was murdered on June 13, 1980, allegedly on order from Burnham (*Global Research, February 23, 2016*). Such were the machinations of political militants in the Caribbean.

Hearing of the Bishop coup in 1979, I marvelled that an anti-American communist who had stingingly criticised the "CIA and US capitalist pigs" would allow St George's University—an epitome of US capitalism in education—to survive his putsch. I was disappointed to read of events in Grenada, and stunned by the Reagan invasion, Bishop's capture, and the role of his deputy, Bernard Coard, in his execution.

In the next two decades, private American medical schools, copies of St George's, would spring up in several places: Barbados, Dominica, St Kitts, St Maarten, and in Guyana, joining others in Latin America, where the school in Guadalajara, Mexico, catered almost entirely to foreign, mainly US students. The Ross school in Dominica, and St George's, had "honoured" me with an offer to teach a 3-month Pathology course each year. I politely declined. Later, I learned that several UWI faculty in the EC had been enticed to participate in these and in the many others that mushroomed in the islands and Guyana. The current PAHO director, Dr Carissa Etienne, a Dominican, had studied Medicine at UWI in the years I was Dean, and was once an Associate Professor at Ross.

The University of Guyana had also opposed the foreigners, to no avail, as they had contacted Burnham directly. Bribes seemed to have oiled their way, and lubricants regularly repeated. These schools were hypocritically "condemned" by US authorities and medical mandarins, but secretly welcomed as they spared NA schools the greater expense of expansion to meet market needs. They have become so much a part of the NA medical school alternatives that students and parents speak of them in the same breath as they do prestige University medical schools.

The UWI did not have the resources to oppose these "businesses," whose graduates, mostly North Americans, would pay heavily for their education — despite claims by the schools' owners — and must wait years to enter a Canadian or US residency. While Dean, and tempted by several founders of these schools, I had examined their learning plans, all copies of US curricula, and regarded them as weak, and pre-Flexnerian in organisation. I reported this to the UWI Academic Board, and argued in favour of UWI accepting foreign fee-paying students to pay for our expansion schemes. But interest was low, and my suggestion soundly derided, in and out of the Faculty, as mercenary. However, attitudes have changed since, and foreign students were welcomed two decades ago into the Trinidad Faculty, and recently in Jamaica.

In the next decades, I was surprised to see how US medical schools had multiplied in the anti-capitalist *Organisation of Eastern Caribbean States (OECS)*, which had emerged in 1981 from the *West Indies Associated States*, formed in 1967 by Antigua, Dominica, Grenada, St Kitts-Nevis-Anguilla, St Lucia, and St Vincent. Maurice Bishop and Bernard Coard had many sympathisers in the others, and were copied in St Vincent, where Ralph Gonsalves (pp 207, 257, 259) had become Prime Minister. Grenada achieved independence in 1974, St. Kitts-Nevis, in 1983, while Anguilla chose to remain a separate state, associated with Britain.

In February 1975, while we were debating at Howard issues re health of Black populations, a trade pact was concluded in Togo, West Africa — the Lomé Convention (Lomé I) — between the European Economic Community of 15 states (EEC) — which Britain had just joined — and former African, Caribbean and Pacific colonies (the ACP countries), now struggling economically. Lomé I came into force in April 1976, but was soon in trouble, as more colonies became independent, requiring adjustments. By 1992, the single EU market had led to major changes. These were tough for the Caribbean, and entities like the UWI. Then, on Jan 1, 1995, the GATT morphed into the WTO, allowing greedy US businesses to bleed poor countries, while failing to lighten the heavy subsidies given to US farmers that made them undersell all competition. The immorality and unfairness of this practice were lost on Americans.

Lomé IV was new. It was the prototype of later, more voracious deals sponsored by the USA and endorsed by the *International Monetary Fund*, which gave US and Rothschild banks the freedom to empty the increasingly shallower pockets of poor countries. IMF policy demanded divestment of public property and enterprises, and encouraged "development" loans; when the inevitable failures occurred, harsh measures were used to recoup. The US and allies thus watched the poor starve, as the WTO gave lending Corporations full control of borrowers' economies and trade. Defaulters were pilloried by the IMF's *Structural Adjustment Program (SAP)*, and could lose ownership of entire islands.

Structural Adjustment for Developing Countries, 1990 version

The Deal:

World Bank/IMF grants large development loans in exchange for

Currency Devaluation
Smaller Budgets
Reduced Government Role in national Economy (privatisation)
Removal of price subsidies (note, however, that the US maintains their own)
Staff reductions in public sector
Open trade policies
Other concessions, as dictated by borrower and lender(s)
to achieve Economic Renewal and Growth!
(BUT, growth of what or whom?)

Who benefit?

Foreign investors
Wealthy locals
The politically preferreds
Dunce nations (world bank principals)
Other opportunists and entrepreneurs (carpet baggers)

Who lose?

The borrowers,
All others not involved in deal
The local taxpayers and cosumers (i.e. everybody!)

In 1988, Davison Budhoo—his surname is Indian—a Grenadian economist on the staff of the IMF—wrote to Michel Camdessus, head of the Fund, announcing his resignation, as follows: "*Today I resigned from the staff of the International Monetary Fund after over twelve years, and after 1000 days of official Fund work in the field, hawking your medicine and your bag of tricks to governments, and to peoples in Latin America and the Caribbean, and in Africa. To me, resignation is a priceless liberation, for with it I have taken the first big step to that place where I may hope to wash my hands of what in my mind's eye is the blood of millions of poor and starving peoples...The blood is so much, you know, it runs in rivers. It dries up, too; it cakes all over me; sometimes I feel that there is not enough soap in the whole world to cleanse me from the things that I did do in your name.*"(from *The Indelible Red Stain Bk 2, vi*)

Jamaica and Guyana's economy, and others in the 1980s, wilted, as they fell, under SAP, to US Corporations, Rothschild organisations and the Bilderberg group. Currency devaluations wrecked many economies.

But the University survived, as I had always expected, largely because there was no alternative as reputable. The financial stringencies of the eighties showed at UHWI in peeling paint; damaged walls, windows and ward furniture; and shortage of equipment and supplies. The SAP had another victim! The thoughts of many turned on possible relief from donors to the Faculty. The fledgling Alumnus register we had started in the early 1970s, had been neglected for lack of staff, time and leadership. Ms. Costa and Mrs. Jung, assisted by Mrs. Young, had been swamped with work in the Dean's office, as student numbers had increased, from 1968; yet, by the time I left, they had collected names and addresses in the Caribbean and North America, the majority culled from requests for transcripts! Ours was a shoestring operation, compared to the well-organised and specifically- and professionally-staffed funding factories I had seen in Chicago, New York and Miami. Squeezing anything from alumni needed trained and dedicated staff, especially in an environment without the tradition of "giving back," or where people still felt like aliens, as they had been made to feel in British colonies.

The VC had endorsed the Alumnus idea in 1972, referring me to the Guild of Graduates, and later suggested that our new administrator, Mr. Cato, a law graduate, might organise it. Cato had been expected in early 1975, but arrived five months late, a week before I left, when I was busy with the Conference of Ministers of Health. But I briefed him and took him on a tour of key contacts and left it to Mrs. Rainford to fill in details. Later, I would hear that his settling had been difficult, for reasons I was not fully given; it seemed that he had often disagreed with Sam on spending issues. The Alumnus portfolio, one of the responsibilities and priorities we had discussed at his interview, had stalled. I had stressed its aim of building a reserve fund for education and research, and had referred him to Dr John Homi, the new anaesthetist, who would help.

What I had discussed with Mr. Cato, who did not last long enough to have done much, was to select specific high-profile Faculty projects, e.g. student assistance, essential diagnostic equipment, skill training, critical research, awards etc., and campaign to fund those, while maintaining a steady fund-raising drive. He was keen to work with the Registrar and VC to establish a centre for this, of which the Faculty of Medicine would play a main part, spread throughout the Caribbean, targetting graduates, businessmen, professionals, academics, foundations, well-wishers etc., and recognising their gifts publicly. But progress in the formation of an Alumnus association stalled, in the depressing years of the eighties, and as Jamaica's economy declined, under the SAP.

About that time, Dr Dinah Hony, an English physician, who had been a registrar in anaesthesia at UCHWI in 1955 (I had worked with her as a clerk), stayed on, married a Jamaican, and practised until 1975, in

Kingston, then left for the USA. Visiting her daughter, Dingle Spence, a medical student, she saw the signs of decay in the hospital, and assumed the task of contacting peers and graduates in the USA, an act that led to the formation of "chapters" of the UWI Medical Alumnus Association.

They have not achieved what Dr Hony had hoped, lacking a strong and prestigious central force, with resources to coordinate the operations of many branches, and recruit new members in North America, the UK and elsewhere. The centre at Mona was understaffed and underfunded, and its profile low. The chapters were essentially cliques of physicians who connected to the Centre and benefitted from tax breaks and holidays at annual conferences held in various resorts in the Caribbean, whence they dispensed gifts and prizes: stethoscopes, otoscopes, books, a little cash to bright students, the occasional microscope, and plaques to favourites, friends and associates. The Canada chapter is an example; it is really a Toronto group with the same unchanging executive and nuclear membership. I have never been one, or contacted to join, perhaps because I'm outside of Toronto, and in other ways an outsider, since my 1990 "enlightenment" letter to its perennial president, Dr Massiah.

In mid-1977, in Simcoe, ON, CML Labs dismissed our Chief Technologist, Pat Lycett — a competent and admired leader — without warning me or discussing the reason. Already restless with the lack of challenge in my CML job — apart from the problems of maintaining accreditation of the two district hospital laboratories under my care, the forensic cases from district coroners, and getting to meet the Ontario Provincial Police (OPP) contingents in the several small towns along Highway 3, from St Thomas to Hagersville — I accepted, in November 1977, a position at Chedoke Hospitals, Hamilton, and a professorship at McMaster University, with a prominent role in Education, and opportunity to develop my interest in Community Medicine and health services systems. For this job, I was interviewed by all the laboratory heads in the city, one of whom was Dr E A (Ted) Belle, head of the Hamilton Public Health laboratory; he was a virologist, friend, and former co-worker in the Department of Microbiology, UWI, under Professor Grant, now settled, as noted, in a Public Health post in Simcoe, about fifty miles from Ted, and two from me. Small world, indeed!

In 1978-9, I became Chair of an *ad hoc* committee to develop a plan for a model of health care delivery, covering all levels of services for the entire region related to the hospital, about 1.5 million people, and with linkages to the other four teaching, and several district hospitals. At Chedoke, I had introduced the initiative of the hospital's highly-regarded Southam Laboratories "mothering" two community hospital laboratories to ensure maintenance of proficiency This idea was novel, and, not surprisingly, resisted by the more sequestered Mc Master purists who shunned contamination by non-university units, but the Ministry of Health and Lab Proficiency Testing Program welcomed it, wished us success, and if so, would urge other teaching hospitals to do likewise.

The clinical model, based on the UWI's modified Community Medicine plan *(Appendix 16, p. 372)*, was approved by the Hospital Executive and favourably reviewed by the same Asst. Deputy Minister of Health for Ontario who had reviewed our laboratory supervision program for district hospitals. But before the Chedoke Board could approve it, the Hospital was amalgamated, by Government fiat, with the unpopular McMaster Health Sciences Centre (HSC), whose departmental hostilities were only slightly relieved by the welcoming attitude of its Hospital Director, Mr. Ray Walker. He too liked our model, but advised that HSC heads were, incredibly, not kindly disposed to Chedoke initiatives, even those approved by the Health Ministry! For vague reasons, some of them, as at Mona, saw it as threatening their authority, though I could not understand why, unless they stood on shaky ground.

The Director promised to nudge it forward, but that was the last we heard of it, from either him or the Ontario Government. The staff Associations of the two hospitals merged, and I became its Secretary, retaining my seat on the new Board, with the President and VP of the Medical Staff. (In 2007, one Local Health Integration Network [LHIN] – Ontario's political contribution to healthcare administrative sinecures – was thinking of a CM model like mine; and by 2017, some diehard McMaster hospitalists had begun to think of offering ambulatory care.)

In 1998, at an alumnus meeting in Jamaica, a group that had spent an hour or so at the Pegasus bar, reminiscing, disbanded, and I was left with Mickey Walrond; I felt awkward being alone with a man who had worked closely with me, then, in my absence, assisted my successors and opponents to effect my exile, and to deny my work, even my very existence. He hardly ever used my name, and, like others, probably found it painful to do so, an effacement that has endured. But alcohol had disinhibited him, made him unusually friendly, and he related in detail, as if to shed a great burden, how grant funds for Community Medicine which I had worked so hard to obtain, had been diverted by Sam Wray, to uses "not relevant to the purpose of the grant," while the work languished (see Bibliography, *Review of Community Medicine Project,* Faculty Paper, June, 1979).

Minott had meekly accepted, and Standard elated with the gift of the *Department of Community Health,* the thing that the latter had long silently craved! It mattered little that an innovative concept, agreed by him and others, and promising greater benefits to the Caribbean, had thereby died, and alienated Kellogg, a potential ally. It brought to mind Karl Smith's message to me in late 1977, after my resignation, "Your program was cancelled, as soon as you were out of the way!" Walrond confirmed what I could only infer from Wray's evasive behaviour at meetings, and comments by the Dean's office staff, as early as mid-1976.

Walrond had "left a sinking ship" in 1976, when everyone felt that Jamaica was going Communist. I had expected him to be appointed Dean, but the political turmoil unnerved him, and he chose Barbados, not unreasonably, as it was his home, where he would soon become top dog. The UWI sustained curriculum reform and the PGME program through the vicissitudes: they had gained enough momentum to survive the new Faculty leaders' axe, and Manley's misjudgement and flirtations with the economy, the crippling devaluation of the Jamaican dollar, and the subsequent IMF intervention in Jamaica's economy with its devastating *Structural Adjustment Program*. Community Medicine gave way to CH, a program disparaged by many elsewhere, even at the WHO.

We talked of the EC scheme. PM Barrow had lost the 1976 elections, and that had left me few friends there to speak kindly, or make a difference. The EC Scheme had been enthusiastically greeted by students, staff, and more cautiously, by government doctors. Eric Williams had remained aloof, and cool to me as an Indian. He had snubbed the EC scheme in 1967, but PM Barrow, a more objective influence, had made him change his mind. Williams' early reactions reflected his wish to have his own medical school, and for a time it was felt that he would withdraw from the UWI, frustrated with the politics of Michael Manley and his reluctance, inability really, to put any capital into structures in the EC. Williams had started that trend, when he cancelled the paltry amount (US$48,000) promised for the PG building at Mona.

In meetings with his Minister of Health and senior staff, we had sketched a teaching plan for Trinidad, based on principles of adult learning, modified from the integrated organ system approach of Case Western Reserve University School of Medicine, originally proposed for Mona in 1969. We emphasised self-directed learning, problem-solving, early study of demographics, social and behavioural sciences, ample exposure to all clinical disciplines, at all levels of care, in community clinics, ambulatory and inpatient settings, with electives each year, to provide coverage of all levels and complexities of care, prevention and health promotion. The program would span five years, merging seamlessly (p. 56) with further specific training for primary or family care (2 years), or specialties (4-5 years), which had already started in both POSG and QEH. GMC conditions would be satisfied. He had agreed to the multi-professional nature of the *School*: Medicine, Dentistry, Veterinary Sciences, Advanced Nursing, Allied Health and ancillaries.

He had questioned and approved the medical curriculum, and conjoint basic sciences and clinical facilities, to permit integrated teaching of all disciplines, wherever appropriate.

It remains a mystery to me why PM Williams fumbled the plans so badly thereafter. In 1974, he had welcomed the decision to expand in Trinidad, starting in 1975; but dithered, ostensibly waiting for the economy to "recover," a mere excuse. It is even more intriguing why he discarded UWI plans that his Health Ministry and advisers had meticulously screened for 2-3 years, and approved, in favour of a French open model, with a French curriculum that even the French would have liked to change! The waywardness of this decision baffled many, including PVC Braithwaite, the Principal at St. Augustine, but was consistent with PM Williams' intransigence at meetings, which, some said, was a pose, to cover his deafness. Williams died in 1981, and his successor, George Chambers, started construction, six years late. The new buildings were completed in 1985, and left empty for five years, a playground for fungi, spiders, other insects, and rodents, during which railings and steps, made of French West African soft wood, rotted *(fig 22-2, p. 208)*, as did the French curriculum, with its rigid linear teaching over six years, and three *competitive* examinations.

When the T&T Faculty of Health Sciences was finally opened by PM ANR Robinson in 1989, fifteen years after its approval, and five years after completion, it copied McMaster's pricey undergraduate curriculum, without the corresponding staff, offered space to foreign students and patients, and hired a novice McMasterite to implement the teaching plan! Ironically, as a new McMaster professor in 1978, I had helped to evaluate and revise it! By 1980, its high cost, sub-optimal results and growing requests from students and staff for objective in-course assessments, to allay anxieties, had forced changes in evaluation. By the 1990s, the early evangelists that Wray and his team had met, had fled!

Up to then, McMaster's "education leaders," including the non-medical head of the education program, often had near-panic attacks on hearing the words *"test"* or *"examination;"* I had routinely tested my own tutorial and elective students, with question sets I had used at the UWI; later, I had used the same test tools in the program we had developed for the CPSO, under my direction, to test the competence of practising physicians. Their success led the Faculty to introduce two of the tests: MCQs and short problems, under triumphant stylings: *Personal Progress Index* (PPI) and *Objective Structured Clinical Examination* (OSCE)!

Barbados developed a full Faculty in 2007, expanding from the previous 3-year clinical program. Each site thus acquired a campus and a local Dean. This might in time necessitate the creation of a University Dean, or PVC Medicine, to set central policies, coordinate the work of the three faculties, serve the fourth, or "Open" campus, and cope with long-standing demands of other islands for a physical medical faculty, which private US for-profit medical schools have relentlessly cultivated, in non-university settings, reminiscent of pre-Flexnerian America.

The development into four campuses was foreseen. In 1960, when Gool Khan and I toured the islands, we heard the wistful speculation, even in St Eustasius, that one day the University would be more than just a name, and have a local presence. The extramural department hardly touched Medicine. When Philip Sherlock was head of ACURI, and the extramural leader at Mona, I had discussed with him the possibility of our Faculty sponsoring CME, Nursing and other courses in the Antilles, perhaps annually in rotation, such as were needed locally. Drs Davis of Bahamas, Comissiong of Grenada, and PM Compton of St Lucia were, by 1973, optimistic that this could happen. But interest waned, as staff left.

At the UHWI, newer policies and financing led, in 1987, to the development of a full Emergency department, as we had proposed *(Appendix 15.8, p 363)*. It obtained donor funds to add private wards, named the *Tony Thwaites wing* (p. 44), after one of the businessmen involved. Pushed by funding shortages, as costs of independence rose and contributors' economies flagged, the UWI began to rethink the commercialising of its expertise. It began to appraise marketable assets and examine possible revenue streams, to fund expansion, as some of us had advocated in the needy 1970s: e.g., medical services; laboratory tests and consultations; radiology; scientific, engineering, legal, management, business, language and other consultative fields. It reviewed roles, curricula, examination methods, Community and Family Medicine, adopted a divisional structure, and other administrative changes.

The new buildings at Mona exemplify this new approach. The campus would be almost unrecognisable to the early entrants, save for the preserved aqueduct, the old dramatic theatre, library, and outdoor concrete sinks, and the first permanent new structures: Irvine, Taylor and Chancellor Halls; the Registry; the Science and preclinical buildings, and the UCHWI. They would no doubt wonder, too, how so many private American medical schools *(48 so far, p 281)* can thrive on these small islands, competing with the UWI, like so many commodity factories, or expressions of commercial tourism in education. Six of these are accredited by the Caribbean Accreditation Authority for Education in Medicine and the Health Professions (CAAM-HP); six by the state of New York; and four by Accreditation Council for Colleges of Medicine (ACCM), an Irish body that claims equivalence with US Liaison Committee for Medical Education (LCME). The schools have undoubtedly pushed the UWI to emerge from a restrictive socialism and claims of a special morality, and induced it to "join them, since you cannot beat them."

The most impressive Faculty addition at Mona is the new Basic sciences complex *(cover photo)* which fulfils a personal dream and promises for curricular innovation; it should have been there *ab initio*, and was passionately advocated in the early 1970s, as illustrated in our defence of the Report of the Committee on Expansion, 1971, despite the coolness of the official record. How it would please those men to see their wish come true! The building should facilitate curricular changes and integrations that we had craved in the 1970s. Efforts then to co-ordinate teaching had failed for reasons already given. Regrettably, the S&P Medicine department, which became the Division of Community Health in 1978-9, has remained remote, almost aloof, from the clinical departments with which we had tried to integrate it functionally as CM. We had succeeded philosophically, creating an educational model, much admired by authorities in the north and south, especially by our peers in PAFAMS, but scuttled, no sooner had I left, by those charged with its health and validation, to satisfy personal whims and narrower visions. A ship without a captain inevitably founders in a storm.

Most of our graduates know little of the Faculty's formative years, or indeed the University's; some of the official writings about them contain significant errors and biases. Those who know better, speak nostalgically of early years and events. So far, no rich benefactor has spontaneously emerged in the Caribbean, no Ford or Carnegie, however modest – Ray Chang and Michael Lee-Chin notwithstanding – despite the affluence of many graduates, and their influence in the highest offices in the supporting territories. Some graduates admit a lack of attachment, and feel like outsiders, some citing my experience as an example.

But there is a bright side. By century end, the University had developed a fund-raising program, vested in the *Office of Institutional Advancement,* located in the Regional Headquarters building, Mona, under its charming director, Elizabeth Buchanan-Hind, and has already raised large sums. It has held annual gala events in Toronto, and New York, attracting philanthropists like the modest billionaire Ray Chang, now sadly passed on, and his friend, the equally philanthropic but flashy Mike Lee-Chin, with bases in Ontario and Kingston, Jamaica.

When I received Prof Wilks' request in early 2004 to give the *Jeffrey Wilson Memorial Lecture* to the *Association of Consultant Physicians of Jamaica* (ACPJ) on Sept 11th that year, I thought it was a hoax, and only agreed when my great friend, Rabin Sahoy, now no more, confirmed it.

Mary and I arrived in Kingston on September 9th, two days before hurricane *Ivan*. Its fury was awesome, Category 4 over land and 5 where the eye passed 23 miles south of Jamaica, dumping a foot of rain as it went; we spent his passage in the ballroom of the Pegasus, with many well-off locals, who had fled their homes to shelter in the sturdier hotel building. We listened all night to the winds slamming and rattling the doors and windows, rain whistling through every crevice, and to the frightened cries of children. The damage to the structure was slight, but to the country, enormous, totalling some US$360M.

The lecture and presentations were postponed to December 4th, at a gala event, where I felt honored to hand out awards, some to eminent men and women whom I had known as students, some well, others fleetingly, or by name only, in my years at the UWI. What a bright array of specialist physicians our PGME plan had produced! The UWI should be justly proud of that program. Our detractors of 1972 should have been there to eat their doubts. It warmed my heart to see members of the old COPMED, Drs Sahoy and Ashley. It was good to see the Vice-Chancellor among the persons to receive an award; I had met Nigel Harris once before, when I visited with Dean Gibbs in 1998; but I knew his father, the memorable and enigmatic Guyanese writer, Wilson Harris, who occupies a few pages in my book, *The Indelible Red Stain*.

On the occasion, Dr Amza Ali, a neurologist, secretary of the ACPJ, one of four medical doctor sons of Dr Emran Ali, a contemporary and fellow Guianese, retired orthopaedic surgeon, asked, "What do you think of the DM now? Nobody told us you were responsible for it!" I chuckled.

"*I'm* not surprised; they forgot me the day I left. They swept all I did, like so much litter, under a rug, and trampled over it, like bulls trashing rice, until it was flattened, and my name erased; they kept the PGME and EC parts but discarded CM and other innovations, like so much chaff!"

I told them how I had heard that the Dean or an associate had been overheard to say, "Now that he's away, we'll see that he stays there!" And in 1977, Sam Wray had written advising me not to come back, as that might lose him several senior staff! I had been booted, *oboted*! (*Milton Obote, Uganda dictator, deposed in absentia, 1973*). Prof Cruickshank had warned me of this, despite innovative and selfless service in the harsh 1970s, when I did the duties of three professors. I had been forgotten also by Dr Wilson's successors in the Ministry of Health, and in the EC. So the UWI was not alone in my side-lining, barring the brief and unfulfilled attempt by Deans Raje and Gibbs to correct that omission.

In 1998, I was surprised with a 50th anniversary medal that added to tokens of appreciation from others: Chancellor Hall, UWI, KFAFH, Jeddah, Saudi Arabia; PAFAMS; two Canadian Professional Colleges; several community organisations, and readers of my books and articles. The ACPJ added a splendid plaque and although not a Faculty or

University act, the invitation did come from its professors. So my Chancellor Hall *Super Lion* now has these two for company.

ACPJ members asked what Dr Wilson might say of today's UWI. Two decades after his retirement, Jamaica's Health Services were divided into four *Regional Health Authorities (RHA)*: Southeastern, the parishes of Kingston, St. Andrew, St. Thomas and St. Catherine, with 47% of the population; Northeastern, St. Ann, St. Mary, and Portland, 14%; Western, Trelawny, St. James, Hanover, Westmoreland, 17%; and Southern, Clarendon, Manchester and St. Elizabeth with 22%. Each was given responsibility for public health and general services, while the Ministry of Health retained charge of planning, policies, and regulations (shades of Ontario's LHINs). In 2008, the UWI opened a medical faculty in Montego Bay, about the same time as a full 5-year program was started in Barbados: three at Cave Hill, and two at QEH. I think Dr Wilson would have mourned the loss of CM and approved the rest. In 2009, the TMRI became a member of USA/Canada section of INCLEN, a body it could have joined *ab initio*, with benefit, had Sam Wray been more alert.

The social inputs into medical training seem muted, and graduates I have met over the last decades appear to be more like North Americans: commercial, snooty, and drug-oriented, as affirmed by a retired UWI professor of agriculture. Few engage in integrated community work, and most seem ill-adapted to their resource base. Community care in several islands has fallen into the laps of foreign doctors: Chinese and Cubans, who do not speak the language of their patients, the very thing our CM plan had sought to avoid. On 5 Feb, 2011, the POS *Daily Express,* writing on the importing of doctors to Trinidad, when the local university was training 100 per year, asked *"Where have all the doctors gone?"*

With regards to this and Community Medicine, Dr Wilson would have regretted that his successor, Dr Patterson, was unfamiliar with the novel, more economical and promising role of the CM specialist planned for Jamaica (and the Antilles) — still viable today — that PAHO's Horwitz had accepted as worth trying, in that unique setting. But it was brushed aside by his successors, who did not grasp its unique concepts. My PAFAMS colleagues would have sympathised; they too spend scarce resources on US methods. To some of their people, as to ours, "foreign" was better; so salt fish and potatoes "from foreign," as Jamaicans say, were superior to local fresh fish and yam. The Caribbean feeds on foreign foods. So too, a foreign method and teacher, especially if "white", were *de rigueur* in a Commonwealth Caribbean University. British honours remain coveted; almost everyone in Barbados is a "Sir Somebody!"

END

PART 2: APPENDICES

Appendix 1: PAPERS On Manpower and Education

1.1 Structure of Postgraduate Degrees in the UWI Faculty of Medicine; Extract, University Regulations, 1969-70

Postgraduate Training Plan for Specialist Qualifications in the Faculty of Medicine, UWI, approved by University Board for Higher Degrees, 1969

1.1.1. Specialty Degrees by Residency Training

(i) Doctorate in Medicine (DM)

Anaesthetics; Family Medicine; (Internal) Medicine; Pathology and Microbiology; Psychiatry; Radiology; and

(ii) Master in Surgery (MS): Obstetrics & Gynaecology and Surgery (now also styled DM)

AIM: A four year post internship training program leading to a specialty degree in the chosen discipline.

Year 1: The chosen specialty – at the University of the West Indies;
OR – optional subjects)
OR – Basic Sciences) as applicable

End of Year: Diploma Examination for those enrolled for diplomas in Anaesthetics, Obstetrics & Gynaecology, Psychiatry and others, e.g. Child Health, Public Health, etc., as they become available. Successful candidates may use the abbreviation "Dip." followed by the approved Specialty form, e.g. *Dip.Anaes.(UWI)*

Year 2: The chosen specialty - at the University of the West Indies or approved Institutions in the West Indies or elsewhere;
OR - optional subjects
OR - Basic Sciences

End Year 2 - Part 1 examination in specialty – a test of suitability to continue training. Examination for the Diploma in Laboratory Medicine (*Dip. Lab. Med., UWI*)

Year 3: The chosen specialty at University of the West Indies or other approved institutions in West Indies or elsewhere;
OR - optional subjects

293

OR - Basic Sciences

Year 4: Whole time in the specialty or in a subspecialty at University of the West Indies or in approved institutions in the West Indies or elsewhere.

End year 4: Final specialist examination.

Throughout Course: Regular attendance at:
Journal Clubs;
C.P.C.'s; Special Lectures; Seminars
Death Conferences, Autopsy Demonstrations
Research Meetings at Campus Institutes
Courses in other departments relevant to medicine e.g. biometrics, public health, demography, ecology
Supervision of students, interns and junior residents

NOTES and GUIDELINES:

1. This schedule in no way interferes with supplementary requirements of individual departments, e.g. necessity to do orthopaedics in general surgery course, or general surgery in obstetrics and gynaecology program. Nor does it affect other examination requirements, e.g. case book, operating registers, etc.

2. The four year training period is the <u>minimum</u> required, except for Family Medicine. It is probable and desirable that most candidates for the specialist examinations will have had more than the minimum training.

3. Post-internship experience in Casualty care, Pathology, Microbiology, Basic Sciences, may be a preliminary <u>requirement for some specialties</u>. This would, however, immediately lengthen the period of total specialty training beyond 4 years, which though undesirable from the viewpoint of duration , may be unavoidable for the quality of the course.

4. The schedule envisages graded responsibility during the period of postgraduate training; the syllabus would be structured to take account of this.

5. Yearly progress checks to supplement in-course evaluation (continuing) to determine whether knowledge, skills, attitudes are being acquired at a satisfactory rate and manner, and to determine readiness to continue.

6. Credit may be given for years spent in training for diplomate examinations, if there is a break after acquiring a diploma. This would accommodate trainees sponsored by governments for diploma training only, in the first instance.

7. Credit may be given for time spent in specialties in approved institutions in the West Indies or elsewhere. <u>At least 3 of the 4 years of training should be spent in the West Indies.</u>

8. Specific post-examination experience may be stipulated in certain specialties, e.g. Surgery, Psychiatry, etc.

9. Lists of optional subjects would be available in each department.

10. Residents are encouraged and may be required to complete a research project, done on a "horizontal" plan, and prepared for publication. A supervisor will be assigned to each resident; details will be discussed at the start of the program.

1.1.2. **Academic Degrees by Thesis**

A. MPhil and PhD *done by research only:*
Anatomy; Biochemistry; Physiology; Pharmacology, Public Health; Microbiology; Nutrition, Pathology
MSc Microbiology; Nutrition;
PhD Clinical Psychology (New)

B. *(i) MSc*
Counselling (by Distance Education)
Family Medicine (by Distance ")
Clinical Psychology (joint with the Faculty of Social Sciences)
Nursing
(ii) *MPH* in Health Education/Health Promotion; Public Health
(All in B above are self-financed)
(iii) New Nursing (Didactic) Programs:
Mental Health; Psychiatric Nurse Practitioner;
Nursing Education and Administration; Nurse Specialist.

1.2 Pan-American Conference on Health Manpower Planning, Ottawa, 10-14 September,1973

Report of WORKING GROUP III: NEW HEALTH OCCUPATIONS
(M. S Ragbeer)

Affirming the principle that health is a fundamental right of each individual, the group stated that it is the responsibility of each country to design a health care system appropriate to its needs and within its socioeconomic and cultural-political contexts. Despite significant differences in health conditions and manpower availability between North and South America, both could benefit from the introduction of new technical and auxiliary workers in their health services.

Traditional concepts and existing numbers of health personnel are insufficient for the needs of existing health services and extension of these services to rural areas. Training costs, particularly for physicians and dentists, are high and there is underutilization and maldistribution both geographically and among medical specialties. Many of the professionally performed functions could be delegated to others with less basic education and who are less costly to train and employ.

Only when the decision is made as to types of personnel needed, can training objectives and methods be decided. The process includes an analysis of the roles of existing categories of personnel and the possibility of task reallocation. Local authorities should determine whether existing training institutions should be modified or new schools created.

The group considered the role of the universities and teaching hospitals and suggested that existing practices tend to prepare professionals more for service in metropolitan rather than rural locations. Training should be related to the health conditions and should utilise facilities and opportunities available in the entire community, not just the hospitals. Most important, training should emphasise teamwork among professionals and auxiliaries.

Though admission requirements should be flexible, students should have a sufficient basic education to enable them to cope with program content. Students should be selected from the area in which they will eventually work and be trained there, as far as practicable. If trainees have to be trained elsewhere, it is preferable that periods of absence be kept short. Training should be of an in-service nature but with appropriate didactic content designed to teach the trainee adequate knowledge, skills, and attitudes appropriate to the level of performance desired. Curricula should be flexible and include opportunities for continuing education and the evaluation of performance within the context of the goals already established.

Teachers should be closely associated with the local health services that will absorb the new personnel. Financing of training programs should be the responsibility of the individual Ministry. It would be advantageous if existing educational institutions, government bodies and international agencies collaborated in this effort.

Many countries have already introduced into communities new types of health workers for the promotion of health and prevention of disease, to assist professionals in urban or rural services, and to carry out limited diagnostic and therapeutic services under supervision. They are being trained to perform either single or multiple functions.

The health care delivery system should be suitably modified to absorb the new groups in appropriate staff positions and it should ensure that their roles are understood and accepted by the professions. The new workers should have reasonable opportunity for financial and professional advancement, including promotion by further training. In addition, appropriate legislation should be introduced to permit the use of such workers, and training programs should be adequately financed.

The group recognized that different ideologies and levels of development existed in the health services of the Hemisphere and that in a single country, several institutions or organizations may be involved in health care delivery, public and private. It may not be possible, everywhere, to propose a national health plan, but it is suggested nevertheless that any plan should provide a rational basis for determining the types of health manpower required.

The following Report was also relevant to our immediate interests then:

"GROUP IV. HEALTH MANPOWER REQUIREMENTS

"Four principal methods for estimating health manpower requirements were identified by the working group and are based on economic needs; biologic needs; personnel:population ratio; and service targets. Selecting the correct method depends upon the individual health care system and data availability. Besides using any one method or a variation of one of the basic four, a combination of several techniques can often give satisfactory estimates of manpower requirements.

Selection of methodologies is not the critical issue, however. The lack of skilled planners is often more serious than the lack of planning data or methodology. Many planners are untrained in the application of the techniques for estimating requirements, nor do they attempt to verify past estimates with present available data. Such verification could provide guidelines for improving the techniques employed.

The problem of data is a general one, applicable to most sectors in developing countries; hence the inadequacy is not peculiar to health manpower planning.

Political constraints are of major importance in health manpower planning. Political decisions are taken in the preplanning stage. A political decision to plan is necessary before planning can begin, but even when such decisions are taken ideological differences between planners, politicians, and professional associations could render planning efforts inoperative.

Generally there will be greater support for manpower planning in the health sector of a centrally planned economy than in the market economies which characterise the majority of nations in the Hemisphere. Unfortunately there is still no method for determining the ideal health situation to which a country should aspire."

1.3 Dean's Inaugural Address to Faculty Board, July 1971

I come to this first Faculty Board meeting of my deanship with a feeling of humility as I face the task of Faculty reform and to continue and expand the work of recent deans: Professors Bras, Cruickshank and Stuart. They are not the sort whose shoes can be filled instantly. I shan't try to do so, and instead will rely on their advice and support, already generously offered. I know there is considerable sentiment for the previous administration, of which I was a part. I am deeply grateful for the support, stated and implied, that exists throughout the Faculty.

Our Faculty is starting an era of change, progress and expansion, which may well glorify it, or sink it, if we're not cautious. Professor Stuart recently remarked that the faculty is further ahead today than it was two years ago, and felt sure that in two years' time, further advances would be made. I share that optimism, and will work assiduously to justify it, and prove him right.

That the Faculty—that is, all staff and University officers—has willingly undergone deep soul-searching this past year, is a sign of its academic honesty and maturity, and a desire to evaluate what it has done, where it stands, what needs to be done, and how to go about it.

Last year, our review identified a crisis, discussed it with the University administration, and made recommendations, which we shared earlier this year with the IADB Committee on expansion, whose report is imminent. We agreed on the first two things. But there may be differences of opinion on what needs to be done, and how to do it. Our crisis is a crisis of perception, of method, of inadequate resources and how to get more. For efficiency now, we need to pool what we have, add what you can provide, sift them, and select what is most desirable, attainable, and cost:efficient, for implementation. To do this, I ask for the unswerving loyalty of each of you to Faculty goals, not persons, and for help in whatever way you can give it: to define, refine and realise them.

The Faculty is an academic body that has immersed itself, so far, in building a strong educational program to produce doctors with thorough and up-to-date knowledge of disease, its manifestations and treatment. While this effort has done that, enhancing careers here and abroad, it has fallen short in nurturing the equally important matter of research into the requirements for, and maintenance of good health in our environment, and in the contributing territories. Extending our attention to this makes good sense from several viewpoints:

1. It demands a deep understanding of the environment, in respect of social, psychological, economic, demographic, geopolitical and other factors that affect the lives and health of people, and its maintenance. This in itself will contribute not only to our own knowledge of those things, but would add data to help identify, prevent, reduce, and treat disease early, and to train, more appropriately, professionals and other functionaries to meet health care needs.

2. Much of the load that now swamps our hospital departments consists of "preventable" illness. It is economically smarter to spend money on schemes to improve and safeguard the health of the public, to promote it and prevent illness. This would free hospitals to focus on building expertise to care for the sick.

3. The UH Casualty department is a mix of primary care and true casualties. It can become the organisational base of programs aimed at carrying health care, continuously and at low cost, into communities and homes, to bring benefits to larger sections of the populace, and to enhance education. The identification of illness at an early stage of its development would invariably mean easier and more economical management of individuals and whole communities.

Our students must be indoctrinated in a holistic approach to medical care and schooled in all its facets, to investigate them further, to expand the knowledge needed for the growth of health systems, and to teach others the results of such work. Manpower is the key element; we produce key manpower. The Faculty's role in improving and securing the health of the nation must therefore lie in identifying and training the types of manpower appropriate to form functional health teams. In the training of the physician, the likely head of such teams, the burden on teacher and student is considerable, to master the wide-ranging and demanding roles, which the physician is required to fill, and often all at once: I refer to the roles of healer, scientist, investigator, teacher, community advocate, specialist in a chosen field, with links to, and knowledge of medical technology, forensics, engineering, psychology, sociology, agriculture, communication and so on. If we look at our output of traditional trained doctors, we would see the short-comings in our program. Our medical faculty is today the main source of doctors for the supporting territories, even though the British Colonial office is still responsible for those not yet independent.

Our clinical training is delivered by departments, piecemeal, not by systems, or holistically. Ideally, topics should be integrated, but at this time, this is left up to students. We can assist by increasing interdepartmental cooperation, which some already do. But even within departments the spirit of cooperation may not be well enough developed, perhaps for logistic reasons alone.

Our full time teaching faculty is small, and we do not have enough part-time staff to ease the service load, and help with teaching, as some Faculties of similar size elsewhere do. Staff need to know how the University functions and how those functions affect or can assist them in their career. At present, too few faculty members are fully aware of the processes of university management and faculty administration. Correction of this might conceivably contribute to the feeling of belonging lacking in so many, especially at junior levels.

The office suggests that the cure of the sick individual, which at most times seems the end of all our efforts, is not the prime function within the university, though it is a much needed and demanded professional and humanitarian one, which we must accept and perform assiduously. The education of a medical student in hospitals is dependent upon the study of such sick people, but it should not exclude learning of that major level of care required by the multitudes outside the hospital walls. You know, of course, that the traditional British medical education we follow fails to expose students to about 80% of all medical problems of populations in their communities: transient and minor illness or accidents, the early stages of most diseases, grouped as primary or ambulatory care, nutrition, immunisation and preventive care. In hospital, students learn to handle mainly secondary and some tertiary care, a tiny percent of which needs intensive care, yet these consume the bulk of health spending. We must correct this imbalance. Students must see this wide spectrum and learn its lessons. The Curriculum Committee is studying reforms to this end.

We are proposing a novel entity, a Division of Community Medicine, to be a centre for Primary and holistic care, and Family Medicine education, which should concern each doctor and student; it is the major thrust of World Health systems and activities; the IADB Committee has endorsed this, and its report will be available to you when finalised. It also includes the funding requests for the expansion scheme in the EC. Community Medicine will integrate clinical and preventive medicine and health promotion, in hospital and in related community clinics. Inter-relationships and dependencies will be highlighted, to facilitate learning. The curriculum will be modified, to promote integration wherever possible e.g. basic sciences among one another, and with clinical disciplines. The separation of pre-clinical and clinical facilities, a major original planning error, hinders this process. I know most of you have good ideas of what can be done, and support the aims and initiatives. PAHO has agreed to fund two seminars of two weeks each for all staff: one on *Curriculum Development*, in September, the other on *Teaching of Behavioural Sciences*, later this year.

The Dean's office needs to be re-organised; remember, the dean has always been part-time and head of his own department; files are therefore everywhere. The university registrar, Carl Jackman, has loaned us Mrs. Irene Walter, for this job, and we are reforming the governance structure, starting with the Faculty Board, which, as you already know, now includes all Faculty on 3-year contracts. We welcome all new members, and urge you to join the debate. The major functions of the Faculty will devolve to small Select Committees of 5-9 members, based on Faculty representation, not departmental. Thus we can become our brothers' keepers, and take advantage of all the talent that we have.

Our newest development, apart from the IADB Committee, is Jamaica's approval of our PGME plan, with formation by the Caribbean Health Ministers Conference, of the *Committee for Postgraduate Medical Education (COPMED*, p. 324), with membership from the CHMC, Faculty, and HOPE—our partner in PGME—and the UHWI Junior Staff Association. It has appointed a Task Force to survey the region's needs for specialists, which I will chair, and includes a JSA member.

Despite limitations of staff, this office would like to assist, so please do not hesitate to use it. We will be glad to call on you at such times as suit your convenience, to discuss mutual problems, activities and goals. The office further wishes to act as a centre for information on any aspect of university or extra-university endeavour, for dissemination of news and for news on administrative matters of various kinds. This is a regular item on the agenda of Board meetings.

The office desires to introduce a public relations program to mitigate a further criticism, that of failing to share our educational experiences with the community outside our walls. We would therefore ask you to send us reprints of published work, or typescripts of work completed and submitted. In time, selected items might form the nucleus of a regular display, which I've discussed with Dr TVN Persaud of Anatomy, who edits the WIMJ; it will be located in the library, or in the main lecture rooms. The visit of the BMA audio-visual director next year will provide further opportunity to develop this program.

The office also wishes to mount a display of all the lines of training at the UWI and UHWI, and the work of special independent but affiliated units such as the TMRU, the ERU, and the CFNI here, TRVL in Port-of-Spain, and any that develops elsewhere. There is widespread ignorance of some of these and this extends to all sorts of unlikely people, including leaders in the Faculty and University. We would appreciate the opportunity to discuss your training and research programs and how to display them.

Our office is small and grossly under-provided. We need a fund-raising mechanism, a Foundation or Trust, in addition to personal efforts, such as Professor Bras's that resulted in the Rippel Building. We need endowments, grants, and regular contributions from well-wishers. One of our staff has begun to collect addresses of alumni, and we hope to form an Association for the prime purpose of marshalling their support, through subscriptions, gifts, bequests, volunteering, and so on. We had a preliminary meeting with recent graduates here, who were keen to support. We hope to do the same in the EC, as part of the expansion there. At the moment 50 final year students go yearly to POS and Bridgetown; next year 25 fourth year students will go to POS, as a step towards full clinical training in both Trinidad and Barbados, and preclinical in Trinidad.

A few weeks ago, at my first meeting with department heads, I noted that my personal commitment to the Faculty is a grassroots one; my entire scientific education was obtained here, having transferred from the Faculty of Arts midway in my first term. Most of you were educated elsewhere and so have other loyalties. Not that that diminishes your commitment; instead, it brings the enriching benefits of diversity and external genes. But my attachment is original, and total. When I was a student, some of you were my respected teachers, and still are; you know my faults and my strengths. But I hope we can work together to strengthen this *alma mater*, which a few of you may know that I decided to serve, instead of a more established one at Columbia University. So I make no apology for my enthusiasm and commitment, and ask your indulgence and help.

Thank you very much for your support and attention.

Mohan M.S. Ragbeer
Dean, Medical Faculty

1.4. Paper on **Post-graduate Medical Education in the Commonwealth Caribbean** (*M.S. Ragbeer* 1972, WIMJ 21, 147.)

The case for initiating programs in postgraduate medical education in the West Indies may be simply stated. Technical advances in medicine have been occurring with increasing pace; the body of basic knowledge now available, assimilable and applicable to health care delivery has expanded beyond the content and capabilities of our undergraduate syllabus and have created increasing demands for extending formal education beyond the year of graduation. At the same time changing social, political and economic circumstances in the Commonwealth Caribbean have led to new levels of community and individual expectation from the health services. The services themselves, caught up in the atmosphere of social and technological change, have begun to seek the varied resources of manpower and facilities needed to practise modern medicine.

These considerations have weighed heavily with the Medical Faculty; efforts to plan postgraduate programs at the U.W.I. were begun some ten years ago. In the early period, training was based on strict apprenticeship and graduates were prepared for British professional examinations, the degrees granted being recognized throughout the commonwealth Caribbean for specialist and consultant appointments. A few departments went further and organized courses for such students with commendable results; this was particularly so in Obstetrics & Gynaecology and in Surgery. Various arrangements with United Kingdom Medical Schools and teachers facilitated exchange programs, fellowships and scholarships for this purpose. These, however, had many limitations, not the least of which was the uncertainty of a graduate obtaining one of these awards, as they were few, and went largely to those who had won the favour of the particular department head. Many graduates therefore preferred to enter formal residency training programs in the United States or in

Canada where these factors did not operate. They were influenced, too, by the structured nature of these programs and by the fact that the British system – except in Pathology, Anaesthesia and Radiology, was not geared to produce a skilled individual, rather someone with a theoretical degree; the acquisition of practical knowledge and documented clinical skills came after. The loss of graduates into North American residencies increased rapidly to the level of just under 50% of individual graduating classes. Those who remained behind began to press for formal training in all disciplines and many gave up when it seemed that progress was too slow.

In response to pressing needs diploma level programs were begun in Anaesthesia, Laboratory Medicine, Child Health, Psychiatry, and latterly, in Public Health and Obstetrics & Gynaecology. These have had variable success, those in Anaesthesia and Psychiatry having the best response. Diplomates in Anaesthesia and in Psychiatry have begun to fill important places in the health services, not only of the smaller communities, but of the larger hospitals as well.

The efforts to institute full specialty training to consultant level gained momentum and direction in 1969, when the Caribbean Health Ministers Conference requested the U.W.I. to present formal proposals for post-graduate medical education in the disciplines in which full programs for the training of future consultants could with advantage be developed.

PROGRAMS IN POST-GRADUATE MEDICAL EDUCATION

In presenting its case in 1970 to this Conference in Barbados,[2] faculty officers were careful to state the educational, social, economic, professional and other factors that would justify the establishment of such training in addition to the technical ones already mentioned. They referred to the loss of graduates and pointed out that in 1965, 30% of the graduating class had left the Caribbean, 45% of the 1966 class, and 59% of the 1967 class; and that the trend was continuing. They stressed, too, that the in-service nature of much of graduate training would require the involvement of regional hospitals for this training; such use would bring great benefits to the regional hospitals in terms of upgrading facilities and providing dedicated young graduates to work in them at the time in their career when they would give their best service.

At that time there was little precise knowledge of the size of the needs or the relative priorities for training in the different specialties. A joint committee of U.W.I. and Governments, with PAHO/WHO assistance in funding and personnel, was charged with providing answers. It reported to the Conference in February, 1971, submitting ten recommendations.[3] Among these was a list of the top priorities for training: Anaesthesia, Microbiology, Paediatrics, Pathology, Psychiatry, Social and Preventive Medicine, Radiology, Medical Administration and General Practice. The Committee had not been able to provide exact figures on the total need for the different specialties throughout the Caribbean. Whether for this reason, or for others not connected directly to medical education, a decision to implement the scheme was further deferred and a Task Force was appointed under the leadership of the author to conduct a study of the needs of the area for specialists, the ability of the area's resources to contribute to training, the extent to which they could benefit from such training, and their ability to absorb those trained. Again financial support came from PAHO/WHO and from the U.W.I. At this meeting, Jamaica indicated readiness to proceed with implementation, and that she would seek the means to proceed ahead of the others.

The Task Force visited all Caribbean territories except the Bahamas and Jamaica (consent to carry out the study in these was not obtained), and reported to the Conference in February 1972.[4] The information it obtained showed grave shortages of specialists in the priority fields and indeed in others, with disturbing regional and urban-rural imbalances of distribution, severe unmet needs in vital areas such as community medicine, medical administration, patterns and organization of the health services themselves, and general practice; the Task Force reported lack of fundamental resources, physical, manpower and technical, in many of the major health facilities of the Caribbean. Of more serious import was the dearth of medical statistics of any validity or reliability in most of the territories. This lack made it difficult to come to firm conclusions as to what types of professionals would best suit the health care needs of a particular area. It reflected poor direction and planning, much of which could be corrected through the influence of, and demands created by appropriate postgraduate training programs. For example, an important component of programs in Community Medicine or in Pathology would be the investigation of basic health conditions of an area; such research could usefully be undertaken by graduate students and would be vital to the whole educational exercise; for whatever else might be said, postgraduate training could not really be seen to prosper, or indeed be possible in the absence of full research programs.

THE EXTENT OF NEED FOR SPECIALIST PROFESSIONALS

Basically every type of medical professional is required in the Commonwealth Caribbean. Opinions differ on the actual number of each type needed in any one area; this cannot be resolved in advance of appropriate studies into health care delivery. Nevertheless it was possible for the Task Force to indicate the levels of skill needed in various environments in terms of the common problems encountered and the facilities available. It was obvious that whatever else was said, no Government would be willing to accept any "lowering" of the standard they had set for specialty recognition in any of the disciplines. In the smaller communities it was recognised, however, that full specialists were not needed in every discipline and that the prime need was for well-trained general practitioners. A few of these could be further trained for a year or so in one of particular subjects, e.g., anaesthesia, or child health, and they could become responsible for the primary routine needs in these specialties, while basically functioning as general practitioners. Higher levels of skill could be secured by arrangements from a larger island or could be concentrated in one large centre serving several small islands.

The Task Force found that 192 new specialists would be required within the next ten years. This figure did not include the needs of Jamaica, Bahamas and Bermuda.

LEVELS OF TRAINING REQUIRED

This type of arrangement had the support of most health ministries and fitted well with the concept and plans for two levels of formal postgraduate training which the Faculty had developed and presented to the Caribbean Health Ministers Conference.

(i)   Practical training for one calendar year in a particular discipline (except for laboratory medicine, two years) leading to a diploma in that subject.

(ii) A four-year residency training program in each of the major specialties leading to a Master's degree (M.S.) in the case of Surgery and Obstetrics & Gynaecology, or to a Doctorate in Medicine (D.M.) in the other specialties.* (It should be noted that the University already had regulations governing award of degrees earned by research theses viz. Ph.D., & M.Sc. * *Details of these programs are obtainable from the Dean's Office, Faculty of Medicine, U.W.I.)*

RECOGNITION OF DEGREES

The diplomas would not ordinarily confer on the holders any eligibility for consultant status. They should however be able to hold middle grade posts in the appropriate specialty, or to perform specialized service within the limitations of their training, particularly for small communities, which could not afford fully trained specialists, nor which did not need them continuously.

Holders of the D.M. and M.S. degrees, on the other hand, should be eligible for consultant appointments in the Commonwealth Caribbean; the Caribbean Health Ministers' Conference has already agreed to this.

Many persons have expressed reservations on the value and respect U.W.I. degrees would command in other countries and have argued for settlement of reciprocities even before the programs are undertaken. This approach is unduly pessimistic and presupposes the existence of internationally recognized postgraduate qualifications. I know of none. West Indians should be reminded that the recognition accorded to some British qualifications in Commonwealth countries is a legacy of the colonial era, and not an act of "reciprocity". It should be stressed that medical qualifications earned in the U.K. have no automatic recognition anywhere in the U.S. or in Europe. Each qualification is subject to individual scrutiny before its holder is allowed, by registration, to practise. Often, too, residential qualifications have to be met before the foreign-degree holder is enabled to practise independently or outside of hospitals.

Obviously then our primary concern is not to earn reciprocity. However we expect fully that the standard and quality of our training will ensure that those who satisfactorily complete the training programs will have no difficulty establishing their worth. We have no doubts about our capability in this regard; the excellent record of our graduates in foreign lands will attest to this.

ATTRACTING THE GRADUATE

Responses to questionnaires directed to new graduates suggest that there would be no shortage of applicants for training. This is heartening, but the response may vary with the specialty. Individuals tend to be attracted to a particular field not only by its prestige and quality in the eyes of the community and of fellow professionals, but also by the economic gains its pursuit will bring. The concerned practitioner has traditionally been the best advertisement a specialty can have had, persuading others to follow, by merit, precept, example and excellence. While this may suffice in some instances, it is clear that the major instruments for channelling young graduates into the different specialties in a balanced way must be the curriculum itself and the opportunities and practices within the health services.

Young doctors wish, and rightly so, to enter services which allow them scope for improving their education and academic standing while providing satisfactory conditions for patient care. This means that hospitals and other facilities must be adequately provided both in middle-grade and consultant staff so that the former can get sufficient time off for educational pursuits and the latter for assisting in training and planning, without affecting the quality and range of patient care.

The other recourse to attracting staff into unpopular specialties must be the creation of adequate incentives. There is no shortage of persons wanting to train in Surgery, General Medicine, and Obstetrics and Gynaecology. These have, by tradition, been the fields held in greatest esteem by laymen and professionals alike. Perhaps this is related to the drama, emotion, personal satisfaction and economic gains from individual patient care. Perhaps the relationship stems from the fact that these disciplines were in the van of medical specialisation and dominate the medical undergraduate curriculum. The truth lies in both. Most specialties in medicine have come of age only in the last thirty years, and while circumstances may have changed, patterns and attitudes have not. The change can be stimulated by promoting interest in the scarce specialties in some tangible way. I can think of no better way than through salary differentials, or special allowances during the training years, and through enhanced opportunities for academic and financial rewards within the services. Unless some such device were used (in addition to curriculum change), the scarcities in the specialties listed as "Priorities" will continue.

IMPLEMENTATION AND FINANCIAL CONSIDERATIONS

The resources needed to implement the programs are detailed, with supporting arguments in the documents already cited. Briefly these are physical and human. Physical resources are either equipment or buildings; clearly both would be related to the type of program. It is envisaged that existing facilities should be used wherever possible, and in this context the major health facilities – hospitals, clinics, health centres, should be brought into the system by a process of accreditation and affiliation. Similarly, professionals already working in these facilities can be brought into the program according to their talents and inclination. These resources are now in the control of the various health ministries, and satisfactory mechanisms must therefore be established to permit their utilization within the training program. In this way, considerable benefits can accrue to the health services from the viewpoints of efficient use of economic resources, and of meeting consumer needs satisfactorily. The major advance then would appear to be to alter the present structure of government facilities sufficiently, to make them able to contribute to, and benefit from postgraduate training activities. This exercise would cost little, but the advantages gained would have far-reaching impact on the quality of health care that it would stimulate.

Elsewhere[4] emphasis has been made on the difficulties inherent in the present structures of the health services with its "British Civil Service" attitudes, patterns and practices. Administration is weak; there is no freedom to manage or direct finances even in the most limited sense; management of supplies is wasteful of time and money; there is little cooperative or integrated planning; recruitment practices discriminate in favour of the short-term foreigner at the expense of the native who wishes to remain; facilities, ill-managed, deteriorate rapidly; others (e.g. librarians) are not provided. All this points to mismanagement on a massive scale, not through wickedness, but through sheer traditionalism and an unwillingness to evaluate the system in use, or to accept the need for change even when the evidence is as clear as crystal, and the manpower to effect changes available.

The other need, no less urgent than the first (and from some points of view a need that exists because of the former) is for personnel on a recurrent basis. Allied with this is the need for teaching and office space, for supplies for auxiliary staff, and the usual annual recurring expenses. The total investment would be large, but the developments could be phased in over a number of years to spread the costs thinly over the years. Moreover, economies can be effected through improved management and full utilization, where possible, of existing resources. Staff is the biggest single item of recurrent expenditure, and is in short supply everywhere. Substantial assistance in this regard has come from several sources and this assistance has enabled establishment of several programs:

(i)   The PAHO/WHO has provided funds to employ a Senior Lecturer in Social and Preventive Medicine to assist with the D.P.H. program.

(ii)   The People-to-People Foundation of Washington, D.C., U.S.A. (HOPE) has agreed to provide staff— one specialist and up to two senior residents in the 7 disciplines of Medicine, Surgery, Obstetrics & Gynaecology, Pathology, Anaesthesia, Radiology, and Paediatrics—for a five-year period to facilitate implementation, in collaboration with the Jamaican Government. Other specialties can be added upon review, and it is expected that the scheme will be extended to other countries in the region. The arrangement under which this was set up is perhaps a good prototype of the kind of joint investment that is required to implement the programs. The Government of Jamaica has agreed to provide certain recurrent and capital funds that are central to the development of Postgraduate Medical Education, and to provide housing for the HOPE staff. The agreement was signed late in 1971 and since then training has started in three specialties – Obstetrics & Gynaecology, Paediatrics and Surgery. Training is expected to begin in Medicine, Pathology, Microbiology, Radiology and Anaesthesia in July, 1972, or January, 1973. The financial problems are, however not all easily solved; but it is expected that only as the programs develop will we be able to identify difficulties of detail and plan for solution.

(iii)   Other agencies and universities have expressed willingness to assist with staff on rotation; these will be investigated and utilised if they bring advantages.

(iv)   The administrative and clinical staff of the University Medical Faculty has contributed considerably and without pay to this venture. Several programs were begun with funds from individual research or fellowship grants; some were meshed in with undergraduate studies and resulted in no extra expenditures on the budget. Staff time was provided gratis for the day to day teaching and for all the planning, investigative and developmental work done in the past three years. The University bore all administrative costs of planning and continues to carry a burden in this respect.

(v) The University Hospital has contributed generously through use of its facilities: staff, equipment, rooms etc., and continues to do so. Similarly, staff of several Government units have either contributed to teaching or expressed willingness to do so.

(vi) The role of governments in post-graduate medical education is critical. While primary responsibility for undergraduate training rests with the University Grants Committee, postgraduate education should be provided out of funds allocated for health care delivery.

The administration of the programs, like the programs themselves, should remain with the University. This is surely reasonable, particularly in the group of economically underprivileged islands which cannot afford to duplicate the academic facilities of the U.W.I. The U.W.I. in its turn has seen the programs as an investment to meet certain defined needs of the Commonwealth Caribbean. It has people of responsibility, goodwill and a regional outlook on health care matters who can continue to plan, organize and co-ordinate the implementation of the programs if certain facilities are given them. These include the freedom to look critically at the systems in vogue, to suggest modifications that would improve all facets of the services, including the morale of the staff within them, and to define reasonable goals to which they can aspire. For without urgent improvements in crucial areas the services may well continue to lose contact with the profession and with the masses they have been established to serve. Already, morale is low and a sense of accomplishment declining among those who staff these services. A clear re-statement of their goals is needed, and the institution of postgraduate medical education will undoubtedly give a fillip to the many who wish to see these goals attained.

FACULTY ORGANIZATION

The Medical Faculty through its Board has the responsibility for ensuring that training programs are properly organized and conducted. The Board has recommended the appointment of two Co-ordinators, one for the programs at Mona, the other for the Eastern Caribbean. The Jamaican Government has agreed to provide the former and supporting staff to assist in launching the scheme in Jamaica (though up to the time of writing the funds have not reached us). It is hoped that similar contributions will come from the other territorial governments to enable expansion of the programs on a truly regional basis.

The Faculty Board has established a Board of Study to supervise training in each specialty. The Board is made up of Faculty members in that specialty with the Co-ordinator and Dean as ex officio members. (Since a Co-ordinator has not yet been appointed, the incumbent Dean and Clinical Vice-Dean are performing these functions). It has the usual power to co-opt members of Government or of affiliated institutions (e.g. HOPE). In this regard we should note that the HOPE

Foundation has appointed a Co-ordinator of its postgraduate endeavours at the U.W.I. This individual contributes considerably to the functioning of the Boards.

The Boards of study are responsible to the Faculty Board for selection of students from among those who apply, supervision of training, accreditation of teachers and of hospitals and other facilities, and of examinations. The academic functions of all Boards are channelled through a Faculty sub-committee for approval by the Board. A second committee known as the Co-ordinating Committee, made up of a member of each Board of Study and the Dean, and chaired by the Co-ordinator, has been set up to investigate and suggest solutions for problems common to the various programs that require an inter-disciplinary approach for solution. At the level of Government and other funding organizations a Liaison Committee has been established with membership from Government, Foundations and the U.W.I. Their main task would be to review financial arrangements and suggest modifications best suited to fund the programs adequately.

So far this has worked fairly well. Difficulties have arisen because some individuals are, by virtue of their office, members of all of these committees. The educators, however, responded well to the need for these various groups, and in spite of heavy work-loads continue to give tangible support. The novelty of an educational and academic role has perhaps inhibited some Government staff, but it is hoped that their full participation will not be long in coming. Problems are expected in the early stages of any endeavour; we are not put off by them, rather their occurrence is a stimulus to devising ways to overcome them. We hope that detractors and those ruled by timidity will not use the occurrence of problems as evidence of any inherent inability on our part to ensure the success of the programs.

CONCLUSION

The history and development of PGME at U.W.I. is briefly traced. The main features of the programs and the environment of training are described. The mechanisms of implementation, including administrative and financial arrangements, academic demands, the operation of an affiliation system, are summarized. The programs have now begun in Jamaica with the assistance of the HOPE Foundation; it is expected that it will shortly become possible to expand them into the other islands.

REFERENCES

1. Caribbean Health Ministers' Conference – Final Report of First Meeting, Vol. 1, p.7, 1969. Government Printery, Port-of-Spain, Trinidad and Tobago.
2. Caribbean Health Ministers' Conference – Final Report of Second Meeting - Papers 70/6, 70/6a and 70/6 App, (Estimates), 1970. Ministry of Health, Bridgetown, Barbados.
3. Caribbean Health Ministers' Conference, Third Meeting – 7a, b, c; 1971. Dept. Of Health and Welfare, Bermuda.
4. Caribbean Health Ministers' Conference – Fourth Meeting – Papers 17/72, and appendices 1972, Guyana.

PS. We sent reprints to several specialty bodies, in the Commonwealth and Americas. Sir Cyril Clarke, KBE, FRCOG, FRCPath, FRS, President of the Royal College of Physicians of England, 1972-77) wrote the note reproduced below. See also comment on p. 192.

ROYAL COLLEGE OF PHYSICIANS

11 St. Andrew's Place
Regent's Park
London NW1 4LE

Telephone: 01-935 117<
Telegrams: Medicorum Lon

SJA

2 8 DEC 1972

20th December, 1

Dear Dr. Ragbeer,

Thank you very much indeed for sending me the paper on Postgraduate Medical Education in the Commonwealth Caribbean. I am very glad to read this and particularly like the sections on recognition of degrees and attracting the graduate.

Please call in and see me any time you are in London, I am here most of the time.

Yours sincerely,

Cyril A. Clarke
President

Dr. M.M.S. Ragbeer,
Dean of the Faculty of Medicine,
University Hospital of the West Indies,
Mona,
West Indies.

Appendix 2:

Summary of Report of Special (IADB) Committee on Expansion/Duplication of the Medical Faculty, 1971

INTRODUCTION

Preamble

(i)   The Terms of Reference are stated in pp. 4-6 of the Report, which is identified as UWI Council Paper 14/1971.

(ii)   The Committee convened on May 24, 1971 and visited all the territories contributing to the University, and Guyana. It interviewed members of the academic staff in the Faculty of Medicine and in other faculties on all campuses, members of Governments and their advisers in all territories visited, and consulted many documents and papers, in assembling the data for the report. This was submitted to the Vice Chancellor and discussed with the Coordinating Committee in October, by Planning Committee and by Senate. The Committee wishes it noted that pressure of time did not permit the more refined presentation it would have wished.

THE REPORT

As a basis for its major recommendations, the Committee considers the nature of the health services of the Commonwealth Caribbean and examines their major features. This is done mainly in Section B but is further amplified and developed in the chapters of Section C under specific headings.

1.   In Section B (pp. 11-22) the concepts and objectives of medical education in the Commonwealth Caribbean are discussed and certain roles clearly defined for the University and for its Medical Faculty in assisting to remedy the deficiencies noted and so to achieve the fundamental objectives of a health care system, viz: -

(a)   the promotion of health

(b)   the prevention of illness and disability

(c)   the cure, alleviation or arrest of disease at the earliest possible stage

(d)   the rehabilitation and return to productivity of sick persons.

2.   The Committee is concerned that the health services are not effectively meeting these objectives, and considers that the University could materially assist in finding solutions through the following activities:

(a)   the search for new knowledge in both basic and applied fields,

(b)   the transmission of knowledge to students, practitioners, organisers of health services and to the public,

(c)   the utilisation of knowledge by demonstrating how it may be applied, and by giving advisory services to those interested in and concerned with systems of health care delivery.

3.   The Committee defines within the context of these activities the responsibilities of the Faculty of Medicine:

(a)   to produce by appropriate investigation the knowledge needed to solve the health needs of the contributing countries,

(b)   to produce the knowledge required to educate and train health professionals, and to establish the needed training programs,

(c)   to produce health professionals who can meet the objectives set out in 1 (a) – (d) above.

In this context, it is noted that while the Faculty has produced doctors of considerable merit internationally, the emphasis has been on curative and hospital medicine, while programs in prevention of disease, health education, health maintenance and rehabilitation, applied research, and health planning, have not developed sufficiently. Students' orientation into the health systems of the area and into the realities of service in the various territories has not been adequate; the development of departments has been unbalanced, and programs in graduate education have not developed in response to obvious needs. Many graduates are leaving the area.

4. (i)   In various Chapters of Section C, the types and cadres of health professionals needed in an area with 4.5 million people are examined, and the facilities available at UWI to train them. It is emphasised that the current staff and physical facilities, both in pre-clinical and clinical areas, are unable to cope sufficiently well with the current intake of 110 students at Mona. Consolidation measures need to be taken to meet the deficit. The five different types of doctors needed are described (pp. 19-20) in relation to the duties they are expected to perform, in and for the territories. It is emphasized that their training should be relevant to the needs of the area.

(ii)   The Committee considers the curriculum currently in vogue (pp. 44-53) and relates it to the requirements of the health services, discussing at length the strengths and weaknesses of the system. The greatest weakness is the traditional nature with regard to adherence to teaching of medicine in hospitals only, and large chunks devoted to the so-called basic sciences, neglecting social and behavioural sciences. A heavier emphasis needs to be placed on social and behavioural sciences and on environmental studies than is now given. Deficiencies are further noted, not only in the number of professionals produced in relation to the total population (pp. 63-69) but in terms of current needs for applied research that could provide reliable, precise information for planning education, service and research activities. The arguments are presented on pp. 54-62 while an examination of numbers follows on pp. 63-69. Needs are recognised to exist also for new educational developments in community medicine, and for utilisation of community facilities for educational and research purposes; these are described in detail in the chapter on Community Medicine in pp. 54-62 and the role of a division of Community Medicine in undergraduate, graduate and continuing education, in service, and in research is fully explored.

(iii)   On pp. 28-43 and 49-50, the limitations of existing departmental programs are examined as well as the current scheme for teaching in the Eastern Caribbean. Note is taken of the absence of a program for elective study in the associated states, though opportunities for such work exist (pp. 49-50).

(iv)   The "Brain Drain" is discussed briefly on p. 65 and possible causes including university selection procedures (pp. 69-71); conditions of service in the various health ministries (p. 66); lack of programs in continuing medical education (pp. 77-78); and failure to establish multi-disciplinary approaches to education (pp. 93-97), and to solution of health problems; and the inadequacy felt by the young graduate in trying to cope with illness under trying conditions (p. 66).

(v)   The need is examined in some detail on pp. 85-92 for health professionals other than doctors – that is, nurses, dentists and paramedical staff of all types. Though precise studies on total needs in the area have not been done for all of these, it is recognised that in each country significant shortages exist in all cadres. The need for dentists appears particularly urgent (p. 87). A role was seen for the University in preparing programs for the supervising education of the higher echelons of paramedical training, and to collaborate with Governments in all levels of training through the C.H.M.C.

(vi)   It is noted that there has, so far, been little real success in developing collaborative programs between the UWI and the Health Ministries of the region –a necessary prerequisite to developing effective educational service and research programs. However, recently, tangible steps have been taken to improve this through the mechanism of the Caribbean Health Ministers Conference. Chapter 15 (pp. 98-101) is devoted to this important topic, and the broad areas of collaboration are described, viz.: -

(a)   Policy formulation and objective setting
(b)   Curriculum planning
(c)   Contractual relations for teachers and facilities
(d)   Research

RECOMMENDATIONS

These could be summarised under two headings, and emerge clearly from the above discussions:

1.   Those requiring little additional financing – largely matters for Faculty and Academic Boards and for Senate.

(a)   Reorganisation of administration in Faculty of Medicine (79-82)
(b)   Development of a curriculum geared to the needs of the area (44-53)
(c)   Promotion of closer collaboration between Governments and the University, and thereby between health ministries and the Faculty of Medicine (98-101)
(d)   Review of admissions procedures and attempt to identify applicants more motivated to practice medicine in the Caribbean (69-71)
(e)   Improvement of teaching skills in teaching staff by suitable training programs (228-43)
(f)   Establishment of Inter-faculty Committees to study needs for multi-disciplinary programs in health care (Ch. p 14, 93-97)
(g)   Urge Governments to organise health services and improve conditions of service (66)

2.   Those requiring substantial   new funding: Remedying deficiencies in current educational and research programs:

(a)*   Establishment of programs in Postgraduate Medical   Education, to train specialist professionals in demand throughout the area. (72-75)
(b)*   Establishment of a division of Community Medicine based at the Mona campus with responsibility for developing programs for the entire

Caribbean, and with a major role in the curriculum (Ch. 4:54-63); responsibilities: (pp. 57 et seq.; teaching duties, 59)

(c)*   Expansion of the undergraduate teaching in Barbados and in Trinidad and Tobago (p. 30), phased (p. 31) in such a way that first, teaching in all three clinical years is developed in both hospitals, then followed by establishment of preclinical teaching in Trinidad and Tobago. This expansion should aim at a final intake of 110 students and could take place within eight years of the time that funds are allocated for this purpose. Simultaneously, postgraduate training should be developed in these centres. The planning mechanism is described on pp. 38-41, siting on pp. 35-37, and phasing spelled out on p. 105.

(d)   The Mona campus preclinical facilities should be expanded sufficiently to accommodate 20 dental students, and facilities sought either in the area or elsewhere for their clinical training.

(e)   Advanced Nursing training should be expanded to accommodate 60 students annually at the Mona Campus.

(f)   Communication between Campuses needs to be facilitated by various methods, including increased staff interchanges for short periods.

Concurrent activities/developments

Costing was done by the offices of Pro Vice Chancellor, Finance, and Mona Bursary, to indicate the scale of operations (p.108). The Committee commented on but did not critically examine financial arrangements between Governments and University, feeling that this was properly the exercise of another body, even though it was in its remit.

CONCLUSION OF REPORT

It is emphasized that investments in medical education must be seen not as a contribution to higher education but as investments in overall health services development and in social advancement of the peoples of the Caribbean (pp. 103, 104 and 108).

Appendix 3

Communiqué issued at the conclusion of the 7th Commonwealth Caribbean Heads of Government conference, 9-14 October 1972, Chaguaramas, Trinidad and Tobago

<u>Re: "University of the West Indies</u>

"The Conference adopted a Resolution dealing with several aspects of the future role, character and functions of the University of the West Indies.

"It was agreed to retain the regional character of the University. Recognising the importance of Tourism in the Region, Conference took a decision to initiate steps for the University to provide training in tourism and Hotel Management in its expansion program in the present triennium. In the siting of the new training facilities, it was felt that serious consideration should be given to a non-campus territory.

"Immediate training programs should be undertaken by the University to assist in the training of hotel personnel at various levels in existing hotel schools in the Region.

"In order to determine the basis for the expansion of the University a Technical Committee consisting of representatives of the University of the West Indies and the University of Guyana was appointed to assess the requirements for training manpower at the professional, administrative, managerial and sub-professional levels in the Commonwealth Caribbean. The report of this Committee should be completed before the beginning of the 1973/74 Academic Year for submission to Heads of Governments.

"Subject to the approval of the University Council a program of expansion in the priority areas of Medicine, Engineering (including Agricultural Engineering), Tourism and Hotel Management, and Business Management was agreed upon. In addition, Conference also resolved that efforts be made to accelerate the introduction of training programs in the fields of Journalism and Mass Communications.

"It was also agreed that the existing entry requirements should be maintained.

"A new formula for contribution to the University was also approved by Conference.

"With regard to the relationship between the University of the West Indies and the University of Guyana it was resolved that the two Universities should continue and intensify their programs of co-operation, particularly in the fields of scientific and technological research.

"The Conference by resolution reaffirmed its confidence in the Vice-Chancellor of the University of the West Indies and directed that its expression of confidence be conveyed to him. (my emphasis)

"Health: The Conference formally recognised the Caribbean Health Ministers Conference as the body responsible for promoting and implementing programs of Regional co-operation in Health matters, and approved the establishment of a Regional Nursing Body which will be concerned with the raising of the standard of Nursing Education in the Region, as well as other aspects of nursing training.

"1970: The Committees, the Legal and General Committee chaired by the Hon. S. S. Ramphal, Minister of State and Attorney General, Guyana, and the Budget and Economic Committee under the Chairmanship of the Hon. E.H. Lake, Minister of Trade and Production, Antigua, were appointed by the Conference following the submission of a Work Program by the Secretary-General of the Commonwealth Caribbean Regional Secretariat, Mr. William G. Demas."

Chaguaramas, Trinidad &Tobago, 1972

This communique came at a time of deep uncertainty about the future of the University as a regional institution. It was the third year of the Vice-Chancellorship of Dr Roy Marshall, a lawyer by training and an academic, who had commenced his term in April 1969, facing a campus crisis following a Government exclusion order against UWI sociologist CY Thomas, a socialist, deemed undesirable by the Shearer Government. Students and Faculty protests were quick reminders of the action in October 1968, when riots erupted following a similar exclusion of Walter Rodney, Thomas' colleague and fellow Guyanese. The Mona protests had followed about two months after students at St Augustine had refused to allow Canada's Governor General Roland Michener to enter the campus, in retaliation for the expulsion of black students from Ottawa's Sir George Williams University, for rioting. A year later, they refused service to Chancellor Princess Alice. The students also teamed up with Black power forces soon after the mutiny by T&T soldiers. At Mona, students picketed the Creative Arts centre and yielded only on the VC's court order. Three students disrupted Easter service at the Chapel; two were expelled, and one suspended for six months and subjected to a psychiatric evaluation. The Students Union was occupied by "invading" thugs, requiring Police action and beefing up of security, plus enclosing sections. Princess Alice resigned in Feb 1971 and served until Sir Hugh Wooding took over in November. Eric Williams resigned as Pro-Chancellor in Feb., 1971. Staff unrest over salaries, squabbling over inter-campus unity, and revenue shortfalls added to the VC's woes; students and some staff were not kind and quite unfair to him. By comparison, our problems were a picnic. Governments were asked to define the future role of the University, and to recognise that underfunding jeopardised existing and new programs, and induced staff losses.

Appendix 4: Teamwork for Health in developing countries

Paper presented at a Joint Meeting of the Jamaica, British and Canadian Medical Associations, Jamaica, April 1974. Teamwork was viewed as an integral concept in the delivery of Community Medicine, as defined by the study group of the Pan American Federation of Associations of Medical Schools [PAFAMS] and summarised by the CM Director, Dr Julio Ceitlin, in his book (see Biblio.). This paper was published for PAFAMS in Spanish by ASCOFAME, Bogota, Colombia.)

Introduction

Teamwork may be defined simply as the output of a *team*. Everyone on this audience is familiar with the cricket team, how such a body of men is put together and what is expected of them.

In addition to the field of sport, teams have for a long time been operating in various sectors of society. But they have not been sufficiently well developed in health care delivery though they are appropriate to the needs of developing as well as of developed countries.

In most parts of the world, one is accustomed to see health teams efficiently and effectively operating only in times of epidemics or when other severe stresses are placed on the health care system. The professionals and leaders in the field of medicine are largely to blame for this. They have not themselves been schooled in teamwork and their individualistic and conservative approach to problem solving perpetuates the situation.

This week for example two prestigious international gatherings of medical people were held here. The first was the Council Meeting of the Commonwealth Medical Association. None of those representing Commonwealth Countries was, as far as I could ascertain, trained in Public Health and most in their discussions did not appear to have the principles of preventive medicine near enough to their hearts. This body is the major medical organisation in the Commonwealth.

The second meeting was sponsored by the Secretariat of the Caribbean Health Ministers Conference and PAHO/WHO. It concerned itself with Epidemiologic Surveillance. The participants came from many countries of the Americas, anglophone and Spanish-speaking. The majority were schooled in public health and led the administration in their home countries. The few clinicians present were outnumbered and rarely got in a word. Yet this meeting was aiming to formulate recommendations on Caribbean-wide health surveillance. How, I ask, can you really do this without intimately involving clinicians in the planning stages? After all, they are the ones to make the diagnoses and report conditions BEFORE they could be investigated by others.

The fact that this division exists within the profession, in spite of years of acceptance by Caribbean Health Ministries of the principle of integrated medicine and health care, is evidence of the deep entrenchment of the old separatism of the specialties which is the foremost obstacle to teamwork. *Equally significantly our leaders appear to be the ones enshrining it in our way of life.*

Definitions

A *team* is a group of individuals committed to a common goal, who share a common approach and agree on methods to be used to achieve that goal. The members usually have different levels or types of skills or knowledge, different experiences and abilities, different personalities and are often of different ages and from varying socio-economic and educational backgrounds. A surgical operating room team is an example, including, as it does, surgeons, nurses, anaesthetists, clinical assistants, technicians, porters, etc. Despite these differences, they are unified by the common purpose and derive their satisfaction from its achievement.

All teams have leaders. How they are chosen is largely a matter of prevailing circumstances. Their job is to coordinate and direct the activities of groups, signal the onset or end of time-phases, evaluate performance and present results. They should not be autocratic, but rather depend on consultation or participation and the sharing of responsibility with team-mates to achieve the desired ends. Each should have a skill needed in the group, besides that of leader. Those who put in longer hours or make greater efforts than their crews, would invariably enhance the morale of their crews.

As to *Developing Countries*, how does one define them? In every sense all countries are developing. All are trying to improve standards and the overall quality of life. The newly independent countries and several older ones are poor or poorly developed and their economy and society are said to be "underdeveloped" or "developing". This is the ordinary usage of the term. The characteristics of such nations are of great significance to health care delivery and to the growth of teams.

The Nature of Health

Some of us might feel that the WHO definition of health (i.e. "a state of complete physical, mental and social well-being and not merely the absence of disease or infirmity") was conceived by two idealists during a moment of extreme bliss on their honeymoon. Yet though it conjures up visions of a state that is unattainable except to the few, as if it were some *Nirvana*, we must accept the underlying truth that it derives from the interplay of a complex of factors which cannot be understood by study of the natural sciences alone. This idea is better spelled out in the WHO aim of medical education which is:

To provide training for professionals who could perform the following functions within the health system:

  i) *The promotion of health*
  ii) *The prevention of illness and disability*
  iii) *The care, alleviation or arrest of disease at the earliest possible stage*
  iv) *The rehabilitation and return to productivity of sick persons*

None of these goals can be achieved without manpower. This is the single most important and precious resource in any health service. All categories of health manpower are scarce in the developing countries, largely through enticements by developed countries of North America and Europe. Those that remain are concentrated in cities and towns, and are often inappropriately trained for or utilised in rural settings.

Health Conditions in Developing Countries

There is a cycle of ill-health familiar to developing countries and to many areas of developed ones. Unfortunately, health professionals are not generally aware of this cycle. It is this: a poor country with few resources will have underemployed people with bad living conditions, poor nutrition, low economic productivity, discontent, high birth and population growth rates and high prevalence of illness. They will overload health and other welfare facilities and resources. This overload will eventually lead to further failures within the economy and thus consolidate and perpetuate the cycle.

Of major concern to all nations is the rapidly rising world population which threatens to drown existing health, educational and other developmental resources. This inevitable decline in productivity will add tremendously to the flood. It is not difficult to foresee the chaos that will come from such a situation.

Country	Population Growth Rate %		
	1950	**1960**	**1970**
Ceylon	3.8	3.5	2.8
El Salvador	4.9	4.8	4.0
Hong Kong	3.5	3.6	1.9
Jamaica	3.5	4.0	3.3
Mauritius	4.6	3.9	2.7
Puerto Rico	3.7	3.2	2.6
Taiwan	4.6	3.7	2.8

Table 1: Birth rates in different countries over the past 20 years (IPPF)

The general trend is downward reflecting action taken in accordance with this concern. But note that the position of Jamaica – a country where the majority of the population can be classified as poor by any standards – remains virtually unchanged. This was probably tolerable in the socio-economic sense as long as infant mortality rates were high, i.e. over 50/1000 live births. But these rates have shown a downward trend in this same period, following the institution of control measures for many communicable diseases. Continued vigorous campaigns for control and prevention of childhood diseases, particularly malnutrition, will result in a further net gain in population.

Jamaica's population pyramid (source Prof. Roberts/UWI) shows a wide base with some 44% of the population under 14, concave sides and a narrow tip. This is typical of many developing countries.

Figure I: Outline of Population Pyramids: Jamaica and France

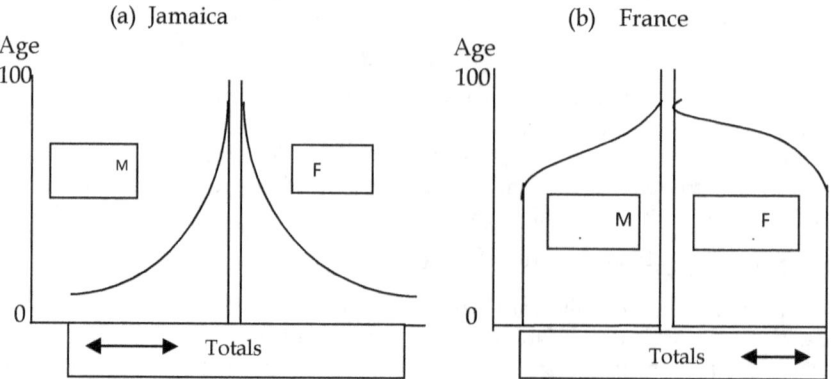

I will not go into the various implications of these distributions except to point out that they indicate profound differences in health care problems and needs, which will call for different approaches.

I would stress that the best approach can only come from a study of the conditions which prevail in the particular country. So often the methods of one, usually developed country, fail when transplanted to a developing country, as when graduates of British Universities return to the Caribbean. We who work in developing countries have seen this happen many times; and what a loss and tragedy it is when it happens. It is clear that such errors must be avoided, particularly when innovations are being introduced to improve the efficiency of health care delivery. Every effort must be made to discover and deal with the opinions, sensitivities and doubts of professionals, of communities, and indeed of the nation that has become accustomed to a certain way, however inappropriate, of doing things. Failure to do this may cause, and have caused, an undue delay or grave difficulties – even amounting to disruption – in the implementation of needed new programs.

I believe there can be no hope for the developing countries unless they break the cycle of ill-health. This can only be done by an increased capacity to deal with illness, i.e. to recognise it accurately and to treat the afflicted; and to remove from the environment adverse and predisposing conditions. These require trained personnel in larger numbers and whose training has correctly emphasised and inculcated in them health promotion and an integrated curative-preventive approach to problems. They should therefore be familiar with the major characteristics of the environment and of the health system, both those which facilitate and those which hinder achievement of health service aims.

The training of health professionals is expensive. Therefore great care must be taken to ensure that they are used effectively and efficiently and are not asked to perform tasks which can be done by someone more cheaply and more briefly trained. The need for widening the scope of training is therefore urgent, if only from considering that the world population is expected to reach 4.42 billion in 1981! *(U.N. 1966.)*In the developing countries, much of this increase will still be rural (i.e. 50% or more of total population). In the Caribbean countries a third or more of populations are in *urban* centres or in suburbs, where slums continue to enlarge and multiply, and overcrowded shanty towns scar the landscape. These, like the rural areas, are the ones in greatest need of medical skills.

This increasing population will make heavier demands too on food production capabilities. By the late 1960s the levels of calorie and protein intake in various developing countries were well below the desired intake (Table 2).

Table 2: Recommended daily Calorie and Protein Intake (Source OHE, UK)

Country	Kc/day	Protein/gms. daily
Desirable Level:	2500	66
Brazil	2500	65
Congo	2250	50
India	2000	45
France	3200	100
U.S.A.	3300	95

As population increases and the years roll on, the productive acreages per head in most countries will fall. In Zambia, for instance, the number is estimated to fall from 40 acres in 1970 to 20 by the year 2000; in Brazil, from 21 to 5, and in Kenya from 5 to 2.

Energy consumption bears a relation to national incomes and productivity, and thereby to the ability of nations to look after themselves. By 1970, the average per caput income for developing countries was less than £100, and energy consumption 500 kg coal equivalent per annum. By contrast, the developed countries had an average per caput income of £1100, and consumed some 10 times the amount of energy as well., thus contributing more to ecologic decline.

In summary, population growth will result in these, *inter alia:*
Unemployment
Overcrowding, particularly in cities, with attendant housing shortages
Reduction of arable land per head, resulting in food shortages
Shortage of places in schools, colleges, universities
Inadequate health facilities and over-taxing of health services
Environmental pollution

Resources for Health Care Delivery

A look at existing facilities for health care shows a concentration of such facilities in the capitals and large urban areas of the world, with only a scattering in rural areas. For example, in 1969, hospital beds in Barbados and Trinidad and Tobago were 18 per 1,000 population in urban areas, and 3.5 in the rest of the country. In Jamaica the numbers are 5 and 4; Argentina 7.5 and 5; Colombia 3 and 2; El Salvador 12 and 1.5; Haiti 5 and 1.

At the same time expenditures on health *per caput* show rates, which, though not entirely accurate, are useful for purposes of comparison (Table 3).

Table 3: Expenditures on Health, 1967 (WHO 4th Report)

Country	Per Caput Expenditure (£)
Sweden	64
United Kingdom	34
U.S.A.	92
Greece	11
Ceylon	2.2
El Salvador	4.5
Ghana	2.4
Jamaica	4.5

The physician:population ratios in most countries show undesirable but probably unpreventable imbalances between town and country areas. In the Caribbean, towns may have one doctor per 1200 population while rural areas range from 1: 4000 to 1: 30,000. The range for African countries in the late 1960s was 1: 2000 for Tomé, Togo (urban) to 1: 190,000 in rural Ethiopia.

The developing countries are short of nurses too. The approximate number of nurses per doctor in Sweden is 3, in Japan 1.2, in Turkey 0.6, India 0.4, Jamaica 2. Unfortunately, capacity to train these and other levels of health workers is low in most countries resulting in a situation where highly skilled workers are often called upon to do tasks that could just as well be done by others lesser trained.

A graphic representation of the skills available in most developing countries would show a figure somewhat resembling an hourglass, but narrowing towards the top and bottom, (Fig. 2a) when what is desired is one more like a pyramid, the base made up of the large groups of the lesser skilled, with the specialist professions forming the apex (Fig. 2b).

<u>Figure 2a</u>　　　　　<u>Figure 2b</u>

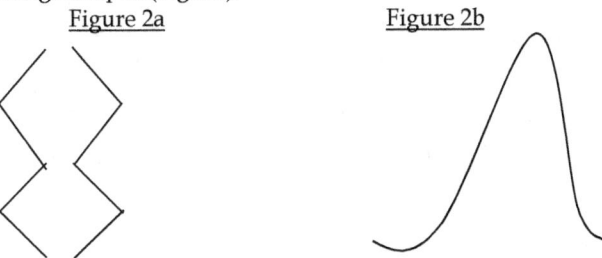

Fig. 2: Skill distributions for developing countries: undesirable (a) and desirable (b); the skew to the left in (b) represents the greater number of ancillaries (sub-professionals p. 292) in health care

Several problems however beset the developing world and prevent the establishment of a proper health services: poor leadership, weak administration, outmoded organisation, inadequate training opportunities and facilities, inadequate research, and imprecise or no definition of goals.

The Advantages of Teamwork

In the prevailing system of health care delivery in most developing countries, a central administration controls a series of departments or other units which inter-communicate little, if at all. They jostle and compete with one another for everything — staff, money, supplies, favours, preferment. The rivalry is intense and often all-pervasive. Output is seen in narrow departmental perspectives, which may or may not relate to the realities of the location. Change is resisted. The system is hierarchical — sometimes benevolent, sometimes authoritarian — and oriented to the individual, with little emphasis on group action or commitment.

Many factors contribute to the prevailing biases - upbringing, social class, patterns of training, place of training, conditions of work, the health system itself. Many of the educated classes in the developing countries were schooled according to the systems and norms of the developed countries, which had, not so long ago, been their colonial masters. These were, and are, perhaps more so now, materialist societies which emphasised individualism and competition. Friendliness and cooperation with others were seen as sure signs of weakness, and any thought of delegation of a duty was a clear indication of incompetence or decadence. These attitudes still prevail, permeate many activities, and dominate many professionals even at the highest rungs on the ladder of authority. Indeed it sometimes seems that these are the worst afflicted.

We all know that two men pooling their efforts and using a stretcher can carry as much weight as 4 men working separately. This simple illustration demonstrates how teamwork can achieve synergism, potentiation and increased efficiency. The administrative framework must facilitate such action through inter-communication, joint planning and the setting of global objectives. For effective teamwork, each team must have an unbiased leader. The members need not all agree—that would be tedious and perhaps undesirable. But they must share a common goal, each having a skill, which s/he can contribute to functions within the team, and even outside of it in other related teams needing his/her skills; this further spreads the habit of cooperation, reducing costly rivalries and disseminating skills and knowledge not only to team-mates, but to others in society. Teams should include consumers to provide a steady feed-back in addition to assisting with planning, and to facilitate acceptance of modifications.

Some Examples of Teamwork, particularly appropriate to developing countries.

The Sectors of Health care Delivery which must become the first team is shown in *Figure 3*, below:

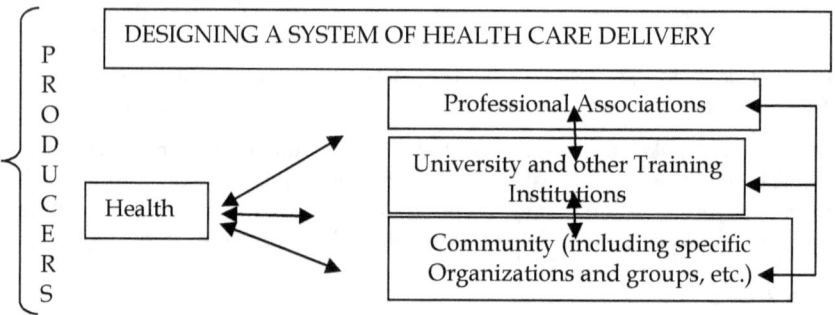

All key groups must come together for the common aim of planning for effective Health care Delivery. Sad to say, this *team* does not quite exist in many countries. It would be possible and desirable for this large team to spawn many smaller ones for specific purposes and activities within the system, using whatever skills may seem relevant to its purposes and creating multidisciplinary groups so badly needed to tackle the varied problems in the environment.

Thus we can have teams whose members are drawn from different sectors or professions within the society or its institutions; these are multidisciplinary as they would bring together skills of various kinds needed for investigation, planning and effecting health care delivery. Teams drawn from a single sector would form a distinct group for general tasks within that sector; teams made up of a group of like professionals could be formed to discharge specific functions within a sector. Several other possibilities exist, the guiding principle being the need to establish a goal and identify the skills needed to accomplish it.

In developing these teams it would be desirable that they receive a certain core of their training together before they differentiate. Later on they should be brought together again for problem-solving in the field, in settings that will show how participation and group action, where each team member is au-fait with the role of the others, can achieve ends not possible before.

From the cost viewpoint, gains will come from redefinition of functions and delegation of particular duties. As an example, the cost of training one medical student at the University of the West Indies, Jamaica, is about J$30,000, exclusive of pre-university costs of about 7 years of high school or college. The West Indies has been schooled to accept health care as the province of the medical professional only. To achieve a doctor: population ratio of 1: 2000 in Jamaica alone in 10 years will mean training an additional 500 doctors at a cost of some J\$ 15,000,000; and to maintain them for 20 years thereafter would be \$ 300,000 each, at least! This is a huge bill and even this will not resolve the problems of the rural areas, nor produce the pyramid of skills that is desirable to perform all the tasks that must be done to bring effective health care to all. Tanzania is tackling this problem by training medical assistants to fill a need at the middle level. Approximately 20 medical assistants can be trained at the cost of one doctor, each would cost half as much as a doctor to maintain over a 20 year period. That country is aiming to move from a ratio of doctors to medical assistants to rural medical aides of 2:1:2 in 1972 to 1:2:4 in 1980. This is to be achieved by training an extra 300 doctors, 1300 medical assistants and 2,600 rural medical aides.

Our own studies in the Commonwealth Caribbean show that we must develop a similar strategy and expand the ranks of middle grade professionals in order to round out our teams.

The poet, Shelley, in lamenting the death of fellow poet, John Keats, remarked that the gentle and human spirit that was Keats had

> *...outsoared the shadow of our night,*
> *Envy and calumny and hate and pain*
> *And that unrest which men miscall delight*
> *Can touch him not nor torture not again,*
> *From the contagion of the world's slow stain*
> *He is secure ...*

The spirit of teamwork reiterates the hope that we can secure the *living* from the contagion that the poet laments, (Keats died at 24 of *tuberculosis*, a disease that ravaged populations globally, before the discovery and synthesis of anti-mycobacterial agents, which emptied sanatoria world-wide, until smoking and lung cancer and degenerative lung diseases replaced Tb!). Perhaps *we* can do it with the same passion and with conviction. There are advantages and benefits to be gained, though our progress has so far been slow. The obstacles are largely matters of personalities and of attitudes, which can be overcome with goodwill and a sense of justice. What is needed is the impulse to start. Once conviction takes over from doubt, the achievements would be truly astonishing.

As I said at the beginning, we have seen teams at work in many sections of society, though not much in day-to-day health care delivery. We must develop them, and hopefully they will become truly creative and successful, so that we could dream of better things, as another poet of that prolific era, Robert Browning, surmised,

> *All we have willed or hoped or dreamed of good shall exist*
> *Not its semblance, but itself; no beauty, nor good, nor power*
> *Whose voice has gone forth, but each survives for the melodist*
> *When eternity affirms the conception of an hour...*

M.S. Ragbeer, Dean, Faculty of Medicine,
The University of the West Indies,
Mona, Jamaica; St Augustine, Trinidad; and Cave Hill, Barbados,
25 April, 1974

Appendix 5:

CARIBBEAN HEALTH MINISTERS CONFERENCE, 2nd **Meeting, Bridgetown Barbados, 1970**

Resolution 4: Approval of PGME program; formation of Committee on Postgraduate Medical education (COPMED), Monday, Nov. 15th, 1970 AGENDA Item I (v)

THE CONFERENCE

Having considered the papers presented by the U.W.I. (Document 70/6 and 70/6 app.)

RESOLVES

(1) to congratulate and thank the University for the excellent and comprehensive document prepared on its behalf;

(2) to approve the basic concepts of the flexible program of postgraduate medical education therein described;

(3) to request the University to seek in collaboration with the Ministers of Health the means of implementing these programs;

(4) to recommend to the Governments that support be given to these programs in the interest of protecting expenditures made in undergraduate training and at the same time of keeping middle-grade staff in the area (along the lines set out in Document CHMC 70/Sub Com.1);

(5) that the following be appointed as a Committee to study the needs of Postgraduate Medical Education:

One member each from Jamaica, Trinidad and Tobago, Guyana, and Barbados; one member representing Bahamas, Bermuda and British Honduras, if agreeable to British Honduras; and one member representing the Leeward and Windward Islands and British Virgin Islands who shall be nominees of the Ministers of Health of these territories; and one representative of the Pan American Health Organisation.

Appendix 6

MEMORANDUM to Members of CHMC on POST GRADUATE MEDICAL EDUCATION, UNIVERSITY of the WEST INDIES, from Dr L. Comissiong (See University Paper C.H.M.C. 70/6)

1.   The University proposes that Post graduate Medical Education might be provided at different levels depending on the demands of individual territories:

(I)   Refresher attachments

(a)   on an ad hoc basis

(b)   short refresher courses for Practitioners to bring them   up-to-date with recent advances.

(II)   Diploma Training – varying from one year to two years depending on the specialty:

(a)   As a first stage towards full specialty training.

On acquisition of a diploma, the Medical Officer might be assigned to a Regional Hospital or a Specialist Department (Radiology, Pathology, etc.) to obtain the clinical experience necessary towards further training in the specialty. He would at the same time render service to the unit to which he is attached.

(b)   A General Duty Medical Officer (DMO) who has obtained an appropriate diploma may be utilised to hold routine clinics in this specialty in conjunction with his other duties. This would pre-suppose access to a Regional Centre where full Consultant coverage is available, or periodic visits from a Consultant.

(III)   Full Consultant Training – 4 years – provided partly at University Hospital, Mona, Jamaica and partly at other Regional Hospitals.

2.   Individual Units of the Windward, Leeward and Virgin Islands would have to consider to what extent they can utilise the training available and decide on the levels of training they need in the various fields. For example: Those territories which want their Hospitals to qualify for acceptance for Medical Internship would need to have at least one fully trained Specialist in each of the following: Medicine, Surgery, Obstetrics & Gynaecology and perhaps in Anaesthetics as well.

The question of the need for fully trained Specialists in other fields, for example, Radiology and Psychiatry would also have to be considered.

3.   They would also have to decide in which specialties the training of DMO's to diploma level, with a view to providing a routine service, would be applicable.

Possibilities are: -

Diploma in Anaesthetics	)
Diploma in Laboratory Medicine	) already offered at Mona
Diploma in Ophthalmology	)

Diploma in Psychiatry
Diploma in Otolaryngology
Diploma in Social and Preventive Medicine
Diploma in Paediatrics
Diploma in Tuberculosis

Individual Governments would therefore be required to provide specific information under the following heads:

(I)   Applicability - How many of each type are required ?
(II)   Are candidates available?
(III) Will scholarships be provided?
(IV) What incentives will be given to officers on completion of training?
       (a)   Increased salary or appropriate allowance
       (b)   Fees from paying patients
       (c)   Private Practice in the Specialty
       (d)   Revision of existing duties
       (e)   Depending on the Specialty, accessibility of assigned district to the main hospital may be necessary

4.   It would be advisable that all these aspects be discussed with local Medical Officers before policy decisions are made.

(Sgd.) Dr L.M. Comissiong

Special Medical Adviser,
Ministry of Health, Grenada
January, 1971

(Dr Comissiong also drew attention later to CHMC *Resolutions 24/74 and 25/74, which dealt with the training of allied health personnel, the former noting that annual resolutions on this topic had been made since 1969, with little progress, except for Jamaica's positive steps forward; see p. 184)
****

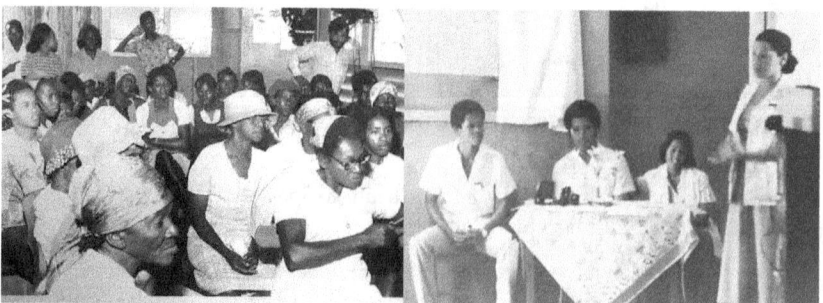

Fig A6, 1&2: Community Medicine Students in an education (prevention) session with community members at Prattville clinic. Dr Comissiong was very pleased with this start, and had wished to visit the Manchester clinics, but I was on my way to Canada just then, so I referred him to Dr Minott and Professor Standard. He was not asked. (Dean's collection)

Appendix 7

Memo to Secretariat, CHMC
From: Dean, Medical Faculty
Re: Collaboration between the University Medical Faculty and Ministries of Health, Commonwealth Caribbean

These are preliminary ideas on the recurring subject of collaboration, which has come up also in the meetings of the COPMED Task Force in the various islands. It was also raised by several witnesses at interviews with the IADB Committee on expansion. The main areas relate to health planning, health care delivery and health education, and health services activities.

1. (a) The University can assist in policy-making and in the setting of specific goals through the provision of advisory services.
   (b) The University can advise Ministries on organisation and utilisation of health services, and of their improvement, as a continuing exercise.

2. Research Activities
   (a) Operational research, analysis of health care delivery, organisation and administration.
   (b) Epidemiological studies into problems of regional importance.
   (c) Evaluation of health programs
   (d) Research into needs for new types of health professionals
   (e) Fund-raising for all activities as defined in the health plans.

3. Education of Health Professionals: (i)   Doctors and Dentists; (ii)   Nurses; (iii) Paramedical Staff; and (iv) Engineers and others

   (a) While the University must be primarily responsible for academic programs at the undergraduate level, Ministries of Health must accept responsibility for programs in postgraduate and continuing education. This is the situation with regard to doctors, dentists and engineers. For the others, Government responsibility spans all levels. But the University could and does take an active part in organisation, planning and implementing higher education in these.

   (b) The results of studies conducted under (2) would influence University and Ministries' decisions about training.

   (c) Government and the University should determine
       (i) whether teaching should be a duty of all government staff,
       (ii) the conditions under which government facilities can be used for teaching functions.

   (d) The education of the lay public in health matters, particularly health maintenance, sanitation, disease prevention, hygiene and public health, although a primary responsibility of Ministries of Health, could be assisted by the and Medical Faculty.

4. Use of Joint University and Ministerial Facilities for Problem Solving

Certain types of diseases have a complex background and a series of causes, for example, abnormal behaviour, accidents, certain organic diseases such as obesity, malnutrition, atherosclerosis and heart diseases, peptic ulcers, respiratory diseases, etc. These cannot be elucidated by the activities of medical professionals alone. Engineers, economists, nutritionists, agronomists, ecologists, and other professionals are needed to find the answers. It is obvious that in these and other areas, governments and university must get together to promote the appropriate investigations and to apply the necessary remedies.

Problems in health care must be seen by governments and university in the light of their economic, social and cultural implications to the nation, let alone those to small communities and individuals. Some of these may be listed as follows:

(i) Effects on national economy and productivity:
    (a) pollution of beaches, soil, air and effects on tourism
    (b) industrial pollution and effects (costs, etc.) on health care systems
    (c) productivity of individuals in different states of health
    (d) effects of preventive programs on national economy
    (e) influence of health engineers on disease, or accident prevention.

(ii) Effects of new industry on disease states, particularly food- borne diseases.
    (a) Manufacturing, storage and handling of food
    (b) Patterns of feeding in infancy
    (c) Use of foods
    (d) Effects of (b) & (c) on development of individuals

(iii) Health Legislation: Effective legislation must be aimed at assisting to achieve the goals of the health services which are:
    (a) to prevent disease
    (b) to treat the sick and restore them to good health
    (c) to rehabilitate those previously sick, maimed or injured
    (d) to maintain health

4.   Ministries of Health can assist the Medical Faculty to secure adequate funds to carry out their part of joint programs:

(i) by influencing their cabinets to provide adequate funding for University programs in medical education and research
(ii) by providing funds from their own resources for specific activities, e.g. Postgraduate Medical Education, etc.
(iii) by supporting applications where appropriate to External Agencies or international organisations for funding of programs.

M.M.S. Ragbeer
Dean, Medical Faculty, UWI
October 29, 1971

Appendix 8:

Postgraduate medical education (PGME) in the Eastern Caribbean: notes on discussions with Ministries of Health, medical consultants, students and HOs in Trinidad & Tobago (T&T) and Barbados, W.I.

In July 1972, Drs. Meltzer and Butler and I visited the Ministries of Health in Trinidad and Tobago and in Barbados. Dr Meltzer and I also visited Guyana.

1. IN TRINIDAD

1.1 Discussions with Ministry Officials

1.1.1.   In Trinidad we met with Minister Francis Prevatt, Permanent Secretary, Mr. Nunez; Chief Medical Officer, Dr Henry; Principal Medical Officer, Dr Elizabeth Quamina; Vice-Dean for Eastern Caribbean affairs, Dr Alan Butler; Associate Dean for Trinidad& Tobago (T&T), Dr Courtenay Bartholomew; Dr Richard Meltzer (HOPE). We spoke about T&T's need for specialists, and of the slow progress in implementing plans for Post Graduate Medical Education, which had been discussed at length at three successive meetings of the Caribbean Health Ministers Conference. *We reminded the Minister that the Jamaica Government had begun supporting residency education in January, and that we had so far enrolled 41 residents (including those from UHWI) in 9 disciplines;* we described the financing that the Jamaica Government has been willing to provide and the basis for this.

1.1.2.   We recalled that the Trinidad Government had indicated interest in the PGME program and, in fact, after the February 1972 CHMC meetings in Guyana, the Minister, Mr. Nunez, Dr Bartholomew, Dr Henry and myself had met in his office in Port-of-Spain; when the Minister had expressed "serious interest" in financing of the program. (At this stage, the Minister being called away to the telephone, Mr. Nunez informed us that no action had yet been taken to put to the Trinidad Cabinet any kind of financial proposal re PGME!) The Minister, upon his return, indicated that he was "completely committed to supporting PGME" and that the Government, and he were awaiting details of the contribution that T&T was asked to make, so that he could prepare a Cabinet submission.

1.1.3.   I was taken aback at this because I had fully expected that by now, with all the information that we had put together, and given to the advisors of the Minister in Trinidad, that he would have had the details. However, it was clear that he did not know our overall plans, the type of project we had gotten into in Jamaica, the objectives, its patterns, in fact, any factor that would influence his making a decision, and to gain his Cabinet's support on financing.

1.1.4.   I may say here that I had had the good fortune of accidentally meeting the Minister at a private residence the day before and we had talked about many things and perhaps had by our talk—though we did not touch directly on PGME—cleared the ground for more official conversation on this very important subject.   Further discussion, to my mind, was almost hazardous because we certainly could not go ahead with any kind of conversation with the Minister, who was not briefed on what T&T needed, to bring the various services to such a point of proficiency that they could contribute to formal specialty training.

1.1.5.   We had hoped that with all the talk over the last two years: COPMED (and its details at CHMC IV, in February 1972), private discussions and the like, that the technical officers in the Ministry, (CMO, PMO, the Permanent Secretary and others) — who had detailed the needs for space, staff and equipment — would have briefed the Minister on the necessity to upgrade facilities, improve basic services like Anaesthesia, Pathology and X-ray; provide seminar rooms, tutorial space, demonstration areas, and audio-visual equipment. These, plus regular and adequate supplies, a review of the organisation and management of the Medical Services, including hospital administration, had all been thoroughly discussed.

1.1.6.   In fact, re-organisation was slowly underway to bring hospitals under regional boards; to integrate curative and preventive services based on common facilities and a "comprehensive" approach to medical care; and to develop Community Medicine. We had indicated these things in various documents to Governments, expecting the local health authorities to verify their needs, and design solutions. We had taken pains to point out trends and outstanding needs, but we did not have the resources to do the work that individual clinical and Public Health departments and Administrative Units should have done already.

1.1.7.   We realised that we had to do something, so we undertook to update the information on the various needs in terms of space, equipment and staff, and to submit these with the appropriate costings to the Minister. Dr Butler, Vice Dean, EC Affairs, agreed to supervise data collection, and present them by the end of September, 1972.

1.1.8.   The Minister repeated what he had earlier said that he was prepared to recommend provision of funds to the Medical Faculty for central PGME facilities at Mona — in fact he said that he would be "foolish not to recognise the need for this." As to amount, we referred to the formula suggested at CHMC II, 1970, which Mr. Nunez had, covering 4 years.

1.1.9.   Despite this, the Minister wished to know from me the basis for the contributions of the Jamaica Government . We explained that Jamaica had based its calculation on the total budget presented to CHMC, anticipating later contributions from others, following the funding formula for the UHWI. Jamaica's Health Minister had also wanted to know the position of the various Governments regarding PGME, because UHWI ought to be fully funded by the region, as PGME was a regional program, and he wished to avoid future confrontations on matters of joint funding of additional facilities for the UHWI.

1.1.10.   Again, Minister Prevatt was aware of the basic issue, and affirmed that the Trinidad Government should have no difficulty in understanding the need to provide a proportion of central costs; he was aware of regional needs but the matter was one for the next Heads of Government Conference (HGC), when they would be asked also to clarify responsibility for regional cooperation in health. (I realised that he was temporising, since T&T had ideas for their own university, and would not commit until the HGC meeting.)

1.1.11.   We left that meeting feeling (or fooled) that the Minister was keen to help, but needed more   information. We were disappointed to note that the technical officers of the Ministry and the Permanent Secretary were made to look as if they had done nothing to inform him in the six months he had been in office, even if they had problems of staff, and disorganisation of services. We were surprised that the CMO seemed unaware of the goals of the T&T Health Services; of Health Services Administration, training and manpower needs. One wondered whether the notion of Civil Service seniority or political connection as criteria for promotion to high offices should not be re-examined in favour of people with ability, drive, dedication and administrative skill.

1.2 Discussions With Consultants

1.2.1. We met with Consultants of the Port-of-Spain General Hospital the following day. Nearly all specialties were represented. We informed them of the substance of our discussion with the Minister. We had earlier had individual talks with groups of Consultants from Radiology, Anaesthesia and Pathology, and examined some of their concerns in general and specific to PGME.

1.2.2. The meeting was, as we had come to expect in Trinidad and Tobago, silent for quite some time, until we suggested that we were encouraged by the attitude of the Minister, if genuine. Most reacted to this, with pessimism; a few optimistic, the rest ambivalent. However, all agreed to assist as far as they could to supply information to Dr Butler. Several consultants said that they had already supplied the required data to the PS. This only served to confirm the view that some of us had already formed on our several previous visits to Trinidad, that there was not really much cohesion or inter-departmental communication within the Ministry of Health. And to think that the major hospital in Trinidad and Tobago — 920 beds, with quite a large quorum of Consultants — did not have ready and efficient access to the ear of the Minister, and that year after year Consultant submissions on health issues would fail to reach the one health advocate in Cabinet, to explain the achievements and needs of the Health Services. I still find this inexplicable, but not surprising altogether in the context of the colonial civil service way of doing things; and Trinidad and Tobago was more British than most.

1.2.3. We did not go to San Fernando because we had visited recently, and the interview with the Minister had given no programmatic reason for a repeat. A serendipitous meeting with one of the Medical Consultants of the San Fernando Hospital affirmed this.

2.   IN BARBADOS

2.1.1.   In Barbados, two days later, we had similar meetings. First, with Minister Ferguson; Parliamentary Secretary Mrs. Eastmond;   the new Permanent Secretary, Mr. H. Howell; the CMO, Dr V. Wells; Dr. R. Meltzer, HOPE; and Dr (Mr.) A. Butler.

2.1.2. We were advised of the Government's commitment to support Postgraduate Medical Education. This confirmed the casual remark made to me, earlier at Mona, by the Premier of Barbados, in his capacity as Chairman of the University Grants Committee, that Barbados was very interested in doing what it could for Post Graduate Education. But again we were flabbergasted by the news that the Ministry of Health or the Minister and Parliamentary Secretary did not have detailed data on the Barbados Health Services to guide their entry into PGME, despite *our* submission of COPMED data on Barbados, originally obtained from the MOH!. Individuals in the Health Services had warned us that the Minister, who was new, might not have looked at that file before our visit, and would bluff his way through the meeting!

2.1.3. We agreed to collate the information on the various specialties and to submit it later to him, with costings, and Barbados' share of the grants expected.

2.1.4. There are significant problems and questions of attitude and inter-relationships between professionals of the same rank and standing in this small country. We have faced these before, and I'm sure, will continue to meet them. An individual's esteem is paramount, and once established, must be paid the proper homage. His opinions become valued and as a consequence no one matters other than established superiors. The maverick might deny the presence of a superior but only for so long as he takes to establish himself and gain sufficient social and professional prestige. Much infighting and behind-the-scenes campaigns take place to maintain the pinnacle positions. These take their toll and the results are easy to see. It's a vicious game. Several of the consultants we have to deal with in the Barbados General Hospital are its victims.

2.1.5. We had evidence of this when we tried to arrange a meeting with Consultants for the day after meeting the Minister. The meeting was held, with only few present, but we discussed the issues, nevertheless, in the same way as we had in Trinidad. Similar reactions occurred, ending in a commitment from those present to provide data. Notably absent was the Chief of Medicine, Dr Haynes, himself a maverick, who later on, after much persuasion privately that evening through the good offices of Prof. Ken Stuart, consented to meet with us. It was significant, perhaps, that he agreed to meet with us at the Hilton Hotel, where he treated us to lunch.

At this meeting we had a thorough discussion of the various issues, cleared the air on a lot of matters—most of which were based on personality clashes between himself and Dr Harold Forde, our Associate Dean in Barbados, an older, wiser, calmer and better-known internist. Problems of communication between Faculty and Hospital, questions of motives and similar matters arose. At the end, we left with the feeling of not only having enjoyed Dr Haynes' hospitality, but of having convinced him that we were both working towards the same general end, and that cooperation and collaboration, not competition, would bring rewards to both. He agreed to help in any way he could with the collection of data, and agreed that if he had any problems he would get in touch with Dr Butler either through the local University staff, or directly.

2.1.6. We ran into an obstacle in the Laboratory concerning a vacancy for a university Lecturer. The local pathologists, Drs. Errol Dos Santos and Harold White, were upset by a letter from Dr Forde concerning the need to advertise the post to attract a Morbid Anatomist (Anatomic Pathologist). It seemed that the letter was mis-interpreted and thought to cast aspersion, if I may use such a strong word, on the quality and range of work done by the existing Morbid Anatomist, Dr Harold White. This was not my impression when I read the letter.

2.1.7. Dr White's reaction to the letter was needlessly vehement, but I should have expected this, knowing how touchy folks tend to be here. After spending some time with him and explaining the needs for the University service to improve the teaching in several areas, e.g. Clinical Pathological Conferences, and to start residency training, all specialties requiring laboratory inputs, particularly an expanded rate of autopsy from the present 15–20%, as fundamental to any improvement of the island's medical services. Reluctantly, but at last, Dr White agreed that it would be desirable to have another Morbid Anatomist than himself. I assured him that insofar as his private work was concerned, our employee should not be a strong competitor, since our conditions of service (or terms of work) would differ from those of the Barbados Government. And we would hope that as far as consultations were concerned there would be no competition, but rather some mutually satisfactory working arrangement would be made. Dr White agreed to this; I believe we can now proceed to advertise the post without creating a furore, and so informed Dr Forde.

2.1.8. A second problem concerned the relationship between our staff and those of the Queen Elizabeth Hospital. Some feel that Dr Forde is uncommunicative. But I do not believe this is entirely his fault. Dr Forde is basically a reserved person, but prompt, efficient and organised. He has, to his credit, begun to publish information via a *Newsletter* to all members of staff. In fact, we were for a minute in one Consultant's office and there saw an *"Extract of Academic Board and Faculty of Medicine Board Reports"*, which contained up-to-date information on many subjects. One consultant argued that he had no knowledge of, nor was ever told anything about specialty training. Yet the Minutes of the Medical Committee of his Hospital contained ample reference to it. It is just that this consultant, like so many others, had not bothered to attend the meetings (and expected things to drop in his lap); nor had he and several others read the minutes. He was silent for a while when he realised that he had been at fault and had sat on the information for some time.

2.1.9. One of the things we did, to avoid some of these problems was to ask the Hospital Director to convene a group consisting of the Hospital Consultants, the University Lecturers and representatives of the Junior Staff, at regular intervals — perhaps every two months or so — to discuss university matters that might affect the hospital and vice versa. Prof. Ken Stuart, who was on holiday in Barbados — a working holiday, as he called it — agreed to take part in discussions and to assist, while he was in Barbados, in getting the group together, explaining the proposals for the Department of Medicine's participation in PGME, and helping to supervise its start.

2.1.10. The visit had accomplished much. I met briefly with the Minister and Parliamentary Secretary afterwards and advised him on the issues. They were impressed that we had ended cordially with Dr Haynes, and settled with Dr

White and the disgruntled physician. They had heard of the dithering in Trinidad and admitted that they had followed cues from them as the lead campus in the Eastern Caribbean.

3. IN GUYANA

3.1.   In Guyana, we spoke to Dr Phillip Boyd, Executive Secretary of CHMC, about matters affecting the next meeting of Caribbean Health Ministers in Dominica, and of his expectation from us in terms of papers and discussions. This was a simple business meeting with no particular matters to report.

3.2.   We had one short session with the Chief Medical Officer; the Permanent Secretary refused to see us, and the Minister was on the point of being replaced, and was not in office, or available.

3.3.   Guyana has in fact really gone backward rather than forward in terms of Health Services development and we were appalled to note that the quality and range of health services had declined since our last visit, and that morale was even lower and staff turnover time was increasing. Community services were badly affected, and tending to rely on foreign aid, mainly Cuban, Philippinos and Chinese. Language was a major barrier to what service was possible.

3.4.   The only person, it seemed, calm, imperturbable and competently trying to do anything constructive was the PAHO Representative, Dr. Samedha Khanna. I discussed with her my views on Cuba's approach to primary and extended hospital care, the decision to base them on clinical physicians, rather than PH specialists or aides, like Russia and China, and the aim to reduce infant mortality drastically, while improving maternal health and life expectancy. I told her of our findings in 1963 re an excess of heart disease in EI (p. 73), and gave her the figures as I recalled them, and suggested she might get more from the Central Medical laboratory (CML) annual reports. I also described our nutrition experiments on rodents, and suggested that Guyana might be ripe for similar interventions, now that Burnham had established his Presidency and dictatorship. She smiled.

M.S. Ragbeer
Dean, Faculty of Medicine, UWI, and
Coordinator of PGME
Mona, August, 1972

REPORT OF THE JOINT COMMITTEE OF THE FACULTY OF MEDICINE, U.W.I. AND THE MINISTRY OF HEALTH AND ENVIRONMENTAL CONTROL, JAMAICA, APPOINTED SEPTEMBER **1977**, FOR FIELD TRAINING OF MEDICAL STUDENTS IN COMMUNITY HEALTH WITH SPECIAL REFERENCE TO THE PROPOSED NEW CURRICULUM.

Fig App. 8-1: How CM became CH (see Epilogue)

Appendix 9:
Teaching of Community Medicine

To: Dean's Advisory Committee (Heads of Departments); Curriculum Committee; Vice-Deans and Associate Deans, Mona and EC; members of Faculty Board, Medical Educator, Student Representatives.

From: Dean, Medical Faculty

Re: The teaching of Community Medicine to undergraduates

INTRODUCTION AND DEFINITIONS

With the successful application to the Kellogg Foundation— through our membership in PAFAMS (FEPAFEM)— for funding of an experimental project on the teaching of Community Medicine, with the assistance of the Jamaican government, and support from the CHMC, we need to promote the concepts and actions on which this is based and which we had agreed. A copy of project document is attached; please feel free to replicate. As a reminder:

(A) Community Medicine involves the application of clinical and epidemiological tools to the investigation and solution of health problems of groups of populations. Since groups of populations are made up of individuals and family units, much of the effort of Community Medicine will be aimed at the problems identified at the level of the individual and of the family group, while ensuring that all public health needs are properly supplied.

(B) A Community may be defined as a group sharing certain characteristics of geography, topography, climate, population size, politics, occupations, activities, physical facilities, communications, professions, beliefs etc. The definition is arbitrary. It can be used simply to mean the people— without further specification—taken as a whole, or in specific age or gender groups. Thus a community may be homogeneous or diversified, each type presenting distinct challenges.

(C) The first indication of an unhealthy state in a community might be the illness which that state produces in a particular *individual*. The task of Community Medicine is to treat the individual, prevent complications, restoring him/her to health, to discover and eliminate the cause, to chart possible effects on family and community, and to protect them from harm. These varied actions will require the help of an active team of health workers. There are many indicators of potential sources and causes of ill-health in a community.

2. GENERAL OBJECTIVES

Community Medicine seeks to provide a comprehensive integrated approach to solving medical problems of individuals and communities and to promote health of communities by extending the work of hospitals (local, regional academic etc.), and integrating it with health promotion, prevention of illness or complications, rehabilitation, and public health practice, such as surveillance and protection, to promote health and prevent disease.

3. ACTIVITIES

A) To achieve these objectives, a wide range of activities is necessary. However the main ones for undergraduates in the final year would appear to be the following – (these are not necessarily in the best order):

i) Diagnosis of the state of health of the chosen community through study of demography, infant mortality, maternal health, anthropometric measurements of pre-school children, mental tests of school children, general mortality and morbidity data, disease incidence and prevalence, attitudes to nutrition, to prevention, immunisation, chronic diseases and to delivery of health care.

ii) The delivery of health care to individuals. This will accomplish at least these purposes:

(a) Consolidation of the knowledge and skills of students and other care-givers in the diagnosis and investigation of individual health problems.

(b) Alerting participants of possible health hazards to the whole community that may attend or follow a particular individual's illness. (sentinel cases at start of outbreak of a communicable disease).

(c) Integrating preventive and curative approaches at all levels of health care delivery.

(d) Early treatment of minor surgical and medical illnesses and obviate hospital visits.

iii) Optimum utilisation of health care facilities so as to bring adequate health care to the people. This would include rational use of health centres, local hospitals and specialist hospitals. A sound system of referral, follow-up and feedback must therefore be set up among them.

iv) Liaison with other community leaders to promote overall objectives.

(B) Undergraduates will be involved in many ways:

i) Assignment to a specific research project designed to fill gaps in medical knowledge about target populations.

ii) Assignment to specific centres of health care delivery to learn techniques of problem-solving. This will involve choice of one or more aspects of a common problem and could take place in a hospital or health centre or other institution (e.g. Caribbean Food and Nutrition Institute, Polio Rehabilitation Centre, etc.), in an urban or rural setting, and illustrate interaction between them.

iii) Direct responsibility for patient care in designated settings to sharpen diagnostic skills and enlarge experience. They will seek to determine the nature, type, frequency and intensity of individual health problems that have an impact on the community, both medically and socio-culturally, and to learn how environmental factors, e.g. sanitation, waste disposal, animal husbandry, food handling practices, e.g. animal slaughter, vegetable preparation for market, etc., promote health or disease in the individual.

iv) Participation in training ancillary workers to do specified tasks, e.g. to dress wounds, take B.P. and other vitals, chart basic data, complete forms, present information, etc.

v) Involvement in educating the community on an awareness of the state of health, health promotion, habits, diet, exercise, recognising threats and the steps to be taken when health is threatened.

vi) Consideration and application of legal and ethical principles in dealings with individuals and the community, and the legal implications of their work.

vii) Combination of above and additional activities to be identified and developed from time to time, e.g. community advocacy groups.

4.   ARRANGEMENTS

(A)   Where necessary and possible, boarding and lodging will be provided. Attempts will be made to subsidise costs.

(B)   Transportation will be provided where necessary.

(C)   If plans materialise whereby students can be offered a Community Medicine Clerkship or Elective, or both in combination, in non-campus territories, attempts will be made to provide fares and costs, where necessary.

(D)   The "Manchester project" is only one of the areas where students may seek an experience in Community Medicine. This has already been explained to the students of the class of 1976. Further they have been told that arrangements are being made to identify existing projects in other locations that can be used, e.g. Morant Bay (Dr Ron Lampart) and to develop others in several territories of the Eastern Caribbean (See attached letter to Health Ministers).

(E)   Further information is available from the Dean's Office, which will be responsible for the subject until a Director is appointed. (position advertised). Your usual cooperation and help will be greatly appreciated, as always.

M.S. Ragbeer
27 Nov., 1974

Fig App. 9-1: **The Manchester and Other CM Projects**

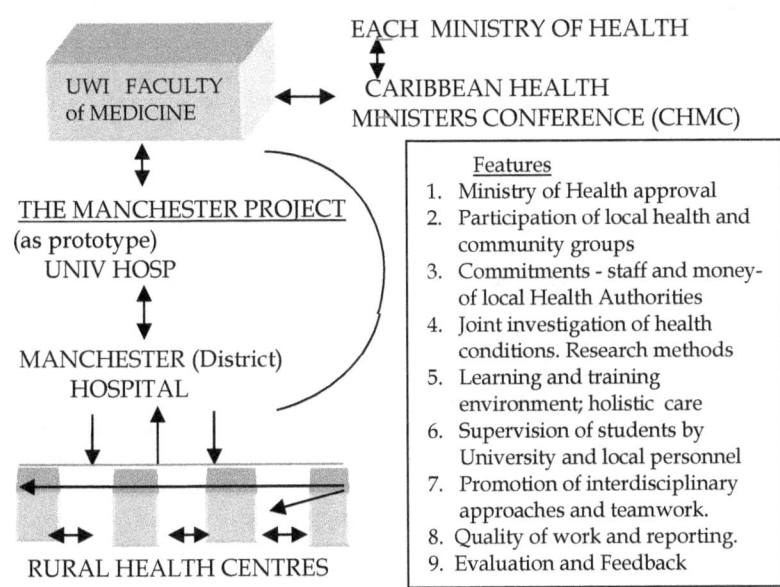

EACH MINISTRY OF HEALTH

UWI FACULTY
of MEDICINE ⟷ CARIBBEAN HEALTH
MINISTERS CONFERENCE (CHMC)

THE MANCHESTER PROJECT
(as prototype)
UNIV HOSP

MANCHESTER (District)
HOSPITAL

RURAL HEALTH CENTRES

Features
1. Ministry of Health approval
2. Participation of local health and
    community groups
3. Commitments - staff and money-
    of local Health Authorities
4. Joint investigation of health
    conditions. Research methods
5. Learning and training
    environment; holistic care
6. Supervision of students by
    University and local personnel
7. Promotion of interdisciplinary
    approaches and teamwork.
8. Quality of work and reporting.
9. Evaluation and Feedback

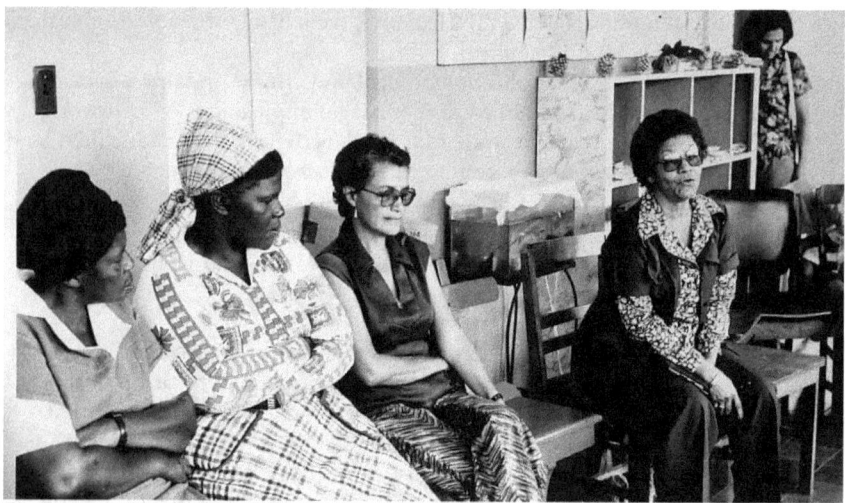

Fig App. 9-2: CM: Health Educator Ivy McGhie (R) conducting session at Manchester Clinic CM project. Dr McGhie was one of several educators in para-medical disciplines engaged to expand student learning in non-hospital and community disciplines, essential for the CM program. Others included sociologists, nutritionists, public health inspectors, laboratory and sanitation specialists, pharmacists, forensic scientists, agriculturalists, water engineers, and others. (Dean's Photos)

Appendix 10:
Community Medicine, PAFAMS statement

In 1973, as we were developing the Kellogg Latin American and Caribbean projects in Community Medicine, Dr Andrés Santas, President of FEPAFEM (PAFAMS), in outlining the concepts agreed by the Administrative Committee, stressed this caution:

"When one speaks of Community Medicine in general, there is a tendency to consider exclusively what applies to a group of people, and among them, the ones more deprived economically, socially, or culturally." This is no more than the result of transferring the concepts and actions fundamental to departments of Social & Preventive Medicine. This leads to two basic mistakes:

1. To limit severely the aims and content of Community Medicine that are inherent in its nature, and

2. To confuse it with the extramural programs of those same departments, which are united in displacing the hospital (community, regional, social security or academic) as a basis to practise it...(giving birth to) deep rifts between true doctors and public health bureaucrats.

"In reality, what you need is for the hospital to be seen as the true medical core in the health field and it becomes the place where intra- and extra-mural activities are planned and coordinated. Motivated by these imperatives, the community would learn to value and prefer the institution and its integral parts, operating inside and outside (the hospital), not only for recovery from illness, and rehabilitation, but also for advice on prevention of disease and promotion of health." *(Translated from Boletin FEPAFEM, IX, 4, July 1973)*

The Committee of Assessors for Pan-American Federation of Associations of Medical Schools (PAFAMS or FEPAFEM) for projects in Community Medicine is named in Box below

PS: Note that when CM is discussed with Americans, and with officers of PAHO, they hear "Community Health"(CH), which is confusing, or as the WHO (Bull 533) states, is an ambiguous term as some equate it with "Public Health and Social and Preventive Medicine", as Dr Santas had noted, above. WHO used it to mean the totality of health care given a community, including public health. Public Health training includes health administration, epidemiology and statistics, environmental health and sanitation, microbiology, behavioural sciences and others, depending on the school.

The UK has supported training of practising physicians in the above subjects for a degree in Community Medicine by the Royal College of Physicians. The UK Royal Commission on Medical Education, 1965-8, favoured a model which has features like ours and PAFAMS', which is endorsed by the CHMC. The Faculty Committee on CM has warned that **we should avoid the use of Community Health for this reason, and to preserve the concept of Community Medicine as a holistic, integrated plan.**

I had briefed Dean West also re this, and urged him not to miss the opportunity to create a boon for poor countries, as Cuba is doing, having already proved with its hospital extension model of primary care, and health statistics bettering anyone else's, including the US, which spends 10 times as much. I urged him to avoid the schisms inherent in the American model, and stressed that our S&P friends had accepted our model. Our field studies through the Kellogg projects, if completed as detailed, should provide a model of how to deliver total care effectively, efficiently, and economically. The Committee was urged to ensure that all students understood this, the changes involved and the opportunities for innovation; each participant should receive a copy of the Project plan.

The project is at a delicate phase (1975), and calls for close attention to the details for implementation and maintenance, as grant features match these. Most Faculty critics have not taken the time to understand the concepts and why poor countries want the integration rather than a continuation of the old British model. Dr Chavez is aware of the social and Faculty hindrances; I have agreed with him and the VC to be available to return for reviews, general and specific, and revision, as needed. **The choice of a new dean is critical: (s)he should be a clinician, oriented to disease prevention and health advocacy.** The references I've left in the office re this should help considerably.

The Committee of Assessors for PAFAMS* (FEPAFEM**) projects in Community Medicine, consisted of

Christina Palma, Pres., *Exec Secty., Chilean Assoc. of Medical Schools*
Miguel Barrios, *Exec Secretary, Mexican Association   ""*
Mario Chavez, *Associate Exec Director, PAFAMS*
Kurt Deuschle, *Chief, Dept. of Community Medicine, Mount Sinai, NY*
Jose Felix Patiño, *Executive Director, PAFAMS*
Gabriel Velasquez Palau, *Dean, Division of Health, Cali, Colombia*
Jorge Villareal, *Chief, Population Division, PAFAMS*

*Pan-American Federation of Associations of Medical Schools
**Federacion Panamericana de Associaciones, Faculdades y Escuelas de Medicina

---

Appendix 11:

UWI faculty relationship with territories, and organisation for teaching of community medicine

UWI MEDICAL FACULTY

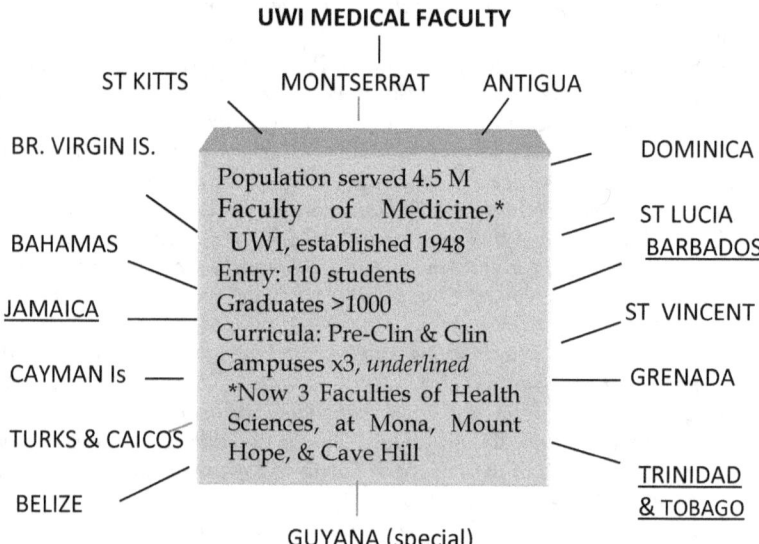

ST KITTS   MONTSERRAT   ANTIGUA

BR. VIRGIN IS.   DOMINICA

Population served 4.5 M
Faculty   of   Medicine,*
UWI, established 1948
Entry: 110 students
Graduates >1000
Curricula: Pre-Clin & Clin
Campuses x3, *underlined*
*Now 3 Faculties of Health
Sciences, at Mona, Mount
Hope, & Cave Hill

BAHAMAS   ST LUCIA
                                                                BARBADOS

JAMAICA   ST VINCENT

CAYMAN Is   GRENADA

TURKS & CAICOS

BELIZE   TRINIDAD
                                                                & TOBAGO

GUYANA (special)

Fig App.11-1: A capsule of the relationships of the current UWI Medical Faculty

DEAN'S OFFICE

↑↓

FACULTY COMMITTEE→   Dean (Chairman)
↑↓   Medical Educator
                     Heads of Departments of
FACULTY BOARD   - Paediatrics
                     - Obstetrics & Gynaecology
                     - Social & Preventive Medicine
                     +Co-opted Members

Planning and Development of Projects *
Curriculum Development
Supervision of Students
Program Implementation
Program Evaluation
Training of Health Personnel other than Medical Students
Liaison with Cooperating Groups
         - Government
         - Communities
         - Others

* *Simultaneously in Jamaica, T & T and Barbados*
Fig. App.11-2: Relationships of Faculty Committee on Community Medicine

Appendix 12:

PLANNED PUBLICATION, IN ASSOCIATION WITH PAFAMS: the challenge of medical education in developing countries of the Americas: an analysis and future perspectives

1. Preliminary Project Statement

   We propose to compile material for publication as a book with the following aims:
   (i) To present briefly the history and evolution of medical education in the developing countries of the Americas and of the Caribbean.
   (ii) To describe to date the successive changes and identify the various factors that have influenced trends, characteristics and styles in medical education and Health Care Delivery in the continent up to this time.
   (iii) To analyse the consecutive strategies, techniques and educational methods that have been employed by different medical schools, universities, health institutions and countries, to accomplish the goals of effective medical education, and to record new programs, such as Community Medicine, training of Family Doctors, and new technology.
   (iv) To analyse some of the models and schemes currently in use and others proposed for the future, e.g. computerised and robotic systems.
   (v) To discuss and evaluate the various characteristics which have emerged from the above and in particular with reference to achievements and failures.
   (vi) To make recommendations for future action

   The work will provide meaningful data which will be important to medical educators charged with developing education and training of health professionals in the different countries of the region, and whose background of professional training frequently omits exposure to, or training in medical education. The collaboration of two medical educators from countries whose economic conditions are similar, but which differ in historical, ecological, cultural, political and social characteristics, should enable presentation of a more comprehensive view of the subject than that which might be obtained from studies in a single country. Their different experiences would enable them to highlight the variations that have emerged even in countries which have similar socio-cultural conditions or share fundamental common principles of education for the needs of society.

   The native languages of the contributors are Spanish and English respectively, and both are bilingual; it would thus be possible to produce simultaneously a Spanish and an English version at the first writing and so avoid the difficulties and problems inherent in translation.

   The planning, development and conclusion of this work make it mandatory that the authors spend a period of time together in a place where, relieved of their normal duties, they could work without interruption, with adequate library and secretarial support. The Medical Library of the Americas in Sao Paulo, Brazil

(BIREME) has tentatively agreed to provide the necessary library support, both in the initial stages of data collection and in subsequent stages of analysis.

Both authors will be eligible for leave of absence of several months from their Universities between June and October 1974.

A submission will be made to the Rockefeller Foundation to support a Fellowship program which will enable them to spend from four to six weeks of intensive collaborative work at the Villa Serbelloni, Italy, under the Fellowship scheme of the Foundation.

2.   Proposed Contents

1. Foreword – by a distinguished Medical Educator from the Americas

2. Prologue

      (i)   Geographic and Socio-economic description of the Region
      (ii)   Patterns of Health Care Delivery

3.   History and Evolution of Medical Education in the Americas and Caribbean

      (i)   The Colonial Era
      (ii)   The Age of Independence – the derivation of medical education systems in the Americas
      (iii)   (a) Prior to the Flexner Report
                  (b) The impact of the Flexner Report
                  (c) Medical Education before World War II

      (iv)   Modern Medical Education

                  (a) Systems of Medical Education
                  (b) The introduction of Social and Preventive Medicine in Medical Education since World War II
                  (c) The Todd Report and its influence
                  (d) Education Technology in Medical Education
                  (e) Other reports and their implications
                  (f) The education of minority groups

4.   University Systems and their Influence on Medical Education

      (i)   Institutions of Medical Education
      (ii)   The North American pattern
      (iii)   The European (Continental) pattern
      (iv)   The Open University
      (v)   The Selective University
      (vi)   Socio-Political influences on University Reform

5.   Health Care Delivery Systems and Medical Education

      (i)   Traditional Medical Curricula and Instruction; principles of adult learning
      (ii)   Innovations in curricula and information technology
      (iii)   The emergence of the concept of Community Medicine in Medical Education

      (iv)   The Team Concept of Health Care Delivery; the structure and functions of teams

      (v)   Health Care financing; private and public systems

6. The Relation between the Ministry of Health (or Federal or Local Health Authority) and the University

7. International Institutions

      (i)   Inter-university

      (ii)   Inter-governmental

      (iii)   Funding Organisations (Foundations, etc.)

8. The Inter-American Influence on Systems and on Manpower Development

      (i)   Patterns of influence

      (ii)   Newly emerging trends

9. The Role of Non-Governmental Institutions

      (i)   Private Medical Institutions and Practitioners

      (ii)   Research and Funding Organisations

      (iii)   Drug Firms

10. Postgraduate Medical Education

      (i)   Preparing graduates for Academic and Teaching Roles ("Teaching teachers how to teach")

      (ii)   Professional education

      (iii)   Continuing Medical Education

11. The Education of Nurses, Paramedical and Ancillary Health Workers

12. Epilogue - Perspectives for the Future

Alberto Cristoffanini	Mohan S. Ragbeer
Dean, Faculty of Medicine	Dean, Faculty of Medicine
University Austral Valdivia, Chile	UWI, Mona, Kingston 7, Jamaica

December 1973

PS. Political upheavals, the ascent of General Pinochet, and ouster of Salvador Allende in Chile, led to the confinement of many academics, including Alberto, who didn't do well, his diabetes worsening. Similarly, social disruption and deadly violence in Jamaica caused my wife to flee to Canada, in summer 1974, with our five children, with the ultimatum, "You can stay, if you wish!" I followed fourteen months later, when the Jamaican Government ended my permit to send money to Canada. I went on two years no-pay leave. Attempts to contact Dr Cristoffanini failed. On a South American tour in late 1976, I visited Chile, hoping to contact Alberto and to revive our project, towards which we had done so much, only to learn that he had been under virtual house arrest and incommunicado, until that year, when, much enfeebled from poor treatment, confinement and unstable diabetes, he was allowed on medical grounds to emigrate to Australia, to join his daughter. In 1979, PAHO published Jorge Andrade's "Marco conceptual de la educación médica en la América Latina", covering some of what we had planned.

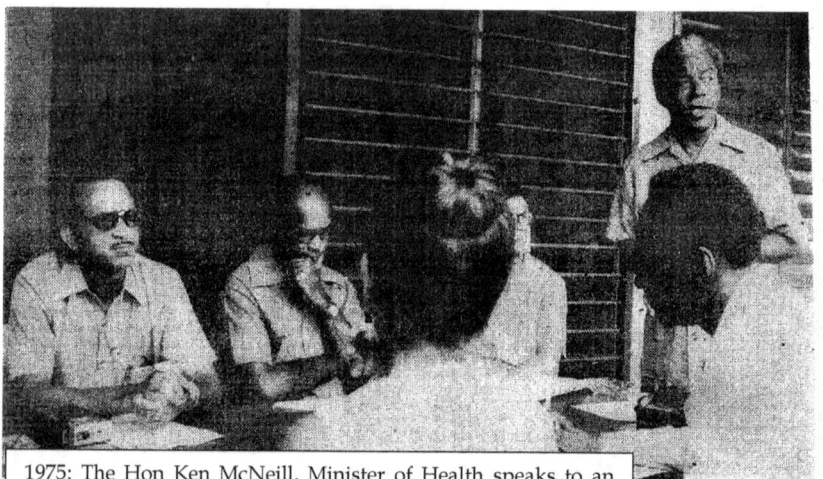

1975: The Hon Ken McNeill, Minister of Health speaks to an assembly at the Cornwall Regional Hospital, Montego Bay on its role in education and levels of service. Earlier at a meeting with GMOs in Kingston, he had outlined plans for the Health Services, but regretted that they were not yet able to participate fully in PGME; His Ministry had provided for a building and trainees to start the program, which graduated its first specialists in1974. It supports a new program in Community Medicine that has started experimentally in Manchester, with elective students, followed by a compulsory clerkship in 1976. Priority lies with upgrading KRH, and other hospitals, and planning to train a novel specialist, with clinical and public health skills, to take charge of district hospitals, and to start teaching at CRH and others, as the economy recovers; see p.247.

—JIS Photo
THE MINISTER OF HEALTH and Environmental Control, the Hon. Dr. Kenneth McNeill, (standing, right), speaking on the role the new Cornwall Regional Hospital in St. James, will assume when it opens later this year. Dr. McNeill was addressing medical specialists and newsmen, shortly before he took them on a tour of the Hospital. Others at table are (from left) clockwise), Dean M. S. Ragbeer, of the Faculty of Medicine, UWI; Dr. Ludlow Burke, Senior Medical Officer, St. James Hospital; Mr. William Peters, Consultant in Hospital Administration; Mr. F. Ducanson, Hospital Administrator; of the new Hospital, and Miss Edna Clarke Hospital Secretary,

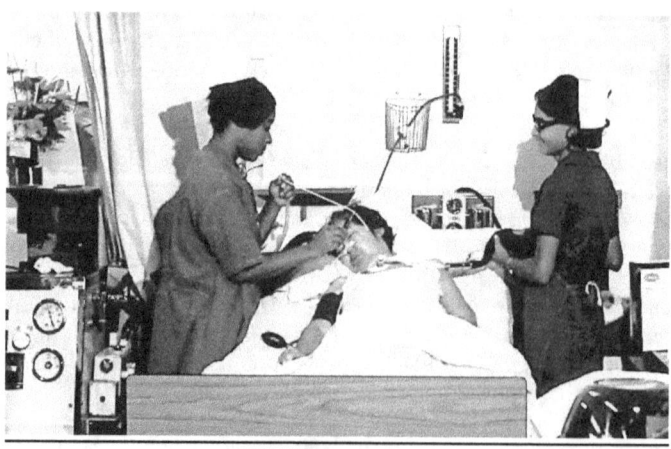

UHWI Recovery Room

Figs App 12-1&2: examples of the educational range we covered: governance to intensive care

Appendix 13

MEMO TO VC PRESTON RE PROPOSAL FOR USAID

To: Mr. A.Z. Preston, Vice Chancellor, U.W.I.
From: M.S. Ragbeer, Dean, Medical Faculty
Subject: Role of Medical Faculty in Community Development,

After the meeting recently with USAID officials, you had asked for material supporting a role for the Medical Faculty in Community Development. The submission below is hurried, but covers the main points.

1.   The Governments of the Commonwealth Caribbean have identified many projects that aim to improve the quality of life in the region. They range from the further development of the petroleum industry in Trinidad and bauxite industries in Jamaica and Guyana, to agricultural development and improvement of food production throughout the area.

2.   Health is an important component of social, political, economic and cultural development. Any program aimed at improving conditions of populations must bear this central fact in mind. The IADB Committee had stressed it.

3.   The West Indian population is some 4.5 million, of whom 44% are under 15. More than 20% of that total lives in rural or in deprived urban areas.   An unknown but large percentage of this population suffers malnutrition, which , with its complications are a heavy drain, not only on health institutions, but on the future potential of the afflicted. Studies here have shown that early childhood malnutrition results in sufficient brain damage to retard intellectual development, thus affecting the nation's efforts to promote economic development and improve the quality of life.

4.   The Caribbean Health Ministers Conference (CHMC), a body made up of the Health Ministers of all contributing territories, has, since its first meeting in 1969, repeatedly emphasised the fact that the region does not have sufficient manpower with the specific skills needed for development, nor for comprehensive and effective health care delivery.

5.   Most of these countries have accepted that Government should provide adequate health services to the total community, and each wishes to make increasing use of skills in *their* regional Medical Faculty to assist them to achieve this aim. (Some have reluctantly accepted the necessity of a parallel system of privately-delivered medical care.

6.   Independently, and in response to this reality, members of the Faculty have conducted several studies in specific aspects of the problem. Their enquiries have shown that the following areas of Government or Faculty affairs must be improved if the Faculty is to make the sound contributions it wishes to total development:

(a) Organisation and management of health services

i) The ministry in each country is responsible for policy making and for implementation of these policies. Most do not have the technical capability to plan appropriately, to manage institutions properly, or to implement policies effectively. Indeed, policies are often are laid down, and no action follows. This is frustrating, particularly as many politicians are known to announce initiatives prematurely to the public, even in spite of knowing that prompt implementation is not possible, in view of the shortage of skills and facilities in the particular country.

ii) The Medical Faculty has been asked often in the past by various Governments to assist them to meet deficiencies. However, the Faculty lacks spare capacity, and its resources, depleted by staff losses, are over-extended in efforts to meet current demands for education and service at the University, the University Hospital (UHWI) and EC teaching units.

iii) The University Council has requested the Governments, particularly of Jamaica, to make adequate provisions for service work at the UHWI so that the faculty could respond to the needs of the region for technical help.

iv) The CHMC has in turn urged member Governments to make funds available to the Medical Faculty to improve infrastructure to meet their varied needs. However, Governments appear unable to meet the costs of enabling the UHWI to offer consultant services to the territories, and in those special areas in health care where needs have been identified.

(v) The CHMC had, in 1972, proposed guidelines for Faculty–Government collaboration (prepared by Dr M.S. Ragbeer and Mr. C. A. Burton) to promote effective health care delivery to the total population in each member country. The concept envisaged that the Faculty should have the capability to provide research services; full consultant services, particularly in special areas where duplication is either not necessary or extremely costly; services which can be regionalised, and based upon a single institution, and where distances are not an inhibitory factor to development of regional organisation; educational services for professional and post-professional levels; advisory and supervisory services for training of auxiliary health workers; programs aimed at development of health schemes; attitudinal studies, etc. The activities of value to Governments will remain dormant, to a large measure, due to lack of the appropriate facilities in both Faculty and Ministry levels.

(b) <u>Delivery of health care: problems and concerns</u>
  i)   outstanding weaknesses in Government programs
  ii) maldistribution of skilled personnel, particularly doctors, between rural and urban areas, and even within urban areas, their concentration in hospitals and in the more affluent areas;
  iii) inadequately developed physical facilities and concentration of expenditure on curative services, especially hospitals, and relative neglect of rural health centres, dispensaries and other facilities, and of programs to prevent illness and promote health. The countries have been unable to develop, organise and operate a comprehensive health care strategy.
  iv) inadequate provisions for supplies, particularly in rural areas and in deprived urban areas (slums).
  v)   poor, obsolete or inappropriate equipment in institutions;
  vi) the University Hospital is short of equipment and space for the services demanded of it, especially specialist units needed to provide consultant services to the region and for the needs of the Faculty's postgraduate program. Much of the equipment is run down; much is obsolete or in need of repair. Maintenance services are inadequate, due to loss of skills, and the cost

of replacement has increased tremendously over the past year. This need for space and equipment has impeded the growth of the UHWI and Faculty in critical areas. It has been catalogued and repeated each triennium to the UWI Senate Committee on Estimates and to the University Grants Committee.

(c) Medical Education

i) The Faculty is a traditional one. It produces medical doctors only, and in 1972 began to train specialists. Before that, several departments had, either taken the responsibility for, or assisted in the development of training programs for medical technologists, community health aides, radiographers, physical therapists, and other auxiliary workers. Many members of the Faculty contribute to the training of nurses; others assist in the program of the West Indies School of Public Health; yet others in Jamaica cooperate with the College of Arts, Science and Technology and teach in some of its programs.

ii) Manpower studies have shown a need for more professional and ancillary staff, including generalist physicians, our prime output, which falls short of regional needs. Ancillary workers are needed in quite large numbers to fill simple roles in health care. Their training is outside the remit of the university, but its teachers need to know their role in health teams, and can contribute extra-murally to their training, and encourage other Governments to undertake it, as the Jamaican Government is doing.

iii) The development of postgraduate training requires substantial new facilities at the UWI, including specialist teachers, and is supported by the CHMC. The requests are before the UGC.

(d) Medical Research

i) The Tropical Metabolism Research Unit (TMRU), the Epidemiological Unit (ERU), the Caribbean Food and Nutrition Institute (CFNI) are well-known research institutes located on the Mona campus of the University. The first two are MRC units, the third PAHO. The TMRU has been handed over to the UWI, and will become a fully funded UWI facility from 1977.

ii) Apart from these institutions, medical research is largely the task of the individual members of the Faculty and, to a lesser extent, small research units in Ministries of Health. Our enquiry has shown that very little research has been done in Ministries of Health and what data repose there, are, for practical purposes, lost. Much of the available medical data have come from Medical Faculty efforts.

iii) There is an increasing need for investigation into health problems of the Caribbean region, as well as for basic data on general morbidity and mortality patterns in the various countries, to facilitate planning of health care services. More data are needed in areas like nutrition, zoonoses, ecology-related health problems, industrial problems, influences of consumer factors including the use and abuse of drugs, and investigation into local remedies. Unless these data are available, heath care resources will continue to be expended in a speculative way.

iv) The lag is too great between production of new knowledge and its application, where relevant, by individual Ministries of Health. This lag is largely due to shortage of appropriate personnel and materials.

v) The most significant areas of neglect in our health care system are at the rural level and the social determinants of health. In some areas inadequate transportation leaves rural communities isolated from health centres and urban hospitals. In any event, hospitals are costly and were not designed for primary care, nor is it the best atmosphere for it. Its access involves, too, the additional expense of moving people in large numbers from rural to urban areas, with loss of earnings to the individual. The further heavy losses of total man hours in the waiting rooms of hospitals throughout the Caribbean and its effect on national incomes must be computed in the cost of total health care if a true picture is to be obtained, but this in fact is not done. These factors, plus the way professional and general health services are utilised, would be a fruitful one for operational research studies, as those data are not available. We are very short of skills in this epidemiological and multi-disciplinary field, though we are very willing to assist in such investigation.

(vi) The areas mentioned above are general though yet specific in the sense of what is required as the educational component of development. I can add others, but I would emphasise in this resume of Medical Faculty needs, our desire to improve our ability to deliver a sound medical and professional education to our students, both undergraduate and graduate, by amplifying social, cultural, dietary, behavioural, economic and like studies in our medical curricula; to increase our ability to train or to assist in training all other levels of health workers and to develop in them the good habits of teamwork; and to contribute to the improvement of health in the region, through research, service and education. A major need would therefore be adequate physical facilities for housing staff, producing materials and for teaching.

7 (a) The development suggested in the above comments can be accomplished by the creation within the Medical Faculty of a Division of Community Medicine responsible for developing the research potential, the teaching instruments and the extension of Faculty programs into rural and urban communities. Our Faculty is seeking Government assistance to develop such programs, but Governments are limited in the extent to which they can contribute, as experience so far has shown.

(b) The Faculty has recently received a grant to establish a Community Medicine demonstration project to test ideas and procedures that can be later used as routines by UWI and others in the Caribbean and Latin America. The project can cooperate with other disciplines in a variety of ways e.g. in the area of food production it would be able to contribute:

 i) to reaching primary targets of increased availability of locally-grown foods, by safe storage, sterilisation or avoidance of spoilage; sanitary food preparation;

 ii) toxicological studies: medical effects of chemical fertilisers, herbicides and pesticides;

 iii) to define the most nutritious foods grown in the area, and those that can be grown economically and organically; food composition; food fads;

 iv) studies on nutritional patterns, attitudes to various foods; preparation techniques and medical effects of these;

v) knowledge of food-related diseases, e.g. malnutrition; other deficiencies; obesity; food poisoning, idiosyncrasies and allergies; properties of "fast" foods, etc.

vi) to ascertain and improve community awareness of good nutrition practices; to control, eradicate and prevent food-related diseases,

vii) to programs for specific conditions e.g., from needs of the diabetic patient, with complications, lying in a hospital bed, to those of the marginally malnourished one, in a distant and remote rural area.

viii) to probe other areas of interest e.g. food handlers, as carriers and victims of food-borne illness; dehydrated foods; and by-products of the food industry.

ix) to improve dental health; a close relation exists between the condition of teeth and gastro-intestinal and nutritional diseases. The Faculty has been for a long time keen to develop dental education. This is now a part of its over-all expansion proposal. It should be noted that the Faculty has continued to take a keen interest in the operations of the Dental Auxiliaries Training School of the Jamaican Government.

8. (a) Looked at in perspective, what the Faculty of Medicine needs then would be funds to give it the physical and equipment base from which it could develop and expand health programs aimed to contribute to any integrated plan of community development, rural or urban, set up by, or in any one country, either by its Government, or by the University as a model project.

(b) The Faculty needs this infrastructure very badly. This should include a learning resource centre with all its implications, and with facilities to extend the Faculty's operations into various communities, not only in Jamaica, but throughout the Caribbean. This would give the Faculty the ability to produce teaching materials using modern audio-visual techniques, to apply recent advances in medical education technology to our needs, to improve and extend the capacity of each individual staff member in the total educational and research initiative. Such facilities require substantial investment, but the benefits gained from its multiplier effects would amply justify the cost.

(c) With such an investment, Community Centres can be developed in which ideas can be tested, projects developed and results evaluated and channelled back into the main project pool of the University and Government for modification and/or dissemination throughout the area, as indicated.

(d)   There is no doubt of the need for these things. The IADB Committee has stressed the role of health in the social advancement of peoples. The Caribbean Health Ministers Conference has repeatedly asked our help, but cannot fund the schemes. It is up to the University now to assist to identify the source(s) from which the needed funds could come to give the Faculty and the University a sound basis from which to develop community programs in many areas which could really contribute to local, national and regional development.

(Sgd.) M.S. Ragbeer, Nov. 19, 1974
cc   Vice-Deans, Dean's Advisory Committee, Faculty Finance Committee

Appendix 14:

ADDRESS TO NEW CLINICAL STUDENTS, MAY 1974

Good Morning, Ladies and Gentlemen, and Welcome to clinical medicine. The euphoria you may feel as you begin this phase is no doubt the same as my class felt in October 1954, excited by the new ambience, the smells, the sights, the casual stethoscopes dangling from the pockets of smart white tunics, which we had craved for two years; the nurses eyeing you, and you them, the formidable professors and ward sisters; the blasé senior students...; you're floating on air wafting from place to place, kings and queens of your universe, eager to cure your first patient. No fooling; it's a great moment; enjoy it; keep it alive.

But I must discuss with you briefly the essential structure of medical studies in our system, derived from the British, and having to conform to General Medical Council licensing standards. These are fairly rigid, and we recently had a rigorous examination by the Council before approval of our revised curriculum. Even though innovative, it is still not half as radical as many experimental curricula and styles coming out of North America, the USA mainly, where the system of health care is essentially a business. Until the last decade, US medical schools had followed the Flexnerian model based on Johns Hopkins of Baltimore, and Case Western in Cleveland.

The technology of WWII, including the Manhattan project, spawned a wide range of medical discoveries, not only in the traditional sciences, but in mental health and drug therapy, with appraisals of how medical care is dispensed, and how it copes with society's many problems. Flush with money from Foundations and Government after WWII, US medical schools developed strong clinical departments, or fortresses, especially Internal Medicine and Surgery, which made many scientific advances, and dominated curricula. By the mid-sixties, this lop-sided dominance of research led some students and teachers to demand more studies in the neglected social, behavioural, economic, demographic and other aspects of Medicine, requiring a less departmentalised, more coordinated or integrated model of education, research and delivery of care. Indeed, if it were not for the requirements of the US National Boards of Medical Examiners, some subjects might not have received any attention there.

Our system differs from that of the US, but we cannot escape the trap between free enterprise medicine and the socialised systems of Europe and here. You must keep this dichotomy in mind, as it affects education, and not fall in too readily with our NA neighbours, as they struggle to come closer to our way; this may explain why they take pleasure in stealing our graduates, who seem more and more easily enticed, and many have gone over to their side, each defection saving them some $200,000 in real terms: 5 years at $40,000 each. The total for the average yearly loss could finance our expansion and graduate programs!

We are poor. Nevertheless, we have done much on slender resources. Want stimulates creativity. Our clinical curriculum, of which you should have a copy, aims to give you a wide coverage of the essence of general medicine, and prepare you for further study of whatever branch excites your fancy. The way ahead is unfortunately full of thickets, more nuisances than hindrances, which you should be able to negotiate. You entered medical school with an image of what you would become and how you would function. Most first impressions are either heroic or romantic, strongly oriented to doing good, scientifically or socially, though more and more tainted by pecuniary goals. Even so, the aim of serving people at the noblest level of human interaction will guide you to right action. Although all of you will follow the same curriculum, each can develop unique interests and emphases that fit your personality and goals; your tutors can guide you, and help you assess your progress to these ends.

The physician has evolved dramatically in the last century and a half; we in these ex-colonies are tied to British models, which in their earliest days may have done more harm than good, in the transition of the doctor from wizard to scientist and sociologist, from blood-letters and vectors of death to Jenner, Semmelweiss, Lister, Pasteur, Koch, Morton and the panoply of early change-makers, to today's Nobel laureates, George Crick et al., probing the secrets of DNA and the creation of life. I happen, by heritage, to know of a half-forgotten tradition, at least 2600 years old and championed then by one Sushruta, whose cataract extraction method is still used, who trephined skulls, removed brain tumours, a technology shared with Inca surgeons of the Andes. The Indians used plant extracts to treat malaria and other fevers, relieve pain and induce anaesthesia; they treated mental illness and hypertension and taught their theories and skills, known as *Ayurvaida*, to all comers, at two Universities and eventually to Arab invaders, who also learned Indian mathematics, science and astronomy, added their bit, and exported that knowledge to Europe, as it entered the Renaissance. The much later industrial expansion of Europe led to scientific discoveries, first in math, physics, chemistry, then biology, with Linnaeus, Darwin and the explosion of new discoveries from the 18th century on. But I must stop. Medical history is a fascinating saga, well worth exploring.

You have already had five terms of basic sciences, unfortunately not with early exposure to clinical problems, to explain why you were learning those things. Our founders made a huge mistake in not building preclinical facilities near to, or on the hospital site, but that was the British model in 1948. Three years ago we argued long and hard for preclinical buildings near the hospital, instead of expanding existing facilities as student numbers grew, but we lost; it is some consolation that the integrated model we sought will be implemented at the coming Trinidad Faculty. So we must make do with the current arrangement.

Besides anatomy, physiology, biochemistry, nutrition, pharmacology, we now include sociology, behaviour, epidemiology, demography, economics, ecology, agriculture, occupation, ethics as basic to medicine. One that we've discarded is Latin, a pity, as 75% or so of scientific terms have roots in Greek and Latin, which, by the way, enabled me, totally new to science, to finish a premedical year in seven months! Clinical practice involves nursing, biomedical engineering and technology, health education and public health. It requires the mathematics that deals with probabilities, norms, modes, reliability and validity, that you need to understand, in order to analyse health data that Governments collect, so that you can draw valid conclusions, and to critique or produce a medical article. You will need these to study a whole person. 2600 years ago, the Indian doctor Sushruta, told students, *"I want someone who can see me as a whole!"*

You will spend most of the next 3 years in this hospital, where ill people – all whole persons, with various illnesses – seek nurses and doctors for relief. You will learn how to identify their illnesses: the art and science of data collection, recording and analysis; how to probe disease causes; assess body defences; make a physical diagnosis from among multiple possibilities, manage the illness, assess efficacy of treatment, prevent complications, and rehabilitate the patient. Central to all interventions is communication, at each stage of the process, in clear and simple terms. As you do this, with guidance, you will learn that patients, like flora and fauna, are a part of their physical environment, with distinct life styles, social and economic underpinnings that affect behaviour and the state of health. So, as you learn about disease, you must face the question: what is health?

Does anyone wish to define "health"? (*Listens to a few offers, all suggesting absence of illness, or disease*). Well, here's how the WHO defines it, in its 1948 constitution (slide): "*a state of complete physical, mental, and social well-being and not merely the absence of disease or infirmity.*" It's idealism makes one feel warm and expansive. I suspect that that this must have been composed by a couple in extreme bliss at the end of the first perfect night of an idyllic honeymoon. But as we contemplate that definition, we realise that it sits at the apex of a pyramid of knowledge that we need to explore, refine and expand.

All of our contributing territories, currently 14, collect data on life expectancy, disease incidence and prevalence, maternal and child mortality, the state of safe water and food supplies, just to name a few, which with others, describe the infrastructure of health in a society. At best, we can hope for an equilibrium between us and the environment, which is indifferent to us, and often quite hostile, as if in self-defence, as mankind seems destined to spoil each sustaining element of Nature. Those of us poorly prepared: socially, biologically, economically, educationally, and those exposed, acutely or chronically, to hostile and injurious influences, will become ill and seek your help, in each of these 14 states. In each of them, the health care system is publicly-funded, generally underprovided, yet expected to give superior service, to save lives and cure diseases. These are pricey objectives, but must be tackled. The logical approach would be to set priorities and goals to match resources, and train students to think of what they must know and do efficiently, to help, *and always to ask themselves: could this have been prevented?* Too often, hospital educators tend to forget this, as they grapple with the imperatives of diagnosis and treatment.

An analysis of data on reasons people seek medical attention will show you a fairly wide spread of conditions, which can be grouped into levels of care, each requiring a set of resources, including personnel, from simple to complex. Ill populations fall into three groups, distributed as in this diagram (*slide p. 53*):

Hospitals will expose you to Groups 2 and 3, that is, about 20% or so of people in need; they consume the most, in time and resources. In every hospital, you'll be under their spell and that of the specialists who care for them.

Specialists have taken over everywhere and are revered among us. They have become entrenched and powerful in institutions, and dominate medical education. For undergraduates, this is not always a good thing. And why not? Simply this: clinical education is like marriage: two weeks of euphoria followed by a lifetime of hard, hopefully rewarding work. It should ideally be under charge of a good generalist, (*slide of cartoon, GM*). Following WWII, US medical schools received large research grants; research encourages specialisation. We are a copy of what metropolitan universities teach, despite the gap in resources. So, medical schools like ours do not have generalists. Not one. None would qualify for any departmental position. Universities too, so far, tend to be associated with hospitals. Hospital work is complex, done by many different specialists, assuring the sick that they are attended by the most appropriately-skilled person.

Before 1910, US medical schools were like market stalls; anybody could have one. The 1910 Flexner report introduced order, proper standards and methods. It stressed disciplined study, proper administration, and a medical program affiliated with a university. Specialists have charge of everything in hospitals and have the responsibility for student learning. This includes curricular design. Specialists usually have narrow perspectives, derived from concentrating on their specialty. This is good for patients and practice, and great for specialty *residents*. But it's not good for undergraduates, who need to see the widest spectrum without selection—at least to start And that spectrum should clearly reflect the realities of their environment. Students must see this. But we leave it up to them, unfairly I think, to integrate their learning; some fumble their way through the program towards an understanding and sometimes get lost. Some never achieve this, but manage to scrape through exams. What we do now is send you straightway into the labyrinth of departments (without any pattern that can be really appreciated) and leave you to the mercies of whatever minotaur you might find there. You're trapped unless you can see the forest, and not just the trees. Each tutor will teach you his/her specialty, and try to make you a mini-expert, in all too short a span of time. And if you learn fast s/he will most likely grab you as a new recruit into that specialty. When each specialty is through with you, you become a *multi-mini-specialist*. Where is the unity then, the biological unity that is woman or man? Why must this single-most important thing be neglected in our education plan, at the highest seat of learning, no less?

Even the evaluation scheme (i.e. exams) is in compartments; and some things are not tested, usually the ones you know best! About half a class becomes specialists, the rest generalists, often by default.

So, back to the majority of patients, that 75-80%, whom students rarely see, except as crowds each day in the waiting rooms of Casualty and Outpatient clinics, rural health centres, or while on community assignments and electives, or in private doctors' offices, and one day, perhaps, yours. If you haven't learned about them, which you won't in hospital, you will try to match them to your hospital experience and diagnostic models, or else start learning *from* them, or as my best friend, Dr Stanley Luck, of Georgetown, class of '56, one of the few great family doctors you'll find anywhere, keeps asking, *why not teach it in medical school?* So finally we plan to start the *specialty* of Family Practice, where the focus will be corrected and directed towards Primary care, that 80%. This will begin before you graduate. If I survive!

By studying the whole spectrum of illness, you can decide what segment of care you would like to provide as a career. Until we can organise non-hospital encounters, you are encouraged to see the folks who walk in to the casualty section with fresh problems, and are triaged by a nursing sister; or use the elective period in your third year for a suitable attachment; or as field work in the Social & Preventive Medicine clerkship; (this is a stop-gap arrangement, since the principles involved in social and preventive practices are common to all types of care, from the general to the super-specialty. The elective is a useful way of learning something in greater depth, or new to suit your career goals.

This hospital is stretched; it has 504 beds and over 300 clinical students; that's at best 2 beds per student, allowing for student dispersion, less than half what it was 5 years ago. We have identified district and community hospitals suitable for education, and we hope that the new Montego Bay Hospital will become a teaching hospital. Others here, e.g., Bustamante Children's, Victoria Maternity, Kingston Regional, the Chest Hospital, Spanish Town, participate in rounds, internships and electives, and are gearing up for full clerkships, slowed lately by economic problems; and so far three in the EC. *See table (p. 165).*

To get this balanced education, the Faculty has approved a program in Community Medicine, to begin this year as a 3-month final year elective, on a grant from the Kellogg Foundation and the Jamaica government. It will integrate clinical and preventive practices, develop primary care, family medicine, and for the Jamaica Ministry, train a unique specialist in Community Medicine to take charge of district hospitals, and perhaps save by eliminating some purely administrative public health physicians.

In this project, students will work, with the district doctor, a team of nurses and aides, in clinics and health centres just outside Mandeville, and get a chance to practice what's been learned, integrate clinical with preventive care, and practice health promotion among the people in the catchment communities. Student research will help to identify needs e.g., protein nutrition. They will use the Mandeville Hospital for referrals and be able to follow patients there; a few needing tertiary care will be referred to this hospital, your home base. Specialist visits from UHWI will be arranged, as needed. Until we get the division going, I will take on the challenge. I've set out in the grant application the details to be followed; it is available in my office and you should read it when your time comes. The experience becomes a regular rotation next year. You will have a chance to devise your own project in association with supervisors. Similar schemes are being developed in the EC, also in the Antilles. Anyone interested in this, say in a home island, could see me for details. We hope that this will help you to see the patient, not as a disjointed assembly of cells, tissues, organs, and systems—as studied in pre-clinical classes—but as a living, breathing whole in whom systems are so inextricably inter-related as to make compartmentalisation a folly, if not a danger.

Last month (April 1974), the Canadian Government suggested that health and health services should shift *emphasis* from curative medicine to *factors promoting health and preventing disease,* and view all the expensive and extensive paraphernalia of disease care as an admission of failure to achieve excellence in health promotion and primary care. This is a timely endorsement of our plan to develop this aspect of medical education in a Division of Community Medicine.

Now a word about specialty training. We are approved for 1-2 year diplomas, begun in 1968, and for full 4-year residencies in seven disciplines, justified by a needs survey which a team I led completed 2 years ago. The HOPE Foundation assists with teaching staff. So, by addressing needs for both primary and specialty care we will have professionals covering the entire spectrum of medical conditions and all modalities of care: health promotion, disease prevention, and illness care and rehabilitation. We allowed hospital residents credit for any training received since 1970. So we expect that three or four of them will sit specialty exams this year and thus our first fully trained specialists will graduate this year; they should be more au fait with local diseases, patterns of speech, and life styles, and therefore better prepared for Caribbean practice than those who learned their clinical stuff in temperate climes. Thus, 1974 is as significant a landmark year as 1954 for the first medical graduates of London-UCWI, and 1967 for the first doctors with UWI degrees. I hope you meet these pioneers and members of the HOPE program. We expect in time that Trinidad and Barbados will commit resources to specialty training. It's inevitable.

Faculty seniors and other staff will tutor you in this introductory course. Social unrest in our milieu is disrupting the growth of our programs, even as it fractures families and defeats national economic goals. We hope for an end to this, and that you are spared its disruptions, as I know that striking unions are keen to get your help. Be aware of these social movements; they have a bearing on health, but try to be as dispassionate as you can, and help where you can. But remember, learning comes first.

About books, although we learn clinical medicine from our own folks, we still get our main textbooks from the UK and tend to quote their incidence and prevalence figures and everything re chronic, non-remitting conditions e.g. DM, HTN, atherosclerosis; we may miss racial proclivities such as Sickling, G6PD deficiency, ABO/Rh disease, and HTN in Blacks, which are studied here, and heart disease and DM in EI, which was first reported by Dr Wattley of T&T in 1959, and by me in BG (Guyana) in 1963; these are my figures, (p. 73), but remain to be explored, clinically, epidemiologically and genetically, perhaps by some of you. Nutritional issues are different here and predispose to disease, especially in poor children deprived of protein, and fed mainly on CHO and a little fat. Our population can get exercise and outdoor exposure all year, so have the potential to be reasonably fit; and, encouraged by you, to keep fit, eat sensibly and avoid most of this.

Be cautious in believing claims of drug companies, all generally reluctant to share critical data; and do advocate strongly for no smoking and moderate alcohol. Some aspects of medicine are exploding, e.g. molecular biology; other micro and imaging techniques are becoming affordable; one good example is in Immunology where advances have led to new groupings of lymphocytes (*T,B, and null*), and new insights into their immune roles and mechanisms of action, the chemicals that trigger them, and how this knowledge aids treatment of the malignancies derived from them. This is just one of the many lights that are steadily illuminating the basis of our profession. In closing, here's one little example of language relevance: a West Indian guest at a British function responded to the hostess's offer of a cigarette or a drink, by answering, *"a duzzen smoke and a duzzen drink"*; he was surprised when she brought six cigarettes and six beers, and said, *"I'll get you the other half dozen when you're done with these!"*

M.S. Ragbeer, Dean, Medical Faculty, April 1974

Appendix 15: Correspondence

1.   Extract from Letter to Professor Eric Back, Paediatrics, Resigned

Professor Eric H. Back
14 Pier Plain, Gorleston, Gt. Yarmouth,
Norfolk, England.   27th December 1972

Dear Eric,
   It was indeed a pleasure to hear from you and to learn that you have – I think quite appropriately – secured a *chair* as the memento of the years spent with the UWI in Jamaica. I really enjoyed the visit with you and your family and have at least one rather attractive transparency to show for it. I shall make sure to get a copy or print for you...
   ...Meanwhile, the Council has decided to expand the Faculty beginning in the 1975-78 triennium, with preclinical facilities placed primarily at Mona and clinical training dispersed in various hospitals. Effectively, this means that chances of developing preclinical facilities in the Eastern Caribbean are slim within a 15-year period unless the Trinidad Government decides to push for an earlier development. A lot of work clearly needs to be done and the problems spiral. I am trying to reorganise this office in order to cope with new trends and demands, and I hope some things will go well for me.
   Again it was really a delight to have tracked you down to Great Yarmouth, and on such a beautiful day too. I hope to see you and your family again sometime, and shall let you know in advance of any visit to the U.K. I shall inform the next meeting of the Board of your choice.
   With all good wishes for Christmas and the New Year,

Yours sincerely,
Mohan S. Ragbeer

   Note: Professor Back was a staunch supporter of integration of disciplines in medical education, and, like Prof. David Stewart, Head of O&G, of the wisdom of moving pre-clinical facilities to, or near to the UHWI, as recommended by the IADB Committee on expansion. He supported Community Medicine as we had conceived it, in line with the PAFAMS model, and regretted the circumstances that prevented his participation in establishing it. He had, like others, testified to the IADB Committee and strongly favoured a Family Medicine program and the training of nutrition and paediatric health aides for home support. He might have taken the Directorship of Community Medicine, or encouraged Colin Miller to take it, had the rising violence and general social deterioration not forced his departure, as they did that of Andrew Masson and Jim Cross, neurosurgeons, Ron Browne, anaesthetist, Louis Grant, microbiologist, Val Young, clinical chemist, Colin Benjamin, Chief Laboratory Technologist, and others (1974).

2.   Letter to CFTC, London

UNIVERSITY OF THE WEST INDIES

Faculty of Medicine
Mona, Kingston 7,
Jamaica, WI
Dean's Office

Cable and Telegraph: University
Phone P.B.X. 76621, Ext 270

June 21, 1975

Mr P.D. Snelson
Asst. Director, Education & Training
Commonwealth Fund for Technical Cooperation.
Marlborough House,
Pall Mall, LONDON, ENGLAND SW1Y 5HX

Mr Snelson,

Enclosed is a copy of my Report on the trip I took in September and October 1974, to Bangladesh, India, Kenya, Nigeria and Tanzania. I would have liked to have edited the report at least once more to eliminate repetitions, improve the style and perhaps add to the substance as there are issues and ideas incompletely covered. I leave, however, in a few days for one, or most likely, two years of no-pay leave which I will spend in Canada working in two rural communities and studying the Ontario system of health care financing through a compulsory pre-paid and Government-run insurance scheme.

I believe that some such type of pre-paid scheme might appropriately meet the financial needs of health systems in the developing countries, but I am extremely sceptical whether a scheme run by a Government could, in view of the nature of Government bureaucracy, be anything but top-heavy with 'administration', inefficient, and unnecessarily costly. The expensive fat that pads Government methods everywhere is well enough known to be a fundamental truth of our times. I am therefore eagerly anticipating what will unfold before me in the months ahead.

I am hoping that by the time I return, the UWI will have decided its future policy in health manpower training, especially in regard to the expansion of medical education to take place in Trinidad in the near future. I have made arrangements to provide as much assistance with the Community Medicine education project I started as the new project directors would wish. I am sure with continued careful attention to the details as set out in the document that this project will achieve its aims and be a model of University-Government cooperation.

I would have welcomed a somewhat longer visit, say two extra days each in Bangladesh and Tanzania and two weeks in India, if only for the fact that it took much time to make local travel arrangements due to the Indian Airlines strike, and settle essential matters such as the changing of the cheques that were given to me in local currency. In Bangladesh, for example, it took one whole day to get the cheque changed and to get permission to pay my hotel bill in local currency: it also took a considerable amount of argument and finally shuttling between, and pleading to high officials of the bank and Ministry to get them both! It seemed my being Indian and not from India — with whom relations are still cosy from gratitude for India's role in their achievement of independence and continuing protection — puzzled them considerably.

Nevertheless the visits were extraordinarily stimulating, and have strengthened my view that the University in a developing country, especially with only one university, must become the innovator, the catalyst, the implementer, the evaluator and quality-controller. It must therefore deviate from its current perceptions and interpretations of what a university role should be; this requires both vision and courage, which ought not to be beyond the reach of those given positions of authority; indeed they should be prerequisites for wielding such authority. I am hopeful that the UWI can display these qualities in the times ahead, and that I can be allowed to use the knowledge gained on this series of visits and my coming studies in Canada, to expand the scope and depth of manpower training in the territories served by the UWI and its affiliates.

I am grateful to the CFTC and the Foundation for the support which made these visits possible.

Yours sincerely,
(Sgd.) M.M.S. Ragbeer MB, BS, DCP(Lond), MRCPath.
                              Dean, Medical Faculty
MMSR/ac
cc PVC L.R.B. Robinson
NOTE: *The report was used as basis for the PAFAMS book chapter on "World Trends in the Education of the Family Doctor (see Bibliography)*

3. **Memo to VC Roy Marshall, 25, Sept 1973** *(This was unanimously supported by the Faculty Board as one of the incentives to staff retention)*

To: Vice Chancellor Roy Marshall
From: Dean, Medical Faculty
Re: Academic Staff in affiliated (accredited) hospitals

Recent resignations in the Faculty of Medicine have created grave problems in the implementation of the faculty's teaching program for the Academic Year 1973-74. The faculty is disturbed at the delay in the revision of academic salaries, and feel that this further aggravates the situation, and advises that it will be made even more serious if meaningful salary increases are not obtained.

We see as a continuing problem the remuneration of medical academic staff. We feel that fundamental changes in the staffing of the teaching hospital at Mona, such as exists in Britain, the U.S., Canada and other Commonwealth Caribbean teaching hospitals, is mandatory if the University in general, and the Faculty of Medicine in particular, is to fulfil its obligations to the area as a whole.

It is imperative that the Government of Jamaica assume full responsibility for patient care in the teaching hospital at Mona, and that greater use be made of part-time staff. The FGP approves this and recommends two categories of teaching staff:

1)   a small core of adequately paid full-time *clinical* academic staff in each teaching hospital, and

2)   a wide range of hospital and other consultants as part-time *associates* who participate in teaching the medical curriculum.

We suggest appropriate academic titles for each affiliated Government medical officer and similarly Hospital titles for each of our staff. We recommend the term "Associate," refined by adding "Clinical" or "Laboratory, " and other promotional ones like "senior," as an academic title for Government staff, and "Honourary Consultant" for university staff in government institutions; these can be further refined *ad personam*. The assessments can be done by a joint committee of Government and University officials at each campus site.

(Sgd.) M.S. Ragbeer,
Dean, Medical Faculty
cc Vice Deans / Faculty Appointments and Promotions Committee

4.   Letter from Minister of Health and Environmental Control, Jamaica Hon Min. Ken McNeill, re my "Ancillaries" Paper.

MINISTRY OF HEALTH
& ENVIRONMENTAL CONTROL

Ministry of Health and Environmental Control   21 Slipe Pen Road,
Hon. Dr. Ken McNeill   P.O. Box 478
                                                          Kingston, Jamaica
                                                          November 4, 1974

Dr. M. Ragbeer,
Dean, Medical Faculty, UWI, Mona, Kingston 7

Dear Dean Ragbeer,

        This is a belated congratulation on your excellent contribution to the Conference on a "New Look at Commonwealth University Co-operation," the seminar sponsored by the Commonwealth Foundation.

        Your presentation on Community Medicine and Training of Allied Health Personnel is very much in accord with the stated policies of our own administration.

        I have requested my secretary to try to schedule early discussions with you on this subject, which was accepted by the Commonwealth Health Ministers' Conference.

Sincerely,

(Sgd.) Kenneth A. McNeill
KAM/pmc

5.   Letter to Minister of Health, Trinidad &Tobago re EC scheme

UNIVERSITY OF THE WEST INDIES

Dean's Office, Faculty of Medicine   4th April, 1974
Mona, Kingston 7
Jamaica, W.I.
Ref: 22/1 40/2

Hon. Minister of Health,
Ministry of Health,
Port-of-Spain, Trinidad & Tobago

Dear Minister,
Re: Undergraduate training of Medical Students in Trinidad and Tobago

1.   The present scheme for teaching in the Eastern Caribbean involves the Port of Spain General Hospital in the final year of our five-year curriculum. Approximately 25 students participate each year in clerkships in Internal Medicine, Obstetrics/Gynaecology and Surgery. We have in this year, in achieving our full target of clinical students, i.e. approx. 330, come to the position where the University Hospital at Mona with 500 beds is expected to handle a load of 280 clinical students.

2.   We feel in the best interests of medical education in the Caribbean that the excellent material and potential for education now existing in the Port of Spain Hospital should be utilised and tapped in an increasing way. Unless this is done, the quality of our education may deteriorate.

3.   You have supported the decision of the University Council to expand the capacity of the University to train medical doctors, when funds become available. Such an expansion would have a substantial part of its basis in the Eastern Caribbean.

4.   These two positions are interrelated. The second is a long-term extension of the clinical training already begun with current student numbers.

5.   The University Council considered this matter at its meeting on March 29th and has authorised me to propose for your consideration the development of a scheme to encompass the training of fourth-year medical students (second-year clinical) in Trinidad and Tobago.

6.   The exact manner whereby this may be accomplished would be a subject for discussion among various officials of your Government and of the University, to include, besides your Honour:

> The Hon. Minister of Education
> Permanent Secretary, Ministry of Health
> Principal Medical Officer
> Permanent Secretary, Ministry of Education
> Chief Education Officer

Permanent Secretary, Planning
Vice Dean, Eastern Caribbean and/or Associate Dean (Trinidad),
  Faculty of Medicine
Dean, Faculty of Medicine
Prof. L. Robinson, PVC Planning
The Principal, St Augustine
The Vice Chancellor
and any other person, according to your wishes.

7.   Members of the University will be in Trinidad for meetings at the St Augustine Campus between May 14th and May 18th. May I suggest that we try to meet on Wednesday 15th May, which seems to be the clearest day for those concerned. This would facilitate our travel arrangements as we are making a similar request to the Barbados Government*.

With best wishes,
Yours faithfully,

(Sgd.) M.S. Ragbeer, MB, DCP, MRC Path
      Dean, Medical Faculty
      cc: see list para.6

    * *As a result of these discussions, the Barbados government decided on an increase up to 25 students for the final year in Barbados, starting in 1975. This would consolidate the existing arrangement of 10-20 final year students that had begun in 1969. The new arrangement was expected to increase to fourth year students as soon as Government facilities were ready. At the same time a commitment to the clerkship in Community Medicine was made starting in 1975, and agreement given to the curricular revisions that would introduce students from year one to the social, cultural, behavioural, environmental and other strictly non-medical issues that determine good health and the occurrence of disease. This would repeat the conclusions of delegates to CHMC V re the multi-disciplinary inputs for Community Medicine: Agriculture, Engineering, Social Sciences, Ecology, to widen the scope of medical knowledge and practice.*
    This theme was discussed with EC students in T&T and Barbados, and the directions generally accepted; a few stated concerns re GMC requirements and were reassured that our new curriculum had been approved. It is quite likely that unless CARICOM governments made specific agreements with the UK, that GMC may begin to "drop" former colonial, now foreign schools from its approved lists. It is quite reasonable that we should develop our own high standards, and begin to think of external examiners from similar clinical settings, geographic and cultural, as the Caribbean. This provoked a lively debate, generally supportive, several anticipating postgraduate training, and later, academic careers at the UWI.

6. Letter from VC Preston re Salary (text only):

UNIVERSITY OF THE WEST INDIES
Senate House, Kingston 7, Jamaica

FROM THE VICE-CHANCELLOR   CABLE: UNIVERS

Telephone: 76661
Sept. 5, 1974
Dear Ragbeer,

In keeping with the decisions of the Finance and General Purposes Committee in June 1964 and November 1973, with regard to the review of the salaries of Professors, I have carried out such a review and I now write to let you know that I have decided that your salary should be increased by J$750 from the 1st July, 1974.

May I take this opportunity to express the appreciation of the University for the very valuable services that you are rendering.

Yours sincerely

(Sgd.) A.Z. Preston

Dr. M. Ragbeer
Dean, Faculty of Medicine, UWI

---

7. Letter from VC Preston re PAFAMS Appointment

UNIVERSITY OF THE WEST INDIES
Senate House, Kingston 7, Jamaica

FROM THE VICE-CHANCELLOR   CABLE: UNIVERS

Telephone: 76661

Our Reference ....

December 2, 1974

Dear Ragbeer,

Thanks for your letter of 28 November, 1974 informing me that you have been elected as the representative for Mexico, Central America and the Caribbean on the Council of the Pan American Federation of Associations of Medical Schools in Caracas. My congratulations on your election.

Yours sincerely,

(Sgd.) A. Z. Preston

Dr. M. Ragbeer
Dean, Faculty of Medicine, UWI

8.   Draft Memo to Mr. Paul Ellis, UHWI Director

To: Mr. Paul Ellis, Hospital Director

From: Dr M.S. Ragbeer, Dean, Medical Faculty; Member, UHWI Board

Proposal for the reorganisation of the UHWI Casualty Department

The Casualty Department, UHWI serves two main functions:
(1)   to handle emergency medical, surgical, obstetric and other cases
(2)   to cater to the needs of the casually ill, ambulant patients, by providing primary care, and referrals for specialist care.

Both are vital services, as in all Commonwealth Caribbean hospitals. We have no hard data however on the distribution of persons between these two functions, nor of the resources devoted to each, at the UHWI or in other hospitals in the region. Dr Carpenter has for some time tried unsuccessfully to launch a survey of the needs and resources of Casualty Departments in the major hospitals in the Kingston/St Andrew area, about 500,000 population, and containing the major hospitals in Jamaica. Anticipating the outcome of such a survey, and indeed its value, I suggest that we examine the structure of the existing Casualty Department to see whether it can logically and simultaneously subserve two functions that require quite different facilities, staffing, other resources and approaches.

UHWI monthly returns show that there is an increasing demand for Casualty Services. The Department is sorely understaffed — having a consultant and three SHOs, with three positions vacant. This level of staffing is quite incapable of operating a 24 hour service, and cannot offer full service on the basis of 8-hour shifts. Part time staff has helped temporarily to meet needs but these are individuals drawn from other services in their off-duty time, or private physicians without a commitment to education.

The Council of the University of the West Indies has recently decided on a program of expansion which includes the creation of a Division of Community Medicine in the University. The proposal is that the new Division of Community Medicine, when it is established — and this is expected by 1975 — should incorporate the present Department of Social and Preventive Medicine.

The Department of Social and Preventive Medicine has, at its head, a professor who is a specialist in Maternal and Child Health; a Senior Lecturer who is an Epidemiologist and specialist in Family Planning; and three lecturers: a medically qualified statistician, and two general medical officers; one of these is a former Casualty consultant, while the other position is vacant. As part of its teaching activities, it runs a service clinic for the residents of August Town, and attempts to provide general medical care for this population, akin to that available at the Casualty Department. This is essentially a field station for the department. It also serves the University Health Centre on Gibraltar Camp Road.

The Department has the following physical sections:
1.   a large waiting area, just off the main entrance
2.   a registration area
3.   six consulting rooms: three "medical," three "surgical."
4.   two inner waiting areas, for post-triage cases

5. a senior consultant's office, and doctors common room
6. service rooms, toilets, etc.

Just inside the main entrance is an emergency bay. There is an upper floor which contains an observation ward of 20 beds and a suite of theatres which are used for minor operations and for fractures. There is no clear separation between the facilities for handling emergencies and those that are required for the care of the more common self-referred ambulatory patients.

It is suggested that the Hospital Board make a policy decision to divide the Casualty Department physically into two main units according to its two main functions: an emergency centre, and a centre for ambulatory care.

1. The Emergency Centre

Exactly where this should be sited will remain to be planned in consonance with the long-term plans for the hospital which the architect is now preparing. Wherever it is sited, it should have the following characteristics:

(a) easy access to the main road;
(b) quick access to operating rooms, x-ray and lab facilities, and patient records;
(c) full equipment for resuscitation and for first aid treatment of medical, obstetric, surgical, psychiatric and other emergencies;
(d) easy access to the wards for admission of patients;
(e) full 24-hour coverage by emergency staff;
(g) it should be separate, if possible (physically, that is) from the area for the care of the ambulant patient.

2. The Ambulatory Care Area

The aim would be to provide a full range of primary care services for the ambulatory patient. There should be a fairly large waiting area (say for 400 persons) and a sufficient number of consulting rooms (10 or more). In addition to providing primary care services, this area and department can take over the organisation and running of certain clinics such as:

(i) the Well-baby and Immunisation clinic; a nutrition clinic
(ii) Maternal and Child welfare clinics dealing with ill patients or those requiring follow-up, particularly nutrition cases
(iii) Family Planning clinics; and consider adding
(iv) clinic services not now available here, for example: Venereal Diseases, Dermatology and other clinics as needs arise.

Staffing

(a) Emergency Area:

Staffing could be from among internes and residents of specialist units, but preferably with a core of permanent staff, trained for emergency work,. This requires more detail, from the educational and financial perspectives. The trend towards emergency medicine specialists will most likely dictate the pattern..

(b) Ambulatory Care Area

This area should be developed as part of a full Department, with the University duties of the training of General (Family) Practitioners, and medical students in their family practice rotation. This could also be the nucleus of the development of specialist programs in training physician specialists in Community Medicine. It is therefore suggested that all University lecturers and ranks above them, who are appointed to the Division of Community Medicine (CM), beginning with those now in the Department of Social and Preventive Medicine, should be appointed Consultants to this area. The resident staff should be provided from among the established Casualty posts in an appropriate number. The present consultant post in Casualty should be attached to the CM Division, with the primary responsibility for administering and running the Observation Ward and adjacent facilities. The Division of Community Medicine could also undertake the organisation of some of the clinics now classified under "Outpatients" but which are really General Practitioner or primary care service clinics, for example, the General Medicine, Maternity, Minor Surgery, Immunisation, Family Planning, and others as decided from time to time, and those not now in place, so that the specialist departments can be free to develop the specialty services within them and to develop joint programs with Community Medicine.

It would be advantageous if the Observation Ward were attached to the Ambulatory Care area, so that this department might have access to some beds which they will need in order to deliver adequate care to a percentage of their patients. Since some of the activities of such an area will impinge on those of specialist departments, it is suggested that the Community Medicine Division have the primary responsibility for their organisation, but that this organisation should be done in conjunction with the appropriate specialist departments. The area should also have its own small clinical laboratory in order to perform simple tests on blood, urine, faeces, and other body fluids. For more complex laboratory procedures the main hospital laboratory would be used.

It is further suggested that this ambulatory care area and the division of Community Medicine would become the nucleus from which the division could expand its activities into extramural district clinics, with the aim of taking health care to the surrounding communities, and thereby relieving the hospital of some of the load that it now comes to it, and save patients much time and expense.

For this to be effective, a clear policy decision must be made by the Ministry of Health, in which a geographic area is to be defined as the primary catchment area for the University Hospital for primary care purposes. A similar decision must be made for other public hospitals in the Kingston/St Andrew areas. This would also serve to free specialist personnel to do what they do best, secondary and tertiary care.

In conclusion, at this stage, what is being asked is that a policy decision be taken to divide Casualty services into its component parts. We are not asking at this stage that a clear decision be taken as to how this should be done; the issue merits the widest discussion within the Hospital among all parties concerned, all consultants and the staff of the Department of Social and Preventive Medicine. I have held preliminary talks with the Casualty Consultant and the Heads of the Department of Social And Preventive Medicine, Surgery, Obstetrics and Medicine, and with several other individuals who are aware of the situation. It would be advisable to resurrect Dr Carpenter's suggestion to survey the use to which all Casualty Departments in the KSAC are put. The results of such a survey would determine the kind of services and the amount of resources appropriate to each activity in each location. The development of the idea, however, does not have to await the completion of such a survey.

The Board is urged to recommend this while considering a decision on policy. If it approves, this draft can be circulated to all department heads as a basis for discussions, now that the University has approved the postgraduate programs, the post of Director of Community Medicine, and is now favourably considering the establishment of an academic Division of Community Medicine.

(Sgd.) M.S. Ragbeer, Dean

cc   Vice-Dean, Clinical;

      President, Medical Staff; Clinical department heads; Dr Carpenter.

9. First two paragraphs of a letter from Paul Ellis, Hospital Director to VC Preston, UWI re Hospital capital needs

UNIVERSITY HOSPITAL OF THE WEST INDIES

AND TELEGRAPHIC ADDRESS
"UNIVERSITY"
PHONE (P B X.) 74431

MONA, ST. ANDREW,
JAMAICA, W.I.

May 20, 1974.

REF.

Mr. A.Z. Preston,
Vice Chancellor,
University of the West Indies,
MONA.

Dear Mr. Preston,

Re: Medical Faculty Problems

The Board of Management of the University Hospital of the West Indies has been for some time concerned with certain pressing problems which have beset the Medical Faculty of the University of the West Indies. Accordingly, the juxtaposition of the Department in relation to the Hospital and the inter-related factors inherent therein, has revealed that these problems will by necessity have a marked effect on the present and future role of the Hospital.

The problems confronting the Medical Faculty have been identified as follows:-

    (1)   Recruitment and Retention of Medical Staff

    (2)   Increasing Service Load of U.H.W.I.

    (3)   Teaching Facilities

    (4)   U.H.W.I. not attracting Interns.

10. Letter from Dr Alexander Robertson, WHO/EMRO, Cairo re proposed project in PGME for Egypt and the ME

I include this as indication of the regard held by a WHO official for our PGME initiatives. Dr Robertson had served on the IADB Committee)

<u>PERSONAL</u>

Dear Rags,

I am writing informally and without, at the moment, any WHO commitment, to enquire whether there would be any possibility of your assisting for a period during 1974, of say, one month to six weeks, in a consultant capacity, in connection with our development program of postgraduate and continuing education in medicine in the Eastern Mediterranean Region.

The Regional Director has recently approved in principle that should start to move during 1974 in developing more intensive inter-country programs in this field, with a view to promoting development of post-graduate and continuing education in medicine within certain countries of the Region.

We feel that such a development would be timely at this juncture because of a variety of factors including:

(a)   The mounting demand for post graduate training especially to man the new and expanding faculties with teachers;

(b)   The apparent overloading of certain of our traditional host countries, especially the United kingdom;

(c)   The gradually mounting acceptance, in at least some quarters (probably more in the Ministries than in the Universities) of new practices to post-graduate and continuing education and (perhaps?) a realisation that British Royal Colleges and American universities with their memberships and Ph.D. do not provide the best answer;

(d)   Our own policy of dissuading long-term fellowships abroad doing something more than we are so far doing, to help preserve opportunities within the Region.

Sometime after the end of the first quarter of 1974, we are hoping to be able to embark on a survey in depth, (lists, descriptions and evaluation, etc.) of existing post-graduate programs in the Region and to assemble one or more small teams of consultants to make the necessary visits and accumulate the required information. We would then hope to produce a background paper for a small working group to meet sometime in 1975, discuss the findings and recommendations with these consultant teams and make definitive recommendations to the Organisation for a suitable program of activities in support of postgraduate education, which might include the designation of high quality and relevant programs as WHO Regional Post-graduate medical Centres.

I should be grateful to have a preliminary indication of your interest in the assignment, with the idea that if you were interested and the matter became subsequently formalised we might ask you to visit one or two countries concerned in company with one other consultant…from the Eastern Mediterranean Region…   Sandy

11. Letter to Professor K.L. Stuart re Committees on which Dean serves

18/3/75
To: Professor K.L. Stuart
From: Dean, Medical Faculty

The following is a list of Committees of the University and Faculty on which the Dean (or his nominee as noted) is a member, or is observer:

1.   EX-OFFICIO

A.   University Committees
        Council
        Finance & General Purposes Committee
        Finance Committee, Mona
*   Technical Assistants Committee, Mona
        Appointments Committee
        Assessments & Promotions Committee
        Estimates Committee, Mona
        Senate
        University Academic Committee
        Planning Committee
        Academic Board, Mona
        Board, Faculty of Medicine
*   Board for Higher Degrees
*   Board for Examinations
*   Board for Postgraduate Studies
*   Board for Undergraduate Awards
*   Matriculation Board
*   Research & Publications Committee
        Admissions Committee
        Nursing Education Committee
        Advisory Committee on Student Health

B   Faculty of Medicine

        Dean's Committee
        Curriculum Committee
        Finance Committee
        Assessments & Promotions
        Higher Degrees Committee
        Specialty Boards (at present TEN))
        Advisory Committee for Sick Students

C   University (or Faculty) representative on Committees or Boards
        CFNI Policy Committee
        Caribbean Health Ministers Conference
        Commonwealth Caribbean – Medical Research Council
        CAREC (former TRVL)

Pan-American Federation of Associations of Medical Schools

D University Hospital of the West Indies

Board of Management
Planning Committee
Executive Committee
Princess Alice Award
Research & Publications Committee

E Governments

Jamaica Government Health Advisory Committee

2. AD PERSONAM

Standing Committee of CHMC
Administrative Committee of PAFAMS
Medical Committee, UHWI
Boards of Management, Kingston and Cornwall Regional Hospitals

Dean or Nominee
**Occasional Member*

(Sgd.) M.S. Ragbeer

The post bypass heart: a symbol of life-saving medical specialisation, now practised in the Caribbean, and, with its companion procedure, "stenting", a tribute to the numerous scientists who have contributed to their current status.

(To be read with Fig 8-1, p.73)

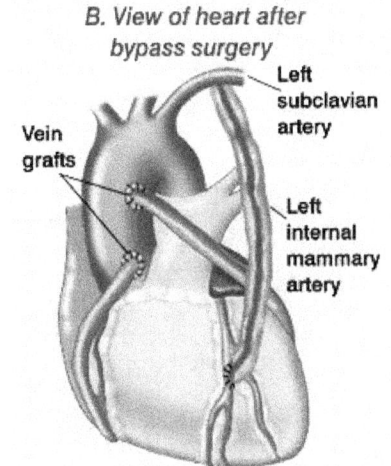

B. View of heart after bypass surgery

12. Correspondence between Editor, WIMJ and Dean: (a controversial issue: the role of WIMJ in medical information.)

THE WEST INDIAN MEDICAL JOURNAL

UNIVERSITY OF THE WEST INDIES
JAMAICA, W.I.
18ᵗʰ June, 1973

Dr. M.S. Ragbeer,
Dean,
U.W.I.

Dear Dr. Ragbeer,

I apologize for the delay in coming to a definite conclusion about your article "INNOVATION AND CHANGE IN MEDICAL EDUCATION IN THE COMMONWEALTH CARIBBEAN."

The Editors looked carefully at it after it was reviewed and the conclusion was that if it were a critical analysis of factical (*sic*) data related to the subject then it would be suitable for publication. Unfortunately it was felt that as it stood we could not publish it in the Journal.*

This does not mean that we will not consider papers related to the area of medical education for publication in the future.

Yours sincerely,
G.A.O. Alleyne M.D., F.R.C.P.
Editor

The Reply:
19ᵗʰ July, 1973

Professor G.A.O. Alleyne
Editor, The West Indian Medical Journal.

Dear Professor Alleyne,

Many thanks for your letter of 18ᵗʰ June, 1973 concerning an article *"Innovation and Change in Medical Education in the Commonwealth Caribbean."*

I think there is some misunderstanding here – as I indicated to you in conversation some time ago. The article I submitted to the *West Indian Medical Journal* was as requested and as modified by Dr T. Persaud, the previous editor of the Journal, and in fact should have appeared in the issue of September 1972. For reasons with which I am not familiar, the publication was delayed. I understand from Mrs. Forrest that the original copy submitted sometime in April of 1972 was not received. This may have accounted for the delay. I am therefore a bit taken aback by your note which indicates clearly that there has been no continuity of information or communication between the previous editor and his successor, nor indeed was any system set up to ensure that this kind of embarrassment did not occur to the Journal's potential contributors.

The previous editor did spend a fair amount of time with me orienting the paper in a particular way to make it provocative to its readership, and it was the specific intent to have this inserted in the Journal as a special article for comment. I feel further that if any uncertainty existed as to its suitability for insertion in the Journal, then I could have been contacted before and apprised of the reason for the uncertainty.

Finally, the article was specifically not intended as a "critical analysis of factical data"; I do not know what "factical" is – presumably "tactical" or "factual" – but as a descriptive one indicating the position from which one wants to move.

I hope this clarifies the position.

Yours sincerely,
M.S. Ragbeer, Dean

* The rejection was final; there was no suggestion for revision, or indication that Journal policy will be re-examined. In presenting the article to the previous editor, Dr TVN Persaud, I had informed him that Prof Eric Cruickshank when he was Dean, and his successor, Prof Kenneth Stuart had endorsed it, but pressure to complete other things had delayed its completion. Prof Cruickshank had put the draft to the old Faculty Board as a Minute Paper for comment. The argument then was that the Journal was failing in its duty to inform readers of policy and education matters in the Faculty, and to invite feedback and comment (e.g. letters), as allowed by most good journals e.g. New England Medical Journal., Lancet, BMJ etc.*

In 1964, I had visited Glasgow, and learned of changes in the medical curriculum, and later read a descriptive article, in a 1969 issue of the Scottish Medical Journal, *which I pointed out to Dr Alleyne. Eugene Garfield, the publisher of* Current Contents, *told me that WIMJ did not match its competition, and should change, unless it saw itself as a research journal, in which case, it had a "far, far way to go. There was no way to tell who was getting what from the journal," least of all the public, and the non-medical academic community, a criticism that educationist, Professor Kassim Bacchus of University of Alberta (and formerly UWI) had also levelled. Prof. Alleyne was not impressed. It is interesting that at a PAHO Conference later, in 1979, discussing Medical Education at the UWI (See* Proceedings, Bibliography*), he would advocate some of the very ideas he had ignored in 1972, on objective examinations (MCQs) and had matured enough in thought to express concern for the Faculty's "responsibilities to the public at large!" That was good to know as it was the same public I was trying to reach with my "Innovation and Change..." article, in 1972, seven years earlier!*

Prof Cruickshank had also noted a difficulty to get cooperation of colleagues. (p 149)

This exchange is included to show how stodgy our young academics remained, less adventurous than their parent institutions, despite constraints by the GMC, which had accepted our innovations. See also comment in box below:

"Much less is done by poor country academics than is required, partly because of their inability personally and institutionally to break from the influence of their training, their inherited syllabuses, and the patterns of thought reflected in rich country journals. The absence of an effective analytical approach has been a weakness in research, extension and policy making."
R. Jolly and L. Joy, *New Directions for Inter-university Cooperation,* Commonwealth Foundation Occ. Paper X IX, p.40, 1973.

Appendix 16:

THE ORGANISATION AND DELIVERY OF HEALTH CARE IN DEVELOPING COUNTRIES, ? A MODEL FOR CHEDOKE HOSPITALS
The Annual Chedoke Foundation Lecture, 1978

Dr Allison, Mr. Hamilton, Mr. Allan, Distinguished Members of this High Table, Colleagues, Ladies and Gentlemen: Good Evening,

I am deeply thankful to Dr Jim Allison, the Director of the Chedoke Hospital, for his interest in my activities in health care research and manpower development, which I have been privileged to experience first-hand in India, Bangladesh, parts of East and West Africa, the anglophone and francophone Caribbean, and Suriname from a working base at the University of the West Indies, where I hope that the plans laid and structures built for health manpower production will survive the fret and fury that forced me into exile.

I also humbly thank the Foundation for the high honour of inviting me to give this talk. It is not often that an advanced country looks off into the less privileged, or so-called third world for a model of anything, since from time immemorial, the other way round has been more fashionable.

To provide background to an understanding of the environment of the work referred to here, I'll show you a series of slides and comment briefly on each to draw attention to particular points. They cover selected developing and developed countries, and show data on gross national product; sources of income; population; population distribution by age and sex; population growth rate; literacy rates; levels of education; fertility patterns; morbidity and mortality statistics; perinatal mortality; life expectancy at birth; health care services organisation; number of hospital beds; types of illnesses seen; infrastructure — roads, pure water, sewage treatment, health care facilities, urban and rural, etc.; training and educational facilities available for health professionals; and other similar and relevant indices.[39]

"These were gathered from United Nations statistical reviews, OECD reports, and similar official documents. The big stimulus for us was the brain drain of UWI graduates, as former colonies were gaining independence and beginning to realise that the buck no longer crossed the Atlantic, and Caribbean Government ministers began to look to the UWI for answers. The demands on the Medical Faculty began while I was an Associate Dean, and intensified during my tenure as the first full-time Dean, from 1971 to 1975.

"From this basis, we developed a comprehensive educational model for manpower, planning to use existing hospitals as training bases for all needs of the people they serve, in such a way that all basic services would be provided by personnel specifically trained to provide them. Complex care was provided at regional or district hospitals, and primary care at health centres and district clinics. Each would organise and deliver care, clinical and public health, for

---

[39] These were covered in about twenty slides; developed countries were OECD members, while developing countries cited were Barbados, Colombia, India, Jamaica and Tanzania, covering a spread in size, population and economy.

individuals of all ages, including promotive and preventive health interventions e.g., immunisations, nutrition education, health education, exercise directives, well baby care, etc., aiming to maintain health and prevent illness. A new Division of Community Medicine, to be based at the University Hospital, is still experimental; it was developed independently by a group of us from the Pan-American Federation of Associations of Medical Schools, of which Canada, the ACMC, is a member. It is funded by a Kellogg Foundation grant. The design hopefully can suit any community. It is similar to the concept of primary care that has given Cuba the best health statistics in the hemisphere, despite severe economic sanctions by the USA. Canada, by contrast, is a developed economy that has gone beyond economising, and may well regard a plan designed for integration of clinical and public health functions for a community, for optimising use of skills, and achieving low cost:benefit ratios as unduly stingy.

But here at Chedoke, a city hospital in a developed country, the attitude is refreshingly more open to innovation, and it is willing to see itself as a comprehensive health centre for this region of Ontario. The principles underlying this have universal validity, and from this basis I would like to show how Chedoke already possesses the elements to become the hub of an integrated system such as I have depicted. You are all very familiar with the following components of health services *(slides on p. 57, figs 5-2 & 5- 3)*:

  i) Problems: primary, secondary, tertiary levels of difficulty and complexity
  ii) Institutions: primary, secondary and tertiary levels
  iii) Personnel: from aides to specialist professionals

Efficiency demands that the most appropriate method be used to address a particular need, in this case solve a health problem: these include sanitary facilities with adequate space; suitably trained personnel; proper organisation and tested methods.

Chedoke is at the centre of a visible and definable community, with established links with sister institutions. It is already involved in primary, secondary, and tertiary care and has units for special functions, which are developed to a high degree: rehabilitation, orthopedics, child and family services, clinical laboratory disciplines, complex seniors care, etc. It has major educational functions in many disciplines, such as medicine, nursing, technology, sociology and psychology. It enjoys community participation in planning, and through volunteer groups. It has *informal* linkages with commerce, industry, agriculture, and education, in relation to the planning of care and delivery of services.

Conditions that would define its suitability to take charge of community care include:

i.   <u>An established plant.</u> Developing countries generally need more physical facilities, and those present are often not easily accessible to the majority of the population, especially in large rural areas with poor infrastructure and inadequate or expensive transport, normal and emergency. The percentage rurality here in Ontario is less than 30; in Tanzania it is more than 80; and 70 in India. The miles of paved roads per unit of population is considerably higher here, and transport is affordable, and mostly private. Health authorities in developing countries often have to start from scratch by building such plants as this, then fan out into construction of the peripheral units in population centres (Fig 5, p. 378). Some argue that the peripheral unit should come first so as to reach the majority. But illness is unpredictable, and peripheral clinics cannot stand alone; they need the backing of a sophisticated medical centre within easy reach. Developing countries often lack funds for adequate staffing and equipment for the various sectors of the system, and may not qualify for loans to the full extent needed for capital buildings and equipment from development banks. Chedoke has a fully functional plant, and a mature administration

ii.   The administrative machinery. This can handle the planning needed, and it already has the manpower, the infrastructure and organisation, to take on the further steps towards implementation of these plans. The North American health system is a loose, often competitive aggregation of units, usually highly sophisticated general hospitals, well-endowed, with many specialised departments. Services are centralised and access relatively easy for those referred to them and from urban or rural areas. Outreach to the population in primary need, somewhere between 70 and 80 % of all care, is not yet an integral part of the hospital mission. Yet hospitals have the capacity to do this, to knit together primary care services into a network, and are probably the only institutions able to develop them (Fig. 5, p. 378). Some have, in addition, enough spare capacity and the creativity to develop integrated models. With its concentration of skills and equipment, what more logical base is there for comprehensive outreach?

iii. The changing age of the population of communities and the higher life expectancies must inevitably affect the pattern of health care delivery. Hospitalisation is everywhere expensive. We have not adequately researched, and therefore remain ignorant of the many physiological changes people undergo as they age, but society thinks that we know. Few among us, lay and professional alike, think of this as a serious problem. Yet we all abandon our old, or appear to do so, and most of us do not think of old age until we get there. It is perhaps human nature, as long as health lasts, to deny the things that tell us how old we are. Some tribes from the Guiana Highlands of South America have dealt with the elderly a little more dispassionately; they simply put them, at their request, each in his own canoe, then point it to the nearest sizeable waterfall; indeed, one of the world's most majestic of such falls, the Kaieteur, got its name from this practice, the word meaning "old man's falls" (Slide of Falls).

Hospitalisation of the elderly is not the answer to our problem. The hospital can be lethal to the elderly, as is well known. It often brings on serious infections, and the isolation and inactivity can be deadly to the elderly mind and body. Being in the company of others and having continual activity are known benefits. Yet they need the services that only hospitals like this can offer as a back-up to long-term community care facilities yet to be provided in sufficient quantity for them. Is the coordinated care of the elderly not a legitimate innovation for this hospital, which has already established itself in this field, these premises providing the central facilities for coordination of such activities and controlling, administratively and medically, a variety of peripheral facilities, private or group homes, in each community, where the elderly can gainfully, naturally and profitably spend their days? How often are the old consulted on what's best for them? We have two duties:

(a) To study their needs more critically

(b) To plan for and meet these needs humanely and effectively, preserving individual dignity and self-respect. This constitutes a large percentage of the primary care that our population now needs and will need increasingly in the future as the population ages. The old and near-old number as many as other age groups, as I have shown you in the population breakdown. Leadership in this area of primary care is sorely needed, as are cooperative actions by community institutions, the public and government.

Chedoke, as I see it, is eminently suited for this function and should be allowed by the Health Ministry to develop into a model centre for the acute, ambulatory and continuing care of the elderly, in addition to the other functions I have mentioned.

iv. Community acceptance and respect. – this is self-evident. The presence of this large audience here tonight is evidence of the respect that the community holds for this institution.

v. A concerned and spirited Board of Management. Administrative wisdom and perceptiveness are crucial in planning and development of innovative schemes. Unwieldy or overly bureaucratic approaches often impede rather than facilitate. Flexibility is key, and careful attention to objectives is mandatory. We have seen the style and method of operation of our Board and feel that they form a body that would be equal to the task of supervising the development and expansion of this institution into a comprehensive community medicine centre for this region and a model for the province.

vi. A working environment that is cooperative and promotive of the best that individuals can provide from their background of education, training and experience. The environment in this hospital is one of cooperation and mutual respect. There are few institutions that I have been to where these qualities are so highly developed, and where morale is at such a high pitch. I know there are many forces at work which will eventually, if successful, erode this morale and destroy this ambience. It is up to the governors of this institution and its directorate to be sufficiently cautious in dealing with these forces, which currently come as suitors with offers. The kind of working environment I am talking about is fragile and can be destroyed very quickly by rumor and falsification, especially when propped up by political manoeuverings. I am convinced however that an environment such as this would be a key factor in assisting the institution to lead the region in holistic thinking in health care delivery, feeding the results of its endeavours into what my Latin American friends call "the National Eco System" as depicted in the following slide (*Fig 5, p. 378*).

The concepts that I've described, began as pilot projects in several developing countries, and are entirely applicable here. The key stimulus in the developing countries has been the need to use resources efficiently and achieve a high quality of care at low cost. This work is in its infancy, hampered by lack of personnel and finances, and more seriously by political storms such as the ones that blew me here. But Cuba has soldiered on, and remains the prime success, envied even by Americans, who currently spend ten times as much for less..

North America has been more fortunate with its resources, as I have shown. But it is now at a stage when it is asked to cut back on services (slide) and to innovate (slide). The striking difference between here and the developing countries is that here we already have in place the most expensive requirements for comprehensive health care: fully equipped hospital facilities in each community, staffed with a wide range of highly skilled personnel of different levels and in nearly all sectors of care. Chedoke possesses that wide range of facilities; activities are well established; it has the respect of the community. It is poised nicely to reach out and give leadership to the municipalities and wider community around it.

It is comforting in this regard to note that members in the immediate vicinity are already participating in this action. And here I should re-stress the importance of a community role in the widest sense — both the consuming sectors and contributors to its functional efficiency: educators, agriculturists (farmers), businessmen, industrialists, men of commerce, professionals, law enforcers, students in general, and others, whose intimate knowledge of their environment and people provide insights that could otherwise be lacking, and so decrease the depths of perception of ideas, or penetration of schemes devised for a particular area. Councils representing broad community interests are invaluable in the overall administrative structure and in the different levels of function of any scheme. It would be short-sighted and imprudent to dismantle these excellent arrangements and cloud the vision so convincingly being developed within this institution. The informed and perceptive leadership, and other attributes already on-site, if dismantled and scattered, would be impossible or extremely expensive to assemble again, like a broken Humpty Dumpty. More important, it has a unique atmosphere of camaraderie and a long history of clinical and academic excellence. With support from its Board fuelling the energies of its staff, only a disaster can impede its development into a prototype of a hospital extending long arms of service into its surrounding communities, uniting them and sharing with them the best of medical care.

I look forward to contributing whatever I can to foster the notion that the General Hospital should be the community's centre of excellence in health care delivery at all levels of care, research and spread of learning. Despite examples of the successful integration of preventive and curative medicine to individuals, and communities to promote health for all, societies continue to divide the practice of medicine into mutually exclusive groups of curative, or hospital, and preventive, or public health, when a merger promises the greatest benefits at least cost to society.

The current division passes off without much comment in rich countries, but poor nations, trained in rich country ways, continue learned habits willy-nilly. Two years ago, a team from the UWI was in this University courting a most expensive curricular plan, and about to discard a superior, home-grown model, which, if implemented as planned, could teach lessons, even to those who may be too wealthy to listen. My research project in Jamaica was in Nutrition, funded by the US NIH; we used a rodent model, and with dietary manipulation alone we could extend their lives by 250%, while they remained healthy, alert and active, maintaining a steady weight of a trim 200-250 grams, one third of their strain's average high body mass on a standard commercial diet. The promotion of health and prevention of illness combined with good diet worked for that biological model. Why not for humans? Why not here?

I thank you very much for being such a wonderful audience..."

Mohan Ragbeer, 1978

Figs App. 16-1&2 are the same as those in Ch.5, figs 5-2&3.

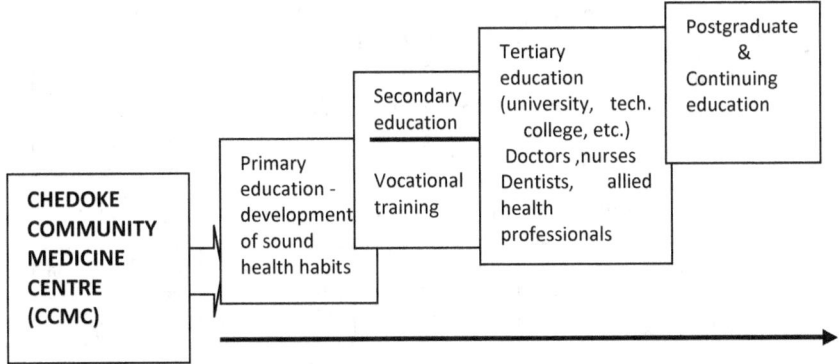

Health Education, Vocational and Professional Training, Continuing Education are conceived in a continuum shown by the arrow ➤

Fig. App. 16-3   *Conceptual Diagram of the C.C.M.C.'s Involvement in Education*

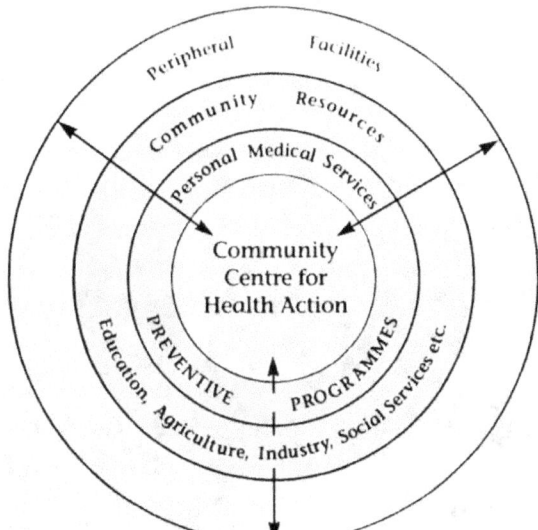

Fig App. 16-4: Inter-relationships of Community Medicine Centre with components of health care (same as UWI's Manchester Project in Community Medicine)

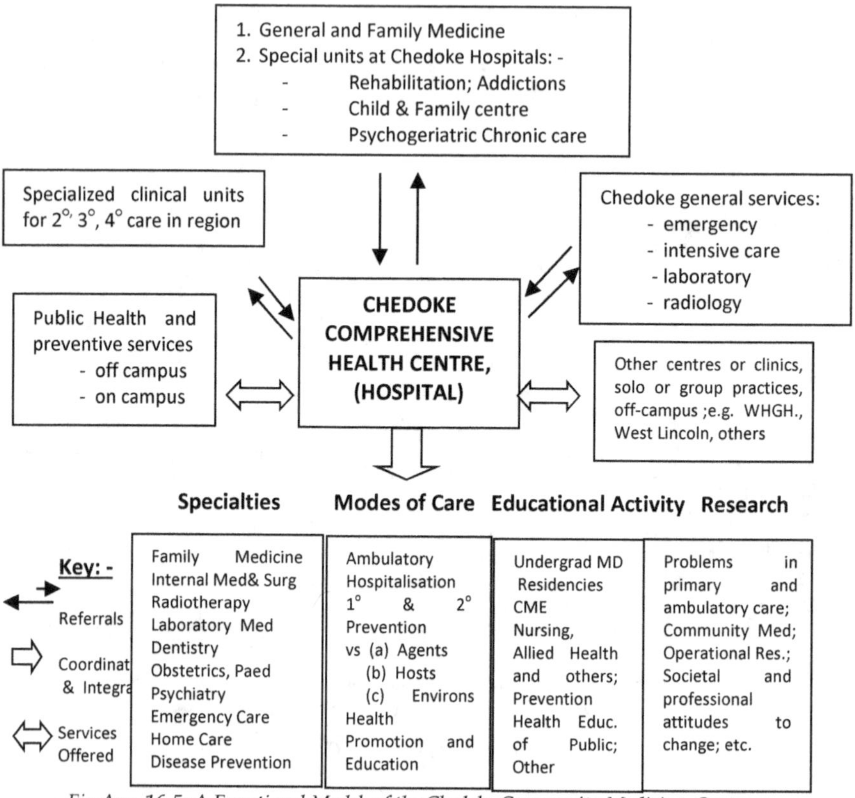

1. General and Family Medicine
2. Special units at Chedoke Hospitals: -
   - Rehabilitation; Addictions
   - Child & Family centre
   - Psychogeriatric Chronic care

Specialized clinical units for 2°, 3°, 4° care in region

Chedoke general services:
   - emergency
   - intensive care
   - laboratory
   - radiology

Public Health and preventive services
   - off campus
   - on campus

CHEDOKE COMPREHENSIVE HEALTH CENTRE, (HOSPITAL)

Other centres or clinics, solo or group practices, off-campus ;e.g. WHGH., West Lincoln, others

Key: -

→ Referrals

⇨ Coordinat & Integra

⟺ Services Offered

	Specialties	Modes of Care	Educational Activity	Research
	Family Medicine	Ambulatory	Undergrad MD	Problems in
	Internal Med& Surg	Hospitalisation	Residencies	primary and
	Radiotherapy	1° & 2°	CME	ambulatory care;
	Laboratory Med	Prevention	Nursing,	Community Med;
	Dentistry	vs (a) Agents	Allied Health	Operational Res.;
	Obstetrics, Paed	(b) Hosts	and others;	Societal and
	Psychiatry	(c) Environs	Prevention	professional
	Emergency Care	Health	Health Educ.	attitudes to
	Home Care	Promotion and	of Public;	change; etc.
	Disease Prevention	Education	Other	

Fig App. 16-5: A Functional Model of the Chedoke Community Medicine Centre

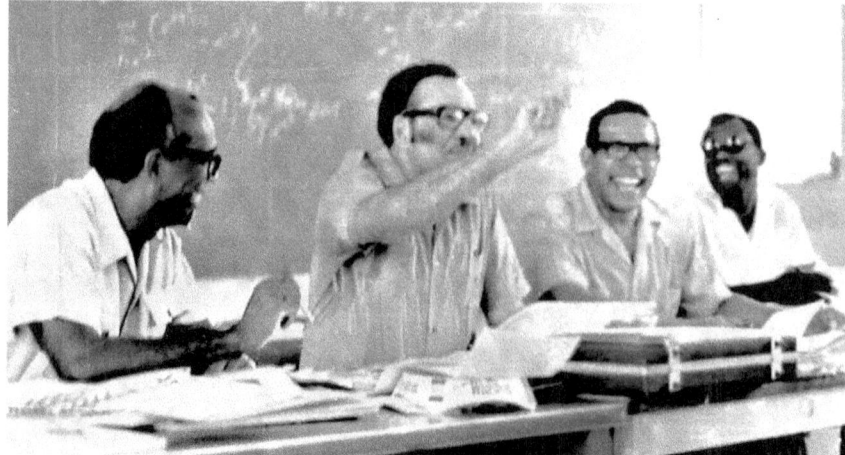

Fig App. 16-6: The UWI Registrar Carl Jackman, VC Preston, Bursar H. Holness, cited often in text above, 1975; fourth person is an official at St. Augustine

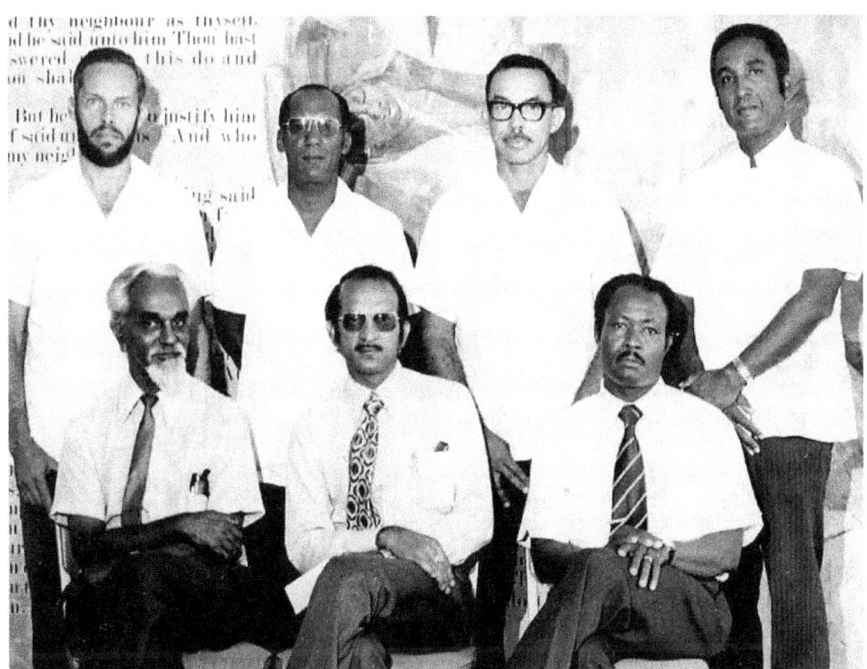

Fig App. 16-7: Farewell, 1975: Back: Colin Miller, Rolf Richards, Owen Minott, Frank Ramsay (B'dos); Front: Sir Harry Annamunthodo, Mohan Ragbeer, Manley West

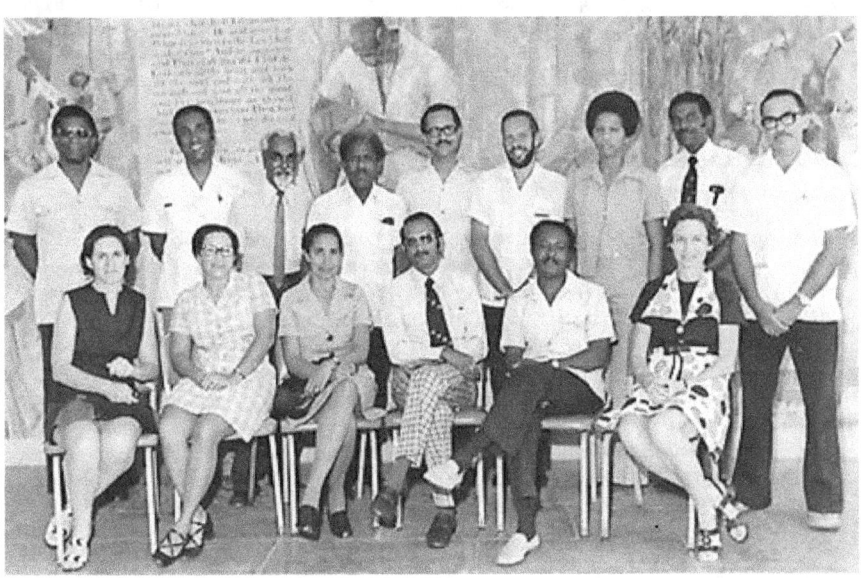

Fig App. 16-8: On my leaving, 1975:
Front; J. Young*, D. Jung*, D. King-Wynter, M. Ragbeer, M. West, A, Costa*
Back: S. Wray, F. Ramsay, (B'dos), H. Annamunthodo, K. Stuart, S. Brooks, C. Miller, N. Rainford,* H. Wynter, O. Minott (* = Dean's office staff)

Bibliography
(Many of my own papers are listed as primary sources for this book)

Andrade J., *Marco conceptual de la educación médica en la América Latina.* Washington, D.C,
PAHO, 1979

Ashley D, and Bernal R., *Poliomyelitis in Jamaica: immunization policies and socioeconomic
implications,* World Health Forum. 6 (3):265-7, 1985

ASCOFAME, El Medico General, una respuesta al Futuro ed. Ruiz HJ, Bogota, 1978

Bobula JA, *Examinations and Decision-Making* WHO/EDUC/73.170

Bowers. J., *Medical schools for the developing World,* Baltimore, Johns Hopkins, 1970

Braithwaite ER., *To sir, With Love,* London, Bodley Head, 1959

Bryant, J., *in Reform of Medical Education,* New York, Fogarty International, 1969.

Ceitlin, Julio, *ed., Medicina de la Comunidad,* Caracas, Venezuela, FEPAFEM/Kellogg, 1978

Clark DW & MacMahon B. *eds., Preventive Medicine,* Boston, Little, Brown, 1967

Crevans JR and Condliffe PG, *eds., Reform of Medical Education,* NIH, Washington DC, 1970

Cyrus, CA., *Clinical and Pathological Atlas: The Records of a Surgeon in St Vincent, WI.* Kingstown,
The Botanic Clinic, 1991

Ibid, *A Dream come True, autobiography of a Caribbean surgeon,* USA, Amazon, 2015

Educating Tomorrow's Doctors, Symposium Papers and Conference Report, 2 volumes, Copenhagen,
4th WMA Conference, 1972

Eldemire-Shearer D & Roberts S., *Doctor of medicine training–reflections on the UWI (Mona)
experience,* WIMJ, 57, 6, 2008,

Feinsilver Julie M., *Healing the Masses: Cuban Health Politics at Home and Abroad,* Berkeley and
LA, USA, University of Calif Press, 1993

Flexner, A. *Medical education in the United States and Canada; a report to the Carnegie Foundation for
the Advancement of Teaching,* Bulletin No. 4, New York, 1910, 1960

Grell G, Ho-Ping-Kong H, Ragbeer MS *et al. Peritoneal Dialysis in severe Leptospiral Renal Failure,*
WIMJ, 20, 76,1971.

Melville GN, Wray SR, Addae J, Young LE. *Progress in medical education in the Faculty of Medical
Sciences, University of the West Indies: implementation of problem-based learning at the St. Augustine
Campus.* West Indian Med J., 42(3):94-100,1993

NIHAE Bull. 10(1):2-4, 1977

Pathak B., *Road to Freedom,* London, Vedic books, 2000 ISBN8120812581

Peter LJ. and Hull, R., *The Peter Principle,* New York, Bantam Books, 1965

Postgraduate Education & Training in Public Health, WHO Technical Report Series # 533, 1973

Proceedings: Workshop on Medical Education, joint PAHO, UWI, Runaway Bay, Jamaica, 1979

Ragbeer MS, *An excess of Heart Disease among East Indians in British Guiana, Report to Ministry of
Home Affairs,* accepted for presentation at MRC Conference, Port-of-Spain, 1963; presented
also at Public Health Hamilton, ON /CICA Seminar on Heart Disease, 1997

Ragbeer MS and Khan GM., *A four-year program for the training of medical technologists at the
University of Guyana and at the College of Arts, Sciences and Technology,* Kingston, Jamaica, 1966.
(Implemented by both institutions).

Ragbeer MS, *Comparison of Objective (MCQ's) and essay examinations for Part I (Pathology) of the
Final MBBS Examination,* UWI, Board of Medical Examiners, 1966, 1967. (Reviewers included
external examiners.)

Ragbeer MS and Jutsum P., *Computer-assisted analysis of multiple choice questions,* UWI
Department of Pathology Examinations Board, 1967

Ragbeer MS, *Performance characteristics of 3300 multiple choice questions tested for Part I (Pathology)
of the Final MBBS Examination,* UWI. Faculty Paper, Mimeo, 1969

Ragbeer MS, EK Cruickshank, Sandison J, Pathak UN, Back E, and Standard KL., *Postgraduate
Training to the level of Diploma (1-2 years) in Pathology, Obstetrics and Gynaecology, Public Health,
Community Medicine, and Child Health,* Faculty of Medicine Paper, UWI Calendar, 1969

Ragbeer MS and Hoyte D., *Objectives of undergraduate medical education–defining performance expectations of the graduate*–Dean's Invitational Seminar on Curriculum Reform, Faculty of Medicine, UWI, Feb.,1969

Ragbeer MS, *The Undergraduate Curriculum, Medical Faculty, UWI - an opinion*, Stethoscope 6,8, 1970

Ragbeer MS, Stuart KL, Butler A, Forde H, and Bartholomew C., *Proposals for the development of Programs in Postgraduate Medical Education in the eastern Caribbean*; submitted to the Ministers of Health of Trinidad & Tobago, and Barbados. 1972, revised 1973

Ragbeer MS., *Plenary Panel Report on "Identifying Determinants of Medical Education,"* in *EDUCATING TOMORROW'S DOCTORS*, Copenhagen, Denmark, Proceedings of the World Medical Association Conference IV, 1972

Ragbeer MS, Wilson J and Burke LM., *The new Cornwall Regional Hospital, Montego Bay, Jamaica, a Report to the Minister of Health with recommendations on its commissioning for a major role in postgraduate and undergraduate medical education*, Kingston, Jamaica Ministry of Health, and Faculty of Medicine, UWI, Mona, 1972

Ragbeer MS,. *Postgraduate Medical Education in the Commonwealth Caribbean*, WIMJ 21, 147, 1972

Ragbeer MS, Bras G & Preston AZ., *Postgraduate Medical Education at the UWI: Detailed Plans and Estimates of Costs*, Hamilton, Bermuda CHMC III, 7a,7b,7c (37pp), (80pp) 1971

Ragbeer, MS and Bras G., *Paramedical Training at the UWI, Information. Paper 2b*, Bridgetown, Barbados, CHMC II, 1970

Ragbeer MS & Burton C., *Collaboration between Government and the University on Health Matters (why the "town" and "gown" should woo)*, (11pp), Georgetown, Guyana, CHMC IV, 18, 1972

Ragbeer MS, Robertson, A, Sahoy R, Arscott P, Comissiong, L et al: *Requirements of the Commonwealth Caribbean for Postgraduate-trained Doctors (the COPMED Reports, 88pp)*, Georgetown, Guyana, CHMC IV, 18, 1972

Ragbeer MS, Hoyte D and Stuart KL ,*The initiation of Postgraduate Medical Training at the UWI - Progress Report*, Roseau, Dominica (4pp).CHMC V, 1973

Ragbeer MS, *Proposals for a Regional Forensic Service for the Commonwealth Caribbean, (7pp)*, Roseau, Dominica, CHMC V, 1973

Ragbeer, MS, Golding J. and Martin F., *The Needs of the Jamaica Health Services for Specialist doctors."* UWI and Ministry of Health, Jamaica, 1973

Ragbeer, M.S *The role of the new university in the training of Medical Ancillaries*, London, Commonwealth Foundation Occasional Paper, XIX, 1973

Ragbeer MS, *Learning Theory and Medical Education in Developing Countries - a Curriculum for Saudi Arabia*, WHO, Alexandria, Egypt, 1973

Ragbeer MS, Smith K., Miller C.G. and Standard KL: *Community Medicine, concept and definitions*, UWI, Faculty of Medicine Paper, 1974

Ragbeer MS and Smith K,*The teaching of Community Medicine to undergraduates*, ibid,1974

Ragbeer MS, *The Medical Faculty, UWI - Twenty five years of Activity, 1949-74*, WIMJ, 1974: 23, 113-128

Ragbeer MS, Stuart KL. Davies A., Alleyne G, &.Standard K., *A model of Health Care Delivery*, CCMRC, Mona, Jamaica and CHMC VI, Nassau, Bahamas, 1974

Ragbeer MS, *Approaches to the Delivery of Health Care in Developing Countries, a study of projects in Bangladesh, India, Kenya, Nigeria and Tanzania*, London, The Commonwealth Foundation, 1975

Ragbeer MS and Smith K, *The Role of Medical Education in Community Development*, Paper for US Agency for International Development (USAID), Washington DC, USA, UWI, 1975

Ragbeer MS and McNeill K., *Designing medical education programs to meet the needs of developing countries: the UWI experience*, Washington DC, USA, International Symposium on Health Problems of Black Populations, Howard University, Feb 1975

Ragbeer M., *Tendencia de la Formacion del Medico general o de familia en otros paises (World Trends in the Training of the Family Doctor)*, chapter in *EL MEDICO GENERAL, UNA RESPUESTA AL FUTURO*, eds. Janer-Ruiz H., de Zubiria Gomez, R. and Restrepo Jimenez, M., 1979, ASCOFAME, Bogotá, Colombia, pp. 281-320

Ragbeer MS., *The Faculty of Medical Sciences, Notes of a Personal Odyssey*, WI Med J, 1998: 47: 5-9

Ragbeer MS., *Community Electives for Residency Training*, Ottawa, RCPSC Bulletin, 1991

Ragbeer MS., *The Indelible Red Stain, Books 1 and 2*, Charleston, SC, USA Amazon, 2nd edition, 2016 *(A comment on the Health Services is on pp. 345-349, Bk 2)*

Ragbeer, MS., *India, under siege, the enemy within*, Charleston, SC, USA, Amazon, 2015

Richardson, SA, Birch, H, and Ragbeer, C., *The behaviour of children at home who were severely malnourished in the first two years of life*. Journal of Biosocial Science, 7, 255-256, 1975

Ross MH and Bras G., *Incidence of Protein Under-and Over-nutrition on Spontaneous Tumor Prevalence in the Rat*. J.Nutr,103: 944-963, 1973

Ross, M.H, Bras G, and Ragbeer M.S. *Influence of Protein and Caloric Intake upon spontaneous tumour incidence in the Anterior Pituitary Gland of the rat*, J. NUTRITION, 100, 177, 1970

Royal Commission on Medical Education Report, 1965-8, London HMSO, 1968

Santas A.A. *Programa de Enseñanza de Medecina de la Comunidad*, Bogota, Boletin FEPAFEM, IX,4, 1973

Singh, WSA, Ragbeer MS, Nicholson CC *The Association of Congenital Heart Disease with maternal Rubella in early pregnancy, Clinical and pathologic features.(Abs.)*, MRC Conference Port-of-Spain, April 1963

Spooner T. et al., *Expansion/Duplication of the UWI Faculty of Medicine, UWI, The Report of the IADB special committee*, UWI CP14, 1971

Standard KL, *Problems of Health and Disease in the Commonwealth Caribbean*, Tropical Doctor, 1,3:131-3, 1971

Stewart, D.B., *A developing medical school in the tropics*, 1962, J med Educ., 37, 1000-11

Stuart K.L, Bras G, & Ragbeer MS, *Proposals for Postgraduate Medical Education at the University of the West Indies*, Paper 6, (36 pp), Caribbean Health Ministers Conference (CHMC) II, Bridgetown, Barbados, 1970

Waterlow JC and Rutishauser I., *Malnutrition in Man and Early Malnutrition and Mental development, pp 13-16, in* J. Cravioto, L. Hambraeus and B. Valquist (Eds.) Stockholm, Almqvist and Wiksell, 1972

WHO. Alma-Ata 1978: Primary health care, Geneva, 1978, ("Health for All" Series, No.1)

Ibid., *Public Health Training of General Practitioners*, Geneva, Tech. Report Series, No. 140, 1957

Wilcocks C & Manson-Bahr PEC., *Manson's Tropical diseases, 17th ed.*, London, Bailliere and Tindall, 1972

Accident 59,159-60,299,328
Accreditation 59,89,265, 289
Achievements 109
Ackee 139
ACPJ 223,276,290-2
Action Group Ch.4,31, 105
Acuña, H., 246,266, 270,280
ACURI 28,34,128, 250,289
Adam, M.,36,216,277,278
Admission interview 145
Adv. Nursing 111,128,137, 287,313
Advances 265
Aides 55,114,186,323,356
AIIMS 229
Aims of Med. Ed.18,30 47, 50
Ali E &A., 291
Alleyne, G., 101,111, 195,254,266,272,362
Alma Ata 271 (Fn. 38)
Alumni 194,250,265,284,300
Alumnus Assoc., 105,150, 230,250,284-6,300
Amin UF., 37,236
Anatomy 19,74,139,143,351
Ancillaries 51-7,70, 158,186, 160-1,229,279,287
Anderson M.,146,152,206
Anglophone ways 242,269
Anguilla viii, 87,282
Annamunthodo H.,64,102-4, 131,182,199-200,258,277
Antibiotics 188
Antigua 94,118,134-5,282,
Appendices 293-379
Applications 62,108,199,220
Arneaud, J., 205
Arscott, P., 36,113
ASCOFAME 85*,279,316
Ashley D., 113,158,291
Assoc. Dean 5,40,70,77,92, 100,147,165,216,
Assoc. States, 246,282,311
Audit 62,269,275
Augier R., 70,108-11,254
A-V supplies 264
Ayurvaida 12,61,230-1
Award 33,194,241,291
Awon M., 87,113,119,176

Back E., 108,207,273,356
Back o' wall 142
Bacchus K., 34,98,117,371
Bahamas 91,93,114,186,289
Balbirsingh M.,204
Bangladesh 93,228-32,357
Bankay C., 8,76,176
Barbados 77,116,120,-2,157
Barrow, E.,48,141,215,251-8, 267,287
Basic Sc.,51,56,139,180,289
Bateson, E., 205
Beaubrun, Mat 184,188,279
Beaubrun, Mike 98,171,198
Behavioural Sc.,55,287,311
Belize 113, 136,154
Belle, E., 37,273,285
Bennett, J., 92,189
Berlin 26,229
Bergoglio, J., 268 (Pope)
Bermuda 77,113,118
Best medical schools,180
Bickering 216
Bilderberg 283
Biochemistry 17,32,101,195
Bishop M., 259,281
Black Power 26,141,198,315
Blocking return 269
Board, Higher Degrees 70,75
Bombing 268
Bowen F., 11,23,276
Bowers JZ., 132,192
Boyd P. 83,114,186,248,334
Brahmam, AP., 73,146
Brain drain 65,78,155, 84-9, 114,165,173,182,192,261
Bras, G., 19,22,32-5,70, 86, 97,99,108,300
Britannic 121-3
Bristol 205
British degrees 81,202,268
British Sp.societies 80
Brooks, S., 36,70,101,109,117
Budhoo D.,283
Buenos Aires 268
Buildings 2-3,51,95,177, 208, 217,288-9,374
Buhbul 216
Burke LM.,126,247
Burkitt's Lymphoma 32,34

Burnham F., 9,12,16-8, 48, 66,141,156-60,215,218-20
Burry Boy 195,222
Burton, C., 52,113,165,187, 209, 346
Butler, AK.,104,188,210,258
BVI 87,95,132,384

Cali 28,128-9,241
Camera 13,268,
Campuses 18,27,66,265,
Campus changes 288-9
"" violence 140
Campus nationalising 210
Canada 73,166,174,186,373
CAREC 74,186, 215
Cargill M., 200-201;221
Caribbean literature 133
CARICOM 179,246
Carmichael, S., 18,187
Carpenter R., 104,255,258, 366
Case Western 51,265,287, 350
Caste 230
Castro F., 16,232, 260,281
Cato 284,
Ceitlin, J., 241,275,316
Césaire, A., 187
CFNI 17,53,74,146,300,347
Chagula, Dr 232
Chambers G.,217,288
Chancellor 44,141,178,223
Chancellor Hall 194,291
Chavez, M., 240-1,275
Chedoke 285-6,372
Chile 268(army); 343
Chicago 26-7,67-8; 98, 139,255
Chimaltenango 241
Chile 188,268
Chin W.,158
CHMC 266
CHMC III, 77; IV,153, Ch. 17; V&VI, 179-
Cholera 185
CIDA 190, 192
CIA 129,268,281
Civil servant 71,136,231
Clarke, Sir Cyril 309
Clinical educ., 76,163,352
CMAJ 189,
CMEC 279

CMH 282,
CML, Canada, 267,285
CML, Guyana 157
CMOs 39,52,157,241,271
CM Specialist 262,274
Coard B., 281
Cochrane W., 188
Collaboration U-G 209
Collections 23
Colonial 204,231,
Colonial practices 183, 233
Colonial service 47,62,82,
Columbia 12,69,98,255
Comissiong, L., 86,94,157,
248
Committees 107
Commonwealth 186,246,
Communism 133,229, 254,
Community Health 269,
286, 339
Community Medicine 128,
148, 161,193,Ch.25 (235-
49), 265 (in peril),271,
274,330,340,361,
Community service 37,334
Community support 243
Competency 89
Complaints, staff 37-8,195-
"" (students) 19,25
Compton, J (St L) 184,289
Conferences 184,186,246,
250, 287
Conferences cancelled 249
Confidence 314 (in VC),
Control Clinic 275
Convention 142 (DNC)
Coordinated teaching 139
Coordinator PGME 82,97- 8,
255
Coore D., 171,247
COPMED 92,Ch. 12, 113,
Copy or innovate 139
Cornwall Hosp. 247
Coroners 263,285
Corporations 283
Corruption 136
Costa A., v;105.Fn; 152, 250,
274,284
Costs (educ.)28;90
Cost of brain drain,; 165
CPSO 5, 288
Creative Arts 315
Credit for training 63

Cricket 9,11,14,23,47,145,
257
Crisis meeting 221
Cristoffanini, A., 188,268,
343
Cross J., 199,204,357
Crotalaria 131,139
Cruickshank, E.,Ch.16,145-6,
151
Cuba 67,116,154,187,210,
219, 280
Current Contents 149
Curriculum 43 et seq,**51**,54,
(new) 58
Curriculum C'ttee., 49-51,
55, 58, 264,280
Cyrus, Dr AC, 113,181,279

Daley R., 259
Dar es Salaam 232
Data, Med Fac., 224-6
Dean, full-time 111,147,372
Deanship 98, Ch.10,
Death threats 211
De Bakey M., 221
Decline 218,224,248,286,320
Democracy 221
Democratic Nat Conv 26,
142,259
Dentistry 45,177,217
Department heads 20,109,
197,235
Departures 277
Detractors 70,101,263,291
Devon House 143
Dew Line Dr 135
Dhaka Univ. 231
Diplomas 56,61,82
Director, PAHO 192,
Director, CM & PGME 191,
236,255,267
Discrimination 102 (appts.),
127(race)
Discourtesy 215
Dismissal 197
Dissent 110,241,259
Division 43,105,184,
Divisive themes 133
Dixon L., 214,15
DNC 142,259
Doctor as civil servant 182,
Dominica 180,
Dorothy (Dean's office) v

Dos Santos E., 205-6,332
Downs W., 185
DPH 270 (derided)
Drayton H., 156
Dreamer 175,189,,261, 262
Drepaul Jr., 156
Drug trade 142,224
DTM&H 61
Dubcek A.,26,259
Dumler I., 268
Deuschle K., 129
Dyer H., 36,166,193,278-9,

East Berlin 229
East Indian Heart, 5,74,183
EC scheme 104,Ch.18 (163-
170), 216, 287-, students
in,194
EC states vi, vii, viii, 210
Economy 210,283
Edness Q., 93,100,154,156
Educating Drs 160
Education tourism, 289
Eldemire, H., 94,143,
Election 98, Dean;
269,272PAHO
Elections (national) 143
Electives (Antilles) 180,248
Elevator incident 215,274
Elliott V., 112,186
Emergency Dept., 289
Embargo 279-80
Enforcers 221-2
Enterprise 138,282,350
Epidemics 64,316
Epidemiology 185
Epilogue 261
Errors 200,273,275,290,319
Essays vs MCQs 28-9
ERU 53,65,74,300
Etienne C., 281
EU 282
Evaluation,148 (Fn. 30),161
EWMSC 208
Examinations 19-30,97-8,
long case 27; objective 23,
oral, 25, PMPs 27
Expansion 131 (IADB),172,
180
Expansion costs 138
External Examiners 81
Extramural 289
Extravagance 28,68

Faculty Board 35-41,,50,55,
70, 97-8,100-1,106-8,110-1
232,239,248,297,308,358
Faculty History,288
Faculty Reform Chs 10 &11
Farewells 130,220,379
Family Drs 166,263,279,353
Family Medicine 38,166,193,
248, 277-9
Family Planning 129,162,
213,231,363-5
Favouritism 67
Feathermop 195,222
Fee for service 205
Fee-paying 118,248,281
Feng P.,25,101,145,147-9
F&GP 42,109,172,360
Field-Ridley S., 155
Fiji 162
Filariasis 61
Flexner A., 248
Flush toilet 230
Force, use of, 211
Forde H. McD 100,148,166,
216,254,332-3
Foreign students118,248,
281; observers 175
Forensic survey 73,185
Francophone 187
French Med Ed.,277,288
Frugality 68
Funds diverted 275 ()
Fund-raising 290

Gairy E., 281
Gangs, 51,195,117,210,
218,277
GATT 282
Gibbs, N., 7-8,36,291
Gilmour J&M.,171-
GMC 55,48,265,359
Gonsalves R.,207,257-,282
GPs 166
Graduates 15, 154,159,
161,174
Graduate loss (see Brain
drain)
Grant L.,50,70,97,112,263,
266, 285
Grenada 65,154,248,281-30
Guatemala 241,243
Guild of graduates 284
Gun courts 221
Gun threat 212,257

Gupta, S., 227-9
Guyana 69,73,88, Ch.17
(153-62)

Hagersville 285
Hagley, K. 247
Hamburg 229,
Hammersmith 32,59-60,79,
264
Hanoman H. 237,248,56
Hansard 246
Harewood, B'dos, 122, 258
Harland E. 275
Hart R., 259
Heads Committee 238
Heads of C'wealth 246
Health and Community
88,182
Health education 162,242,
Health Field concept 187,
Health promo., 30,53, 167
238-9,273,287,299,354
Heart Disease (Masai) 233,
""and rubella 73.
Hijacking 276
Hindu University 231
Holistic 52,271,298,339
Holness H.,36,137,211,378
Homi J., 284
Hony, D., 284-5
HOPE Ch.13, 121, 140
Horwitz A.,91-2,269-72,292
Hospital ships 121-3
Hospitals, teaching 62,90,
106,163-5,358
Howard Univ., 127,244,281
Hoyte D., 51,74,100,132,155,
182-3,195,220,256,
Hull B., 204
Hurricane Ivan,2004, 290

IADB 63, Ch. 14 (131-40)
279; committee photo 132
Ignorance 36-fn
8,228,265,300
IMF 282-3,
Immorality 282
Impeachment 197
Imports (preference)16
Immunology 31
Inaugural remarks 297
INCLEN 279
*Indelible Red Stain,*69
Independence *282*
*India (Book) 45,*Fn9

India 229,
Inequality102,
Innovative 100,233,267,270-
1,363
Integration 51,180,246,262,
265, 270,272,274,278,287
290,299,373
Inquiry 196
Iron lungs 72
Irvine D. 216

Jackman C., v,36,97,100,
106,108, 210,253,300,378
Jagan, C., 9,12,16,66,72
215,232,254,259
Jamaica, PGME grant, 213
Jamaica economy 144,
"" needs, 218
Jamaican doctors 174
JCCS 43, 90,139,140
JLP 143,222 (HQ),
JMA-BMA-CMA Conf. 221
John Hopkins 180,230,248-9
Joint Ctte. with CMOs 39
Jonkers A., 185
Jung, D.,105,152,250,284,379

Kean, C., 195,198
Kebangsaan 104
Kellogg 237-44,275-80,287
Kennedy, R. 259
Kenya 233,
Khan G 112,155,183,186,289
Khanna, S., 154,159,334
Kilimanjaro 232
Killings 221
King, D., 205
King ML 26,259.
Korcok M., 189, 191

Laboratory Director 262
Lalonde M., 186
La Leche league 242
Lalor G., 251-2,254
Lampart R., 248
Lapham Commission 277
Latin America 187,242
Laveran 61
Learning plans 181,282
Lecture theatre 140,172,277
Lecturer beaten 211,
Lee, Byron.,142
Legal suits 85
Let-down (Massiah) 206
Levels of care 52-3

Lewis A.,66
LHINs 292
Lim Sue S, 167
Locke G., 199-204
Lodge, UWI, 276
Lomé 281-2
Luck S.,276,353
Lumsden, Mrs., 204
Lycett, P., 285
Lymphomas 31-34,229

Macedo, C., 192
Malaria 61,72,229,351
Malnutrition 16-7,229,242,
280,293,318,349
Malpractice 85
Martinique 187
Manchester K 195-8
Manchester Project 109, 237
- 244,246-7,269-70,274, 337
"" health links, 243
Manley M.,Ch.19. 171-,199,
210, 215, 219-287,260,
Manpower 36,186-7,246,
Manson P.,61,71
Marketable assets 288
Marshall R.,31,34-7, 43,155,
173,97,156,173-4,210, 220,
235,245, 253,257, 315, 358
Martinique 187,
Mason, Mr., Hosp. Sec 244
Massiah K.,108,206,253, 285
Massiah V., 278 (T&T)
Masson, A., 3-6,107,110-3,
130,152,204,236,273,356
Massop C., 276
Maxine Bennett 32-3(Fn. 7)
McMaster 5,28,92,264-95,
279, 284,285-6
McNeill K.,143,171-7,184,
236,255,266,277,344,359,
MCQs 22-30,106,267,371
Medical assistants 69,
Medal 291
Medical education (aim) 52
(CMOs)
Medical schools for profit
248, 280-1
Medical services 47,60,182
Medicaltech.33,65,78,186
Meetings re CM 270-280,
Meltzer R.,83,114,123-30,
146,263-5,329-31
Meltzer A., 128,239

Middlemiss, Prof. H., 205
Migration of labour 210
Milk cancelled, UK, 280
Miller C., 36,109,114,217,
256,265,266,273-8,379
Millott N., 24
Minott O., 263-6,244,273-6
Model of HCD 285
Modyford J., 121
Montserrat 113,135,154,
Morgan H., 121
Mother's illness 146
Mount Hope 49,78,
180,185,3
MSA 286
Mull, J., 263(CML Ltd),267
Munroe, T., 140,211-2,222,
257,259
Murders 1117 142, 259
(MLK, RK),

Namibia 246
Neglected primary care 53
Negritude 187
Neologisms 264;
Neurosurgeons 201
New Delhi 229
New specialist (CM) 271
Nigeria 234
NIHAE 230-1
Nobbs HH., 9,103,146,
Nuclear nations 13,229
Nurse Practitioners 70,
128,193,295
Nutrition 53-5,242,
Nyerere J., 232,257

O&M 146
Objective tests28-9,98,106,
109, 288
Obote M., 291
OECS 282
Offshore med. school 280-1
Opponents 47
Oral 25
Organisation Chart 96
Organisation(Office) 106,
300
Oriens....9,97
Ottawa 44,186-8,295
Overwork 273

PAFAMS, 5,104,111,127,175,
191, 237,243, 262,,267-9, 276,
292,316,336,340 ,342,345

PAHO 55,178,186,264, 269,
270, 279
Patent 139
Pathak B., 230
Pathak UN., 37,69,273,
Pathik, Dean 161
Patterson W., 277
Paying students 118
Peace concert 277
Pegasus 157,221,286,291
Peru 121,268
PGME Ch. 6 ,59-, Ch.8.71-,
Ch.9, 77- ;141,180,**192**,229
"" building Ch.24, 213-5
PGME (unique) 84
Pharma 188
Photos: heads 152
Picou, D.108,265
Plenty 67-8,
PNP 210
Polio 72, Fn. 13,
Political patronage 222
Politics (instability) 133,187
Poor plan 134
Pope Francis (future)268
Pork shunned 222
POS General 179,205,
Post-internship positions 50
Powdered milk ads 242
Prabhakar Dr 205
Prague spring 259
Pre-med 155
Pre-clinical expansion 139
"" relocation 140
Preston AZ, 83,141,173-
5,198, 213,259,269,
346,364,378,
Prevatt, Hon F 176,215
Prevention, to embed 238,246
Primary Health Care 270,279
Prince Philip 245
Princess Alice 44,178,245, 315
Private med. schools 248,281
Problem-based 126,265
Problems Med Fac., 223-
Professional status 186
Profligate plan 266
Project Review275,284
Proposed seminars 250
Protesters 259
PSC 115

Quality of care 81,116
Queen E 244-6

QEH 170,185,205,287,292

Radiographers 79,186
Ragbeer M., 6-8,39,101,145
Rai BS.,73,
Rainford N.,266,284,379
Ramathibodi 277
Raje D., 6-8,291
RCP (Eng.) 76
RCPSC 6,261
Reading re WI 133
Reagan R.,280-1
Reappointment 47
Rebuttal to St Kitts 181-83
Recognition of PG degrees
    84,246,304
Recruitment 76,82,132,158,
    182,212,236,306
Red tape 231
Reforms Ch.10,97-;Ch.11,
    105-;
Reggae 142
Regional Centre 288-9
Registrar (Univ.) v,36,97,
    108,211,300,378
Registrars 37,64,78,92,102,
    106,115,204,246,278,286
Registration 176,268,304,
    363
Relationships 39,109,141,
    196,205, 06,216,299,332,
    340,377
Research 1,50,65,74,125-6,
    327
Reserve Fund 144,284
Resignation 141,178,245,
    272, 283, 287,358
Resolutions 18,94,184,248,
    361
Resources 28,37,48,65,70,
    65-70,195-7,305,363,378
Revenue proposal 118,248
Revolving loan 142
Richards, R.,36,236,277,379
Rippel J 86,95,126,rds300
Rivalry 18,134.321
Roberts, G.,318
Roberts T., 98
Robertson, A, 35,92,132,160,
    369,
Robinson L,36,45,108,194,
    288,
Rodney W.,142,207,257,
    281 315

Rosenheim, M., 161
Ross, M. 32,53 (Fn)
Ross, R., 61
Ross Medical 281,
Rothschild 282,283
Rubella 72-4,384

Sahoy, R., v,4,36,39, 92,113,
    119,158,236,290-1
Sam's advice 266
Sandison J., 69,236
Santas, A., 262,276,338-9
SAP 283-4
Saudi Arabia 5-6,148,177,
    264
Seaga E., 141-4,171,199,221,
Self-direction
Security 195,210-1,224,315
Self-reliance 85,264,279
Seminars 178 (PAHO)
Seminars aborted 250
Separation 40,272,299,364
Sewage disposal 45,230, 374
Shennan H., 237
Sherlock P., 9,133,145,289
Simcoe 262-3,285
Sinnombre 199-200
Sir Harry 64,102-4,108,130,
    182,200,251,256,258,266,
    277
Sirs 102,292
Smallpox 229.281
Smith, K., 28,34,36,97,99,
    110-12,209,213,215,269,
    276,286
Smoker 207
Social Development 251,
    345
Sociology, clinical 55,351
Somaroo R., 187
Sons of bitches 254
South America 5,13,175,
    268,295,343-4
Spaulding A.,222
Specialty needs 120 (all),
    218 (Ja.),224,201-4
Specialist staff, WI,120
Specialists trained 192,261,
Spence L. 185
Spence G.,*(Feathermop)* 222
Spooner T., 131-3,135
Springer H.,15
St Cyr Dr 187
St. George's 248,281

St Kitts 134, 179,282
St. Lucia 184,282
St. Vincent 279, 282
Staff loss 224,236,247,315,
    46
Stages of a project 149
Standard KL., 97, 264,271,
    276,284
Street, Sam, 52,231
Strike Ch.22, 211-2
Structural Adj. 282-3
Stuart KL.,42,77-96,99-100,
    102,131,146,195,267,277
Student issues (EC) 193
Students 55, 147 (Bd.)
Students suspended, 211
Styling of degrees 144
Super Lion 194,291
Supervision 273 (failed)
Support for PGME 154
Suriname 160
Survival of projects 283,286
Sussex 57,150-2,186
Swansong Ch.27,p.251-

T&T120,174-6,185,194,208,
    215-6,247,329,
Taka 231
Talbot S. 88,89 (Fn.),141,156
Tanzania 14,232,233
    (Masai), 323, 357, 373,
Tapia 18
Task Force Ch.12:113-20,
    153-5,
Taylor T., 10-1,23-4
Teaching hospitals 62,90,
    106,163-5,358
Teamwork 221,316-
Technologists 65,79,86,183,
    263,347
Technology training 158
Tests at McMaster 288
Thanks 149
Thatcher M.,280
The Indelible Red Stain 12,157,
Things Jamaican 142-3
Thompson A (thug)., 277
Thorburn ,M.36,112,236
Three advocates of CM 277
Three Medical Faculties,
UWI, 265,284
Thwaites D., 31,143
Thwaites wing 44
Tikasingh E., 72,185

Tirade 99 (KLS)
Tivoli 142
TMRU 108,195,300,347
Toilet, novel model 230
Tony Thwaites 44,86,289
Town & gown 148
Training posts 67, 74,
Transfer (personal)10
Transient Research 230
Triennium 117,140,172,180,
251,314,347,358
Trinidad campus 176,217,
265
TRVL 72,174,185, 204-5,300
Type of Drs (CHMC), 52

UAWU 211
UG 156,281
UGC 252
UN orgs. 54
Uncertainty 63,301,315,371
Undergrads 162,168-9 (EC)
Union 148,210-2,222
Univ.-Govt. collab.,209
"Unusual Dean", 215
US corporations, 242,283
US litigious 85-6

UWI revenue streams 248
USAID 213-5, 251
UWI disruption 223
UWI vs others 28

Vacancies for MDs 42,47,
82,108,116,153,178,212
Van Kanten 187
VC 35,210,251-2,259,268
Vietnam 26,142,259
Violence 12,18,56,76,104,
140, 176 Ch.22,210,221 249
Viva 25
VOD 72
Vote 107,111,269

Walrond E.,101,256-7,286-7,
Walsh WB.,121,128,139, 146
Walter, I., 106,300
Watergate 127
Welch T., 222
West, M., 215,236,246,258,
379
West Africa,61,185,219,244,
264,282,372
White H., 205,332
White Power, B'dos 257

WHO 229,262, 265,270
WI literature 133
WIGUT 207
Wilks R., 4-5,8,290
Williams, E., 141-2,164,178,
215,245,287-8,315,
Williams, J., 157-8,166,254
Williams, L.,278
Wilson J., 4-5,91-
4,143,,277,292
WIMJ 7,73,119,149,370-1
WMA 160
Wooding H., 178,223-,315
Workshop 161,232,266-
9,275-6
World Trends 279,358
Wray, S., 104,263,267,274-5,
279-80, 286-7,291
Wray's lie to Sir Harry,104
Wright T., 200-4
WTO 282-3

Yippies 26, 142
Young J.,105,284,379

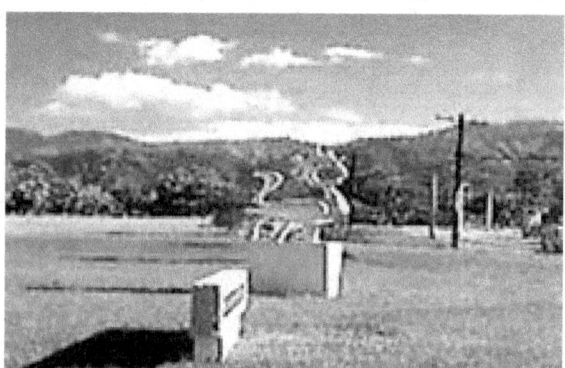

ERU, Mona, with backdrop of foothills of Blue Mountains; the foreground figure is an aluminium sculpture of Savacou (Taino word for "crane"), by R. Moody.

www.ingramcontent.com/pod-product-compliance
Lightning Source LLC
Chambersburg PA
CBHW071248220526
45468CB00001B/36